THE SOUNDS OF FURIOUS LIVING

CRITICAL ISSUES IN HEALTH AND MEDICINE

Edited by Rima D. Apple, University of Wisconsin–Madison; Janet Golden, Rutgers University–Camden; and Rana A. Hogarth, University of Illinois at Urbana–Champaign

Growing criticism of the U.S. healthcare system is coming from consumers, politicians, the media, activists, and healthcare professionals. Critical Issues in Health and Medicine is a collection of books that explores these contemporary dilemmas from a variety of perspectives, among them political, legal, historical, sociological, and comparative, and with attention to crucial dimensions such as race, gender, ethnicity, sexuality, and culture.

For a list of titles in the series, see the last page of the book.

THE SOUNDS OF FURIOUS LIVING

Everyday Unorthodoxies in an Era of AIDS

MATTHEW KELLY

RUTGERS UNIVERSITY PRESS
New Brunswick, Camden, and Newark, New Jersey
London and Oxford

Rutgers University Press is a department of Rutgers, The State University of New Jersey, one of the leading public research universities in the nation. By publishing worldwide, it furthers the University's mission of dedication to excellence in teaching, scholarship, research, and clinical care.

Library of Congress Cataloging-in-Publication Data

Names: Kelly, Matthew, author.
Title: The sounds of furious living : everyday unorthodoxies in an era of AIDS / Matthew Kelly.
Description: New Brunswick : Rutgers University Press, [2023] | Series: Critical issues in health and medicine | Includes bibliographical references and index.
Identifiers: LCCN 2023007667 | ISBN 9781978835078 (paperback ; alk. paper) | ISBN 9781978835085 (hardcover ; alk. paper) | ISBN 9781978835092 (epub) | ISBN 9781978835115 (pdf)
Subjects: MESH: HIV Infections—history | Acquired Immunodeficiency Syndrome—history | Anti-HIV Agents—therapeutic use | Political Activism | Patient Advocacy—history | Community Networks—history | History, 20th Century | United States
Classification: LCC RA643.8 | NLM WC 503 | DDC 614.5/99392—dc23/eng/20230607
LC record available at https://lccn.loc.gov/2023007667

A British Cataloging-in-Publication record for this book is available from the British Library.

rutgersuniversitypress.org

For my family, mentors, friends, and colleagues

CONTENTS

List of Acronyms ix

Introduction: Acknowledging the Everyday 1

PART I: THE SOILS OF UNORTHODOXY: IRREGULAR AND ALTERNATIVE MEDICINE IN U.S. HISTORY 11

1 Situating Unorthodox AIDS Activism within the History of Medicine in the United States 15

2 A Broken Model: Twentieth-Century Transformations in the Social Constructions of Health and Disease 36

3 A Broken Trust: The Changing Character of Health Care 52

PART II: THE SEEDS OF UNORTHODOXY: THE EMERGENCE OF UNORTHODOX AIDS ACTIVISM 81

4 Everyday Unorthodoxies and the People with AIDS Coalition (PWAC) 85

5 Patient, Heal Thyself: The History of Health Education AIDS Liaison (HEAL) 116

Conclusion: Listening to and Learning from the Sounds of Furious Living 142

Acknowledgments 155
Notes 157
Bibliography 213
Index 231

ACRONYMS

Acquired Immunodeficiency Syndrome (AIDS)
Active Lipid 721 (AL721)
AIDS Coalition to Unleash Power (ACT UP)
AIDS-Related Complex (ARC)
Azidothymidine (AZT; Retrovir)
Centers for Disease Control / Renamed Centers for Disease Control and Prevention (CDC)
Cytomegalovirus (CMV)
Dideoxycytidine / Zalcitabine (ddC; Hivid)
Dideoxyinosine / Didanosine (ddI; Videx)
Epstein-Barr Virus (EBV)
Food and Drug Administration (FDA)
Gay Activists Alliance (GAA)
Gay Liberation Front (GLF)
Gay Men's Health Crisis (GMHC)
Health Education AIDS Liaison (HEAL)
Human Immunodeficiency Virus (HIV)
Human T-Cell Leukemia Virus Type III / Renamed Human T-Lymphotropic Virus Type III (HTLV-III)
Institute of Medicine (IOM) / Renamed National Academy of Medicine (NAM)
Joint United Nations Programme on HIV/AIDS (UNAIDS)
Kaposi Sarcoma (KS)
Lymphadenopathy-Associated Virus (LAV)
National Cancer Institute (NCI)
National Institutes of Health (NIH)
People with AIDS Coalition (PWAC)
Pneumocystis Pneumonia (*Pneumocystis carinii* / Renamed *Pneumocystis jirovecii;* PCP)
Treatment Action Group (TAG)
Wipe Out Aids (WOA)
Zidovudine (ZDV; Retrovir)

THE SOUNDS OF FURIOUS LIVING

INTRODUCTION
Acknowledging the Everyday

IMAGES OF AIDS (acquired immunodeficiency syndrome) activism pervade popular culture, emblazoning in our collective memory the pain and suffering endured by people with AIDS, the transformation of this suffering into anger, and the mobilization of this anger into political action. Photographs of protestors staging die-ins on the steps of the FDA (Food and Drug Administration), scattering ashes of loved ones on the lawn of the White House, and occupying offices of pharmaceutical corporations have become allegorical illustrations of health activism challenging the policies and practices of those in power. An encyclopedia of gay and lesbian history names the AIDS Coalition to Unleash Power (ACT UP), the organizer of many of these protests, as the most prominent AIDS activist group of the 1980s and 1990s.[1] By some measures, ACT UP's protests are synonymous with AIDS activism: among the first ten images retrieved through an Internet search of 1990s-era AIDS activism, nine featured public protests organized by members of ACT UP.[2]

ACT UP's contributions to the history of AIDS activism and, more broadly, the history of drug research in the United States, have been well documented.[3] By vocally and dramatically demanding access to treatment, typified by ubiquitous demands for "drugs into bodies," ACT UP facilitated changes in the institutional review of drugs by the FDA. However, just as historians have noted that ACT UP's public protests obscured its less visible campaigns to secure influential positions alongside governmental regulators and pharmaceutical executives, the historical record also masks the heterogeneous nature of the broader AIDS activism movement.[4]

Political scientist James C. Scott has observed that historians and social scientists are apt to focus their attention on "riots, rebellions and revolutionary movements" rather than less violent forms of political action.[5] For Scott, less visible "everyday forms of resistance" constitute open political actions that are collective in nature and possess the capacity to exert tremendous influence on the course of history. In the context of AIDS activism, public protests and disruptions occupy a sphere analogous to the overt forms of resistance typified by Scott's riots and rebellions.[6] However, preceding these outward expressions of anger and frustration is a rich history of contestation directed at dominant professional and governmental bodies responding to AIDS. In many cases, this tradition of political action and resistance centered upon challenges to Western biomedical orthodoxy and dominant systems of drug investigation. Furthermore, it was frequently expressed through avenues of individual treatment and care.

Throughout the 1980s and 1990s, many people diagnosed with AIDS or believed to be at risk actively explored treatment options developed and promulgated by networks operating outside the dominant biomedical model. In some cases, they sought access to chemicals that had not passed the FDA's testing standards for investigational new drugs. In others, they explored treatments derived from traditions and practices historically exempted from rigorous federal review, including herbal medicine, mind-body medicine, homeopathy, and macrobiotics. At times, they directly challenged dimensions of the biomedical model, such as the roles played by governmental regulators, pharmaceutical corporations, laboratory scientists, and physicians. More often, however, they expressed their criticism by silently disengaging from the biomedical model and embracing etiological and therapeutic paradigms that contradicted it.

Because these everyday expressions are defined by their variance from accepted, largely hegemonic biomedical practice, I refer to them under the broad category of unorthodox AIDS activism.[7] Movements consistent with this domain arose from a deep-seated suspicion that biomedicine's approach to conceptualizing and treating disease was flawed and would not provide succor to the sick. For those tapping into this complex and rich tradition, efforts to get "drugs into bodies" could, in fact, contribute to the suffering wrought by AIDS.[8]

Unorthodox acts of resistance are not easily captured in the ephemera of the epidemic, nor do many of their proponents remain to tell their stories. However, one finds echoes of their legacy in many places: in newsletters discussing the benefits of herbal medicines, in detailed recipes for "cooking" experimental egg lipids in Greenwich Village apartments, in macrobiotic information packets describing AIDS as a consequence of the twentieth century's increasingly processed modes of living, and in articles written by people with AIDS rejecting mainstream clinical treatments such as azidothymidine (AZT; Retrovir) and defiantly advancing etiological explanations that rejected a role for HIV (human immunodeficiency virus).

AIDS is, perhaps, the most studied disease in all of history, attracting the attention of historians, sociologists, anthropologists, biologists, physicians, epidemiologists, ethicists, political scientists, and medical geographers.[9] It has taught us a great deal about the implementation of public health practices, the stigmatization of marginalized populations, the establishment of lay expertise amidst professional uncertainty, and the organization of highly visible activist groups aimed at expediting drug approval. In AIDS, we see an archetypal expression of twentieth-century treatment activism, the rise of a voluntarist response to disease, and the self-organization of marginalized individuals in response to a condition ignored by many political leaders. Despite this, the history of unorthodox AIDS activism remains largely unwritten. The most authoritative and insightful volume on the topic remains Steven Epstein's *Impure Science* (1996), but it does not seek to identify the intersecting historical currents underlying the diverse manifestations of unorthodox AIDS activism in the 1980s and 1990s.[10]

The dearth of scholarship exploring the history of unorthodox AIDS activism has important consequences for understanding the history of public responses to epidemics. In both popular and scholarly formulations, AIDS is credited with almost single-handedly instigating profound change in treatment activism, with activists operating "at the vanguard of a larger movement for patients' rights, a movement to revolutionize medical research for all diseases."[11] One recent analysis credits the social movement that arose to combat AIDS with "creating a roadmap for catalyzing significant public policy change" to be used by patients living with other diseases.[12] Yet if we are to credit AIDS activism with transforming the role of the patient activist, we must examine all manifestations of AIDS activism, not just those that promoted mainstream biomedicine.

Furthermore, unorthodox AIDS activism did not develop de novo in the early 1980s but out of earlier social movements—some dating back to the nation's founding era. Therefore, just as studying AIDS activism helps us understand the course of subsequent activism initiatives, so, too, does it provide an opportunity to reconsider our collective past. This brings me to the overarching goal of this volume: to excavate the history of unorthodox health activism in the United States and to use that understanding to contextualize the rise of unorthodox AIDS activism in New York City through the 1980s and 1990s. In researching and crafting it, I have been guided by the conviction that if we seek to remember unorthodox AIDS activism, we must remember anew the history of medicine in the United States and shine a light on the powerful currents that subtended the rise of unorthodox resistance to dominant care systems.

Why, then, has unorthodox AIDS activism been forgotten? I contend that four factors have contributed to its relative elision from scholarly and lay narratives of the pandemic.[13] First, it is easy to construe treatment decisions—an important avenue of unorthodox AIDS activism—as individual and private acts, obscuring their collective dimension. Second, multiple heterogeneous traditions comprise the unorthodox health movement, posing methodological difficulties for scholars endeavoring to map its contours. Third, patients tended to move between these many traditions, complicating efforts to identify discrete systems of practice. Finally, certain strands of unorthodox AIDS activism have been radicalized or stigmatized by scholars and the lay public, making objective analysis of their origins difficult. Because my approach to studying unorthodox AIDS activism necessitates an understanding of these impediments, I shall begin my historical analysis with a brief discussion of each.

FORGOTTEN UNORTHODOXIES: FOUR FACTORS

The first of these factors—the tendency for scholars to interpret treatment decisions through an individual lens—is anticipated in Scott's analysis of everyday forms of resistance. Because his interest is in resistance associated with systems of production, he underscores how seemingly individual acts of protest in this sphere—peasant pilfering, tax evasion, and foot dragging—escape the attention of scholars seeking to chronicle protest movements. Such acts of resistance, performed in silence or within the shadows of individuals' homes, are easily missed in favor of outward displays of group protest typified by peasant uprisings. It should come as little surprise that the conduct associated with unorthodox AIDS activism—individual treatment decisions made in response to a disease associated with deeply personal behaviors—would escape the attention of scholars studying the history of social protest. Indeed, in an era defined by the rise of biomedical ethics and its championing of Kantian self-determination and autonomy, it is deceptively easy to interpret therapeutic choices through an individual lens.

Yet treatment decisions fall into a category of action with overt social and political dimensions. In the case of AIDS, the decisions individuals made to look beyond dominant treatment paradigms were predicated upon the existence of networks of people sharing their experiences, examining the strengths and limitations of their perspectives, providing information for obtaining unorthodox treatment methodologies, and insulating their members from stigmatization. One's decision to pursue a particular treatment plan, therefore, must be understood within the context of larger social relationships.

Furthermore, the collective dimension of unorthodox AIDS activism extends beyond the social forces that sustained its practice. One might concoct a strained hypothetical scenario involving a lone patient making decisions without reliance upon larger networks of support—a hermetic Paracelsus concocting cures in his cloistered closet. Even here, the individual's actions are not truly isolated. For, in choosing to pursue an unorthodox healing remedy, he exerts an effect upon the pool of participants eligible for research trials investigating drugs developed through orthodox channels. In the case of AIDS, we identify many examples of researchers bemoaning their inability to find enough "pure subjects"—that is, individuals who were not using unapproved or untested drugs—for their trials.[14]

This conceptualization of activism may strike readers as surprising. After all, the *Cambridge Advanced Learner's Dictionary and Thesaurus* defines activism as, "the use of direct and noticeable action to achieve a result, usually a political or social one." Yet researchers operating in diverse traditions have challenged such narrow framings. Feminist scholars, whose influence on the history of unorthodox AIDS activism we shall revisit in later chapters, played a particularly important role in the debate. In 1992, Naomi Abrahams argued that scholars should include in their conceptualization of political action those protests individuals pursue in their daily lives.[15] Subsequent feminist theorists expanded upon her analysis, arguing that activism includes actions that reach beyond the public square.[16]

A second factor contributing to the elision of unorthodox AIDS activism from scholarly analysis is the movement's failure to mobilize around one core set of principles. Indeed, the list of historically and culturally-rooted healing systems that have given rise to unorthodox AIDS activism runs the gamut of homeopathy, Chinese medicine, macrobiotics, positive psychology, and Ayurvedic medicine, in addition to diverse interpretations of Western biomedical models that do not ally themselves with any tradition but still challenge mainstream theories. This heterogeneity makes it easy to dismiss the larger unorthodox AIDS movement as internally inconsistent or contradictory. However, as sociologist Rhys Williams has argued, social movements are seldom neatly bounded, internally consistent, or logical in their organization or actions.[17] Furthermore, scholars must attempt to construct their beginnings and endings using archival sources that have the curious tendency of spilling into one another in boundless overflow while paradoxically revealing themselves to be limited and incomplete. It is not always possible to determine, for example, where homeopathy ends and macrobiotic activism begins, or where one divides herbal responses from those advocating contrarian etiological framings of the disease. Therefore, I advocate casting a wide net, considering multiple strands of unorthodox AIDS activism with the goal of uncovering their shared values and themes.

This approach to studying alternative health activism contrasts with an historiographic bias prioritizing the recapitulation of sectarianization in medicine. We see this bias in the very organization of its history—not only is the history of alternative medicine bracketed from that of regular medicine, but it is, furthermore, divided into sundry histories of bounded systems. If we wish to learn about the history of Thomsonian medicine, we consult volumes dedicated to the topic. The same is true of mesmerism, hydropathy, homeopathy, and so on. This historical practice yokes the individual decisions of patients to histories of professionalization, locating them within a matrix of competing philosophies. To capture a more accurate history of unorthodox healing, we must heed the lessons articulated by Susan M. Reverby, David Rosner, and Roy Porter in the late 1970s and 1980s.[18] We must endeavor, in short, to ascertain a social history that moves beyond sectarian battles and professional philosophies to focus on the lives and perspectives of people living with AIDS—the apprehensive, confused, scared, impressionable, demanding, intelligent, irrational, suffering, powerful, and irreverent individuals located at the intersection of these powerful healing systems.

How does one examine the collective mobilization of individuals responding to a fatal condition when they employed mutually exclusive etiological and therapeutic methodologies? What are we to make of the young man who experimented with macrobiotics one day and obtained a supply of the immune modulator inosine pranobex (Isoprinosine) from a Mexican clinic the next, or participated in an AZT trial while secretly taking an experimental egg lipid product? It is easy to assume that such behaviors were abrogative and, therefore, dismissible, or that they proceeded from an irrational "grasping at straws." However, to dismiss as a form of organized resistance any individual's action that is contradicted by his or her later actions is to demand a form of methodological purism seldom seen in the historical record.[19] Furthermore, not all decisions made in desperate times are irrational. Indeed, in some cases, the proponents of unorthodox perspectives demonstrate an avowed commitment to defending their beliefs with evidence.[20] Similarly, in the case of AIDS activism, the scrutiny expounded in the pages of *AIDS Treatment News*, the *People with AIDS Coalition Newsline*, and even the *New York Native* belies efforts to characterize their authors as universally unreasoned.

Thus, I contend that unorthodox forms of AIDS activism constitute examples of everyday forms of resistance. They arose from individuals' disquiet, discomfort, and disagreement with the biomedical orthodoxy—sentiments that were reinforced by historically-rooted shifts in the public's relationship with biomedicine and magnified by perceptions of mainstream antipathy toward communities affected by AIDS. At their core, they sought to challenge biomedicine's control over the bodies and minds of people with AIDS, resisting what Michel Foucault termed the "micro-physics of power" that facilitates institutions' subjugation of individuals.[21]

We must consider one final factor contributing to the relative elision of unorthodox AIDS activism from the historical record. In the case of certain manifestations of unorthodox AIDS activism, lay and academic commentators have contributed to a radicalization of resistance movements. This phenomenon is most apparent in analyses of AIDS dissidence and denialism, movements that maintained that HIV was not the cause of AIDS. It is not uncommon among professional discussions of AIDS dissidence for commentators to dismiss such movements as radical manifestation of fringe paranoia or the projects of rogue professionals.[22] Lost in such treatments are the ways in which dissidence and denialism grew out of and interacted with diverse unorthodox AIDS resistance movements of the 1980s and 1990s.

Readers may grant all that I have argued about unorthodox AIDS activism while still raising questions and critiques regarding my larger project's methodology, utility, and moral underpinnings. Because my reflections on these critiques have influenced my research and analysis, I will briefly examine each here.

METHODOLOGICAL CONSIDERATIONS

The first critique of my project maintains that, while I have defined a category of protest by its variance from a dominant biomedical norm, I have failed to explicitly define that norm beyond vague references. This point is valid. The fact that I have been able to proceed thus far without a formal definition of the model against which unorthodox activism is organized underscores its pervasive reach in society. Here, in discussing the biomedical model, I refer to a broad network of overlapping professional spheres comprised of clinicians, public health professionals, epidemiologists, basic and applied scientific researchers, pharmaceutical representatives, and governmental regulators. It is constituted by the standards of practice and explanatory paradigms these individuals employ in their professional practice along with the values, judgments, and assumptions underlying them. It has grown out of society's systematic integration of scientific empiricism in matters of medicine—a historical phenomenon with deep roots extending to the Enlightenment and continuing through the late nineteenth and early twentieth centuries—expressed, in part, through increasing reliance upon scientific tools and frameworks for diagnosing and treating disease.

The biomedical model provides an explanatory framework for understanding how illness operates, for developing treatments, and for employing those treatments in an organized, systematic manner. It is sanctioned by the state and an expression of its power. Furthermore, just as it provides socially conditioned responses to the catalogue of diseases it has mapped and tamed (e.g., pneumonia), it establishes protocols for addressing diseases it has mapped but lacks the ability to cure (e.g., advanced-stage cancers) in addition to new, unmapped diseases. Its explanatory and therapeutic frameworks are pervasive throughout the structures suffusing everyday life, from the workplace (e.g., in discussions regarding health insurance availability), to schools (e.g., in institutionalized nurse's offices and vaccination requirements), to modes of public transportation (e.g., in health screenings at airports). Its influence further extends beyond the United States, as Harish Naraindas, Johannes Quack, et al. have argued: "Biomedicine has penetrated nearly every corner of the globe, so that most adults living in the twenty-first century know what doctors are and the 'right' way to consult them, what injections are and how one makes use of them, what hospitals are and why one visits them."[23]

UTILITARIAN CONSIDERATIONS

A second critique relates to the societal benefits of studying unorthodox health activism. Critics might claim, for example, that despite my methodology of grouping together different activist traditions under the unorthodox banner, there is no reason to suspect the aggregate movement enjoyed a high degree of support among individuals. Others might argue that the study of this topic is unwise because its practitioners espoused beliefs that have largely failed to withstand the test of time or exert much influence on the course of history.

Disputes regarding the incorporation of underrepresented voices in the historical narrative are not new. They have informed social historical research in addition to the postcolonial field of subaltern studies, which appropriates Antonio Gramsci's framing of the subaltern as an underclass upon whom the dominant class exerts its hegemonic influence.[24] In advocating for the inclusion of these voices, my work borrows from these scholarly traditions. So, too, is it guided by the belief that we ought not dismiss a social movement based upon knowledge we possess today regarding the accuracy of its claims. To do so would welcome into our analysis presentism cloaked in the garb of utility.

If we seek to evaluate unorthodox activism by its success in supplanting biomedicine, then it is true: it failed. However, it is a woefully high standard if, for inclusion in historical scholarship, we demand that a movement topple the dominant forces of society. Is it not worthy of our attention that segments of the population attempted to undermine hegemonic systems to organize and manage their health? Is it not significant that, in a highly technologized biomedical era marked by the promise of molecular biology, biotechnology, and genomics, we find individuals pulled in the direction of contrarian health systems? I maintain that by studying these individuals and their actions, we can better understand the diversity of perspectives and practices that coexist and interact with biomedicine.

ETHICAL CONSIDERATIONS

A third criticism of this project deals with what I shall refer to as matters of professional ethics. Such an objection maintains that any effort to understand the origins and expressions of unorthodox health activism threatens to normalize contrarian health movements. While I take this argument seriously, I ultimately reject it, for historical analysis offers the opportunity to do much more than inculcate or convert. It provides a means through which society can better understand its past and present.

That this philosophy differs from trends we see in journalism is worth noting. In 2014, the British Broadcasting Corporation (BBC) issued guidelines making it clear that it would no longer give airtime to unorthodox views on climate change. In response to these guidelines, one journalist opined, "Were every network to start doing what the BBC is, their unfounded opinions would cease to be heard . . . and maybe, just maybe, they'd all just go away."[25] While I leave matters of professional journalistic practice to those versed in the discipline's history, I contend that such an approach has no place in historical analysis, where our primary concern is not in forgetting, but remembering.

To those who fear that contrarians wait lurking in the shadows to use this historical analysis to further their claims, I am reminded of a discussion I shared with a member of one of the most controversial contrarian groups considered in my analysis, Health Education AIDS Liaison (HEAL). When he learned of my plan to write a history exploring unorthodox responses to AIDS, he expressed hope that the work would clarify what has been a poorly understood history. At the same time, he warned, "Please, if you want your work to be taken seriously, begin by making it clear that you don't agree with any of our ideas. Otherwise, you'll be disregarded and dismissed." This, perhaps better than any material I have unearthed from an archive, speaks to the power of radicalization in discrediting contrarian perspectives and to the potential for historical analysis to move beyond judgment to illuminate and explain.

A final issue of professional ethics warrants consideration. Any historical examination of unorthodox AIDS activism attributes ideas and practices with individuals who have perished from the disease. To the extent that some of these ideas and practices have become radicalized, one might argue that this historical project threatens to besmirch individuals who can no longer defend themselves from the stigma now associated with the movements. This is particularly true for AIDS dissidence but also applies to other forms of unorthodox AIDS activism. It is, therefore, appropriate to ask whether historians have an obligation to protect the historical memory of individuals from the stigma now associated with unorthodox movements.

I maintain that, just as we must avoid using today's standards to judge individuals who lived in a different era, so, too, must we avoid efforts to protect the historical memory of activists by ignoring the contributions they made to social movements. Doing so would be an exercise in historical paternalism—an offense all the more egregious when we recognize that many unorthodox health activists challenged biomedical paternalism.[26] Rather than policing the past, historians have a duty to elucidate it while serving as guides to readers, reminding them of the folly of judging individuals by the knowledge, standards, and practices of the present.

THE SOIL AND THE SEED OF UNORTHODOXY

As I have noted, this volume is an exercise in remembering not only unorthodox AIDS activism but the historical movements and forces from which it arose. To appropriate a metaphor common in discussions of disease, it seeks to understand the soil out of which unorthodox AIDS activism grew and argues that by excavating it, we may arrive at new ways of conceptualizing the history of medicine.

The first half of this volume focuses on the soil itself—the historical movements that helped inform, inspire, and animate 1980s and 1990s–era unorthodox AIDS activism. I begin my analysis in chapter 1 by examining the history of nineteenth and twentieth-century unorthodox, irregular, and alternative health movements, identifying themes that have persisted in them through time. I maintain that dominant presumptions regarding alternative and irregular medicine, embodied in the metaphors scholars use to discuss them, have limited our ability to understand their appeal. In their place, I advocate an alternate conceptual model suited for explaining the persistence of unorthodox health activism through the late twentieth century and beyond.

The book then shifts focus to the specific context out of which late twentieth-century unorthodox AIDS activism grew. Chapter 2 interrogates changing popular perceptions of disease and disease models in the mid-twentieth century, exploring discourse among lay individuals seeking to understand and order their experience of health and illness. Chapter 3 expands upon this analysis by examining transformations in the public's perceptions of physicians and researchers, including allegations impugning the character of the nation's healers.

While the first half of this volume identifies the soil of unorthodoxy, the second half focuses on the seeds that grew within that soil, specifically two New York City–based unorthodox AIDS activist groups. It begins in chapter 4 with an examination of the People with AIDS Coalition (PWAC), one of New York's first and most respected AIDS activist groups formed by and for individuals living with AIDS. Only a handful of scholars, such as Susan Chambré and Martin Duberman, have included the group in their discussions of HIV/AIDS activism, with Duberman noting that the organization is "all but ignored in the standard histories of the AIDS epidemic."[27]

Chapter 5 explores the history of a separate activist organization formed in New York City in the 1980s: HEAL.[28] One of the least studied AIDS service groups, HEAL came to vehemently espouse unorthodox health perspectives and eventually became associated with radically dissident activism. My analysis closes with a discussion of how this project informs our understanding of ongoing activist initiatives questioning biomedicine's authority. I ultimately argue that a greater understanding of the history of unorthodox health activism during the last major pandemic of the twentieth century can aid us in understanding the unorthodox activism that has arisen during the first major pandemic of the twenty-first: COVID-19 (coronavirus disease of 2019).

PART 1 THE SOILS OF UNORTHODOXY

Irregular and Alternative Medicine in U.S. History

If one conducts a Google search querying the cause of syphilis, the results show the bacterium *Treponema pallidum*. A similar search for the cause of pulmonary tuberculosis yields *Mycobacterium tuberculosis*. One for AIDS yields HIV. These results, rendered in milliseconds with a few keystrokes, are the product of generations of scientific efforts to elucidate the cause of disease. They represent not only the triumphs of biomedicine but a turn toward specific etiology that reduces diseases to agents that society can illuminate through microscopy, decode through genomics, and conquer through pharmacology.

Imagine that, upon executing the aforementioned searches, Google explained that these diseases are caused by poverty, structural inequities, and racism. One can picture the querier ogling at Google, thinking, "No, what really causes them?" The fact that a twenty-first century person would expect a search to return the specific microbial cause of each disease is understandable. After all, because we know that syphilis is caused by *T. pallidum*, and we know that *T. pallidum* is susceptible to penicillin, we know how to save the life of someone who presents with syphilis.

However, we also know that poverty, structural inequities, and racism are as much a part of the etiology of many diseases as bacteria and viruses. We know, for example, that these structural factors influence variations in the illness experience across people and differences in how epidemics arise in populations. Similarly, we know that a treatment for a disease that fails to consider these structural factors is unlikely to reach the people who truly need it. And unlike bacteria and viruses, which remained invisible until modern science developed technologies capable of magnifying them, these contextual causes pose unique challenges. Indeed, we cannot develop a microscope to see poverty because it is all around us; its ubiquity renders it invisible.

In the late nineteenth century, Sir William Osler, one of the founders of the Johns Hopkins University School of Medicine, composed a medical textbook that was published at least ten times between 1892 and 1920.[1] In it, he describes the progression of tuberculosis by invoking the biblical Parable of the Seed: "There are tissue-soils in which the bacilli are, in all probability, killed at once—*the seed as fallen by the wayside.* There are others in which . . . more or less damage is done, but finally the day is with the conservative, protecting forces—*the seed has fallen upon stony ground.* Thirdly, there are tissue soils in which the bacilli grow luxuriantly . . . the day is with the invaders—*the seed as fallen upon good ground.*"[2] These contextual factors, which Osler described as a person's material condition, were critical for disease progression and could mean the difference between life and death. "The soil," he wrote, "has a value equal almost to that which relates to the seed."[3]

A similar perspective proves valuable in efforts to elucidate unorthodox AIDS activism, for one cannot appreciate the activism movement (the seed) without understanding the broader social, cultural, and historical movements out of which it arose (the soil). At first blush, it might seem obvious for a work of history to suggest that we ought to study the social and cultural forces that nurtured a movement. However, in the case of AIDS, which has been described as a discontinuous break with history, it is tempting to narrow the lens of analysis by focusing only on historical events that immediately preceded the AIDS pandemic. One analytical approach, for example, would entail beginning with a discussion of the unorthodox AIDS movement, with intercalated discussions of the history and inspiration of the groups' members. This approach would allow for limited excavation of the soils of unorthodoxy, focusing instead on the seed. Yet, ironically, doing so would mean deprioritizing broad contextual factors to study a movement whose proponents critiqued reductionism. Furthermore, failing to consider the broader historical movements out of which unorthodox AIDS activism arose blinds us to these movements' longevity and their continued relevance in the era of COVID-19.

Informed by this perspective, I begin this analysis in chapter 1 by mining the soil—identifying the historical, social, and cultural currents that have attended the rise of unorthodox health movements throughout United States history. In chapter 2, I examine changing lay perceptions of disease etiology witnessed in the late nineteenth and early-to-mid twentieth centuries, arguing that these shifts played an important role in informing unorthodox AIDS activism. In chapter 3, I explore the history of distrust and disenchantment among members of the public toward mainstream physicians, arguing that this history rooted and supported later expressions of resistance during the 1980s and 1990s.

1 ▸ SITUATING UNORTHODOX AIDS ACTIVISM WITHIN THE HISTORY OF MEDICINE IN THE UNITED STATES

IN THE EARLY years of the AIDS pandemic, as physicians and public health professionals struggled to make sense of and respond to the mysterious illness racking the nation's cities, people turned to history for counsel. In the lofty pages of historical treatments, they hoped to find remedies for a modern plague many believed was poised to wreak unbounded horrors as it burned its way through the population. If biomedicine could not cure the condition, then perhaps, they thought, history would offer a salve borne out of past generations' experiences with fatal infectious diseases. This recourse to historical wisdom prompted Allan Brandt to remind readers that history offered no clear or simple roadmaps for organizing a social response to AIDS. All it could provide were lessons to help society avoid the mistakes and missteps of those who came before.[1]

This practice of mining historical experience underscores society's conceptualization of history as a toolkit for aiding and informing our actions. Yet history does more than provide strategies for approaching problems; it fundamentally structures and influences how society defines, thinks about, and responds to them.[2] Our historical experiences reverberate through time in the terms and metaphors we develop to discuss diseases, the structures and institutions we create to respond to them, and the avenues through which values, fears, anxieties, and uncertainties surrounding matters of health propagate between people and generations.

Furthermore, there is no one historical experience or perspective that neatly explains the changes witnessed in society through time. Particular conceptions of the world may be ascendant at any moment, but they typically mask other perspectives, beliefs, hopes, and fears, whose part in historical change we ignore at our peril. By the 1980s, for example, Western biomedicine had established a hegemony over how society responded to disease.[3] However, the dawning realization that a fatal infectious disease had erupted in New York and California and the fear that it would spread through the nation prompted a reexamination of the institutions and disciplines society had entrusted with its health. It was in this context of fear and uncertainty that other voices—those expressing unorthodox and subaltern positions—offered their own interpretations of disease.

AIDS came, then, and the light changed. Now, exposed from the shadows of society was a panoply of subaltern perspectives for conceptualizing and responding to this modern plague. By the mid-to-late 1990s, the light would change once more, as biomedicine reasserted its authority in the form of highly effective antiretroviral treatments. The strands of unorthodox AIDS activism that had persisted through this time appeared increasingly radicalized, and the rich history of a complex social movement became obscured. Through what lens, then, can readers today appreciate the history of a movement society has paradoxically forgotten and radicalized?

There is, perhaps, no better guide when seeking to reconcile paradoxes than poetry, for it renders in black and white the irreducible enigmas and impossibilities of everyday life. In 1980, just months before word came of the first diagnosed cases of pneumocystis pneumonia (PCP) in Los Angeles, the Indian poet Jayanta Mahapatra published a collection of poems titled *Relationship*. In this haunting work, he explores identity formation, interpersonal relationships, death, and disease. To help convey these complex themes, he invokes the loneliness of a solitary traveler "who can sense the brilliant colors of the past / in the ocean's strange and bitter deeps."[4]

To understand the history of unorthodox health activism in the United States, we must focus our attention on the solitary traveler—the patient. For it is the patient who registers the long effects of historical change and contestation in health and medicine. It is the patient who sits at the crossroads of multiple healing systems, all of which lay claim to ordering and managing his or her body. By focusing on the patient, we begin to move beyond institutional histories and, instead, embrace scholarship that interrogates the dynamic position of the frightened individuals who, as Mahapatra writes, were "caught in the currents of time."[5]

In this chapter, I explore the persistence of unorthodox health activism throughout U.S. history, connecting our nation's early embrace of irregular healing systems with the contrarian AIDS health movement of the 1980s and 1990s. I begin by reviewing the shifts in historical scholarship of contrarian health movements shepherded by the social turn in historical research in the mid-to-late twentieth century. Following this review, I argue for a more complete embrace of a "history from below" analytical model, prioritizing the experience of patients located in the confluence of multiple competing health systems. Finally, I identify four historical currents that have helped sustain unorthodox healing systems throughout U.S. history.

UNDERSTANDING IRREGULAR AND ALTERNATIVE HEALTH PRACTICES: THE BORDERLAND MODEL

In her 1929 essay *A Room of One's Own,* Virginia Woolf remarks that history "often seems a little queer as it is, unreal, lop-sided."[6] Woolf's observation is no less relevant today than it was during her lifetime. Historical inquiry is both sanctioned and bounded by historically situated values, assumptions, and patterns of understanding. What we think and how we think are linked processes that are influenced by when we think, where we think, and who we are. The subjectivities of history are more than mere curiosities—they have direct bearing upon how we conceive of our past and present. Which groups, individuals, ideas, and perspectives we include in historical analysis, and how we discuss them, are matters rife with political tension. For at the heart of these questions are queries regarding what counts as history and what deserves remembering. Given such high stakes, it should surprise us little that history will always appear queer and lopsided.

Historical biases and preconceptions are, perhaps, nowhere more evident than in our historical treatments of fringe and subaltern positions—a broad category into which alternative, irregular, and unorthodox health movements have been filed. As historian Norman Gevitz has observed, historical research in irregular medicine was biased through the first half of the twentieth century, with scholars expressing a thinly—and, at times, not so thinly—veiled disdain for contrarian healing systems.[7] It was during these "golden years" of mainstream medicine when the influence and authority of a dominant medical enterprise was consolidated and scholars derided contrarian health movements as absurdities, or worse—as manifestations of psychopathology.[8]

The situation would begin to change in the 1950s and 1960s, as scholars intent on crafting histories of forgotten and marginalized groups branched into the study of alternative health movements.[9] Gradually, the tide began to turn, with historians identifying how alternative healing traditions contributed to the modernization of regular medicine.[10] Irregular sects, once decried as the black sheep of medical progress, were suddenly included in the extended family portrait of contemporary medicine. Homeopathy, with its appetite for infinitesimals, was credited with precipitating the decline of heroic medical measures, hydropathy with establishing a role for female clinicians, and so forth.

In this spirit, the latter half of the century witnessed the publication of more sensitive histories exploring the origins of alternative healing traditions, resituating our nation's experience with Thomsonian medicine, homeopathy, hydropathy, Eclectic medicine, mesmerism, and the positive psychology movement, among others.[11] However, while these historical approaches refuted the more antagonistic treatments that had come before, they often suffered from their own methodological shortcomings. Many, for example, focused on the philosophical underpinnings of healing systems, the colorful personalities of their founders, and the role they played in modernizing regular medicine. For these reasons, they largely maintained an institutional focus.

Here, I advocate a methodological approach that moves beyond institutional histories toward one that highlights the lived experiences of patients caught in the cross currents of multiple traditions. In its focus on the patient perspective, this volume is informed by scholarship published between 1979 and 1985 by David Rosner, Susan M. Reverby, and Roy Porter,[12] in addition to recent works by authors such as Nancy Tomes and Wendy Kline.[13]

My decision to situate this historical analysis in the tumultuous spaces of interaction between healing systems calls to mind a metaphor with its own rich history: the borderland. In the mid-twentieth century, historians seeking to problematize our understanding of U.S. territories conquered from Spain found inspiration in the writings of early twentieth-century historian Herbert Eugene Bolton. Bolton suggested that we conceive of these territories as dynamic borderlands wherein multiple actors engaged in complex exchanges, collaborations, and contestations. Through the borderland construct, developed significantly by Gloria Anzaldúa, historians were able to locate power disputes lurking in the shadows, identifying expressions of resistance and opposition that, in previous treatments, had been masked.[14]

While historians often use the borderland metaphor to discuss geographic areas of social and cultural exchange, its application to the study of unorthodox healing systems is illuminating. Throughout U.S. history, individuals have found themselves presented with innumerable traditions and practices laying claim to investigating, surveying, policing, and treating their bodies. Some of these systems have been hegemonic, analogous to the empires of Bolton's histories. Others were less powerful, but nonetheless found ways to exert influence over individuals. If we hope to construct a social history of health and medicine, we must strive for more than isolated analyses of these systems. We must seek an examination of the experiences of patients living in the borderlands between them.

I present the borderland construct as an alternative to a metaphor commonly used to describe alternative health movements: the fringe.[15] For evidence suggests that there is nothing particularly fringe-like about unorthodox health practice. Surveys by David Eisenberg and colleagues reveal staggering rates of alternative therapy usage by Americans, with 33.8 percent reporting adoption of nontraditional therapies in 1990 and 42.1 percent in 1997.[16] Interviews conducted with over 31,000 individuals by Patricia Barnes and colleagues in 2004 reveal even higher rates, with 62 percent reporting the use of complementary or alternative medicine.[17] A 2005 Institute of Medicine Report estimates that the number of visits Americans made to complementary and alternative care providers in 1990 (425 million) exceeded the number made to primary care physicians (388 million).[18]

Within borderlands, patients encounter myriad systems of healing, each offering its own framework for explaining and treating disease and invoking its own appeals for their patronage. In these borderlands, patients simultaneously embody positions of disempowerment and empowerment. Despite their illness, they are capable, through their migration within the healthcare borderlands, of expressing power.

In this chapter, I task myself with answering a deceptively simple question: What made people move? What attracted them away from the hegemonic system to other systems of healing, many of which had earned the opprobrium of dominant leaders of medicine? To answer it, I first examine the arguments proponents of unorthodox healing systems have made. I then expand this analysis, asking whether these arguments invoked broader objections to the dominant healing system. I continue in this fashion, asking at each stage whether the unorthodox healing systems peppering our nation's history have tapped into deeper anxieties and uncertainties, linking matters of health and disease to broader societal debates.

The result of this approach is a nested explication of the forces underlying patients' movement between healing systems. If we conceive of patients as occupying positions in borderlands constituted by overlapping healing systems, then these forces are analogous to currents that have facilitated their movement. Moreover, while the proponents of orthodox and unorthodox health movements may have marshaled particular arguments to influence patients' engagement with their disease, their arguments generated an effect in complex ways, just as currents interact in difficult-to-predict manners.

Here, I identify four currents that helped sustain unorthodox healing systems through the eighteenth, nineteenth, twentieth, and twenty-first centuries. The first current hews closest to the explicit arguments made by unorthodox health system proponents and was marked by direct reference to the excesses and immoderations of regular medicine. The second current expands the critique beyond assessments of therapeutic strategies to deeper apprehensions regarding the uncompromising stereotype of regular physicians and their dogmatic allegiance to theories. The third current is even broader still, derived from powerful anti-authoritarian impulses that arose at several points in our nation's history, most notably the nineteenth-century Jacksonian era. Finally, the fourth current summons deeper antimodern anxieties stemming from profound transformations witnessed in both micro and macro-level relations through the nineteenth and twentieth centuries.

Before analyzing these currents in detail, two points bear underscoring. First, while I identify common themes subtending resistance to medicine through U.S. history, this should not be taken to mean that the arguments, positions, or perspectives of the players involved were identical. Finding antimodern critiques of medical practice in the nineteenth and twentieth centuries, for example, does not mean that nineteenth and twentieth-century medical practices were similar. Second, in underscoring the relationships between these forces, it is easy to suggest that we may reduce all four currents to a common impulse—that, upon identifying the broadest of currents suffusing alternative healing systems through U.S. history, we have succeeded in explaining their persistence. However, my goal is not a reduction of historical forces but an explication of the ways they exerted their effects on patients. That we can trace a line from antiheroic treatments to antimodern sentiment is interesting, but it does not mean that the mid-nineteenth-century American would say he sought homeopathic advice because he was responding to the soul-crushing effects of modern industrialization.

Here, too, I believe the metaphor of the current is illustrative. That currents flow from one another is certainly true. However, they do much more than that. In the intersections of currents, forces collide in unpredictable ways. Subsidiary currents turn back upon their primary channels, with new currents merging and diverging in ways that are difficult to map. Such is the case with historical currents, whose interactions are, no doubt, even more complex, governed as they are not by the laws of physics but by the impulses of humankind. In the following sections, I task myself with tracing these currents throughout U.S. history, beginning with our nation's earliest experiences with unorthodox health movements and continuing through the earliest days of the AIDS pandemic. For each, I conclude with brief introductory links connecting the current with unorthodox AIDS activism, presaging the analysis that follows in the second part of this volume.

CURRENT I: THE SHADOW OF HEROIC MEDICINE

Historians of alternative and irregular medical sects have noted the distrust, distaste, and fear many patients expressed toward nineteenth-century mainstream medical practice. So-called "heroic medicine," widely associated with the practices of colonial physician Benjamin Rush and his contemporaries, focused on purging, bleeding, and blistering to cure the overstimulation believed to be at the heart of disease.[19] Throughout the nineteenth century, countless regular and irregular physicians questioned the wisdom of these practices. In 1839, for example, Dr. William Fullerton Cumming, a physician in the East India Company's service, wrote of treatment he had received at the hands of his colleagues: "I was largely bled at the arm—had fifty leeches applied to the abdomen, and . . . in addition to extensive mercurial frictions, I swallowed 215 grains of calomel! True, I recovered, or rather, I did not die; whether in consequence of, or in spite of the above heroic treatment, I will not venture to say."[20]

Other physicians shared Cumming's appraisal, challenging the pre-eminence of ancient philosophies of therapeutic heroism. In discussing the standard treatment for congestive fever in the Mississippi Valley, for example, a well-respected regular medical periodical included a piece bemoaning the practice of prescribing calomel (mercurous chloride) in the form of R.A.C. pills: "Would to God that Mississippi and Alabama could be relieved of the curse of R.A.C. quackery! Oh! Ye shades of departed worth! Ye ghosts of Hippocrates, Aesculapius, and Galen, how long will we yet endure such humbuggery! . . . Oh! calomel, and R.C.A. pills![21] Inexorable monsters, who have slain your hundreds, why seek to demolish thousands!"[22] Fears of calomel overuse even played a small but illustrative role in the U.S. Civil War. In 1863, Surgeon General William A. Hammond, concerned with calomel use among the military, issued an order removing the drug from field hospitals. As Ralph B. Leonard has written, regular physicians "rose up in indignation and flooded the Capitol with their vociferous outrage." The result of the so-called "calomel rebellion" speaks to the obduracy with which the medical profession demanded the right to prescribe the drug: in November of the same year, Hammond was removed from office and court-martialed.[23]

Distrust in heroic measures reached its zenith in the writings of Samuel Thomson, the founder of the eponymously named, herb-based nineteenth-century medical discipline. For Thomson, the regular medical system was guilty of committing enormous harm in its recourse to dangerous chemicals, chief among them calomel. Where regular physicians regarded the drug as the "Samson of Materia Medica," Thomson openly lambasted it as the "uncircumcised Philistine of medical science." For those whose recollection of scripture was rusty, he offered a more unambiguous appraisal: the entire mercurial craft amounted to little more than "a monstrous bone rotting, tooth destroying, pain engendering, bile vitiating, skin blistering, blood and life destroying system."[24]

Thomson's criticisms, coupled with similar attacks by hydropaths, homeopaths, eclectic physicians, and physiomedicals, struck a chord among the public, many of whom expressed frustration with regular healers' endorsement of heroic measures over reformers' objections. Popular literature offers an indication of these sentiments. In one 1857 work of poetry, the author criticizes the rigidity of regular physicians, satirizing their perspective on therapeutics: "Let others talk of wind or storm / Or speak of Medical Reform / Against their theories I'll rebel / And stick to good old calomel."[25] Even the country's most revered literary master weighed in on this issue. Mark Twain, whose life intersected alternative healing in fascinating ways, poked fun at regular medicine in his prose, at one point painting a colorful portrait of a regular physician. He was, Twain explained, "one of them old fashioned industrious kind that don't go fooling around waiting for a sickness to show up and call game and start fair, but gets in ahead, and bleeds you at one end and blisters you at the other, and gives you a dipperful of castor oil and another one of hot salt water with mustard in it, and so gets all your machinery agoing at once, and then sets down with nothing on his mind and plans out the way to handle the case."[26]

The turn of the century witnessed a remarkable transformation in the standards of regular medicine. William Rothstein has studied the decline of heroic medicine, noting that its practice had faded by the 1860s and 1870s. As he argues, irregular medical practitioners played a large part in inspiring the abandonment of extreme measures, as regular physicians strove to retain clients in the face of the popular appeal of irregular medicine's more prosaic interventions.[27] However, calomel was not vanquished by the mere threat of homeopathy or even the promise of germ theory. Indeed, in 1902, two decades after Robert Koch identified the bacterium that caused tuberculosis, West Coast physician C. W. Kellogg declared, "Calomel without doubt is the most extensively used preparation within the range of materia medica."[28] Yet by the end of the first decade of the twentieth century, the drug was fading into obscurity, with editorials noting that physicians prescribing it would have to contend with the prejudice and derision of their peers.[29]

While the archetypes of heroic medicine—bleeding, purging, and administrating calomel—have largely faded into historical memory, the legacy of its treatments persisted into the late twentieth century. Many factors facilitated their sustained purchase in influencing public opinion, but one in particular warrants mention here: twentieth-century discourse surrounding mainstream medicine's approach to treating cancer.

As historian David J. Hess has argued, though the early-to-mid twentieth century is regarded as a golden age of mainstream medicine wherein its practitioners identified "magic bullets" to cure disease, its powers were never complete. Many diseases, most notably cancers, defied the efforts of Pasteur, Koch, Ehrlich, and their contemporaries. During this period, healing systems developed by Harry Hoxsey and Rene Caisse generated popular followings.[30] These movements tapped into concerns that, not only was biomedicine incapable of curing cancers, but its ministrations were, themselves, dangerous. Thus, nineteenth-century criticisms of heroic medicine's bleeding and calomel administration gave way to twentieth-century equivalents in the forms of radical surgery, high-dose chemotherapy, and radiation.[31]

Again, popular literature registered these fears. In the late 1970s, *Penthouse Magazine* published a series of articles by Gary Null, extolling the virtues of alternative treatments for cancer and criticizing mainstream medicine's therapies. In them, Null accused physicians of advocating treatments that "knife, burn, poison, and, in some cases, kill you sooner than any cancer could." He went on to claim that "virtually all conventional anticancer drugs actually caused cancer."[32] Lest we conclude that these sentiments were limited to the pages of *Penthouse*, at roughly the same time, feminist scholars openly questioned the "slash and burn" tactics of oncologists, tying their assessments to efforts to empower women to make health decisions.[33]

The ties between unorthodox AIDS activism and antiheroic cancer treatment discourse demand careful analysis given the multiple intersections between the diseases. The first reports of AIDS labeled it a "gay cancer"; one of its early defining conditions was a rare skin cancer; the National Cancer Institute (NCI) conducted a great deal of early AIDS research; Dr. Robert Gallo initially theorized that the disease was the result of a cancer-causing virus; and activists criticized the first antiretroviral developed to combat it, AZT, as a failed cancer treatment. Furthermore, a decade after *Penthouse*'s publisher Bob Guccione published the aforementioned articles, his son oversaw the publication of unorthodox AIDS treatment articles in his own *SPIN Magazine*. Furthermore, Gary Null would carry his allegations of heroic medical excess to his reporting on AIDS treatments, earning fame and infamy as a self-described HIV denialist.[34]

CURRENT II: DISTASTE FOR DOGMA

It is easy to trace antiheroic narratives through the nineteenth century, since sectarian practitioners were assiduous in exploiting them. Harder to identify is a second current that dealt more broadly with perceptions that regular physicians were rigidly attached to theories of disease causation, making them resistant to others' opinions. Sectarian authors frequently discussed this issue using the constructs of rationalist and empirical medicine. While this distinction is of value in explaining the support irregular medical sects enjoyed, its academic trivialities tend to mask issues that were much more germane to day-to-day living. Simply put, sectarian healers painted regular physicians as a closed-minded lot who derogated others' ideas—ranging from sectarian conceptualizations of the world to the everyday experience of patients—in favor of medical theories. As a result, they maintained that physicians were poisoning their patients through their rigid allegiance to unexamined principles.

Historian Richard Shryock has demonstrated that, from the medieval period through at least the eighteenth century, organized medicine was an unapologetically rational endeavor. Medical healers interpreted disease phenomena through their chosen theories, calling upon the authority of figures ranging from Galen (second century A.D.) to Benjamin Rush (eighteenth century). Through the eighteenth and early nineteenth centuries, few medical theories were rigorously tested, with physicians stretching laws of physics beyond their breaking point to subsume the biological within the physical.[35]

In opposition to this long history of rational medicine, empirical healing relied upon experience in responding to disease. As Shryock has noted, even as rationalism flourished in the learned schools of medicine, medical empiricism was alive and well on the streets. We therefore find a curious juxtaposition, whereby learned healers administered treatments based upon the rules of esoteric medical theories, while the population sought recourse in folk remedies. It was a fascinating time in which regular medicine was beginning to professionalize while, as Shryock notes, "even educated men might secure their remedies from the village blacksmith."[36]

Debates between empirical and rational medicine reiterated historically rooted battles regarding the subordination of everyday experience to academic theory. In 1836, a London physician penned a treatise addressing the topic, citing Luther's invocation that "reason should not be held prisoner by words" to decry how clinical theories became doctrinaire over time. Luther's beliefs resonated through the nineteenth century, with many arguing that, whereas theories should bend to observable fact, contemporary medicine seemed to invert the relationship. With exasperation, the London physician noted the consequences of the arrangement: "[O]ur theory, then, becomes our tyrant; and all who work under its bidding do the work of slaves—they themselves deriving no benefit from the result of their labors."[37]

Precisely how this fear of the tyrannical theory—which we might reasonably define as dogma—factored into the history of medicine in the United States is difficult to map. For one, the meaning and valence of the terms "rationalism" and "empiricism" remained contested through the nineteenth century. For example, whereas empiricism was treated with derision in some quarters at the start of the century, at its close, "scientific empiricism" was viewed as an ideal.[38] Even Galen recognized the imprecision of the concepts, arguing that the two approaches shared more than the proponents of either cared to admit and that too much time was wasted trying to distinguish them.[39]

What is important for this analysis is not a rigid articulation of rationalism or empiricism, but an appreciation for how unorthodox medicine proponents could paint regular physicians as dogmatic and inflexible peddlers of broken theories. Reading the literature of unorthodox healing sects, one marvels at the perspicacity with which irregular practitioners presented regulars as elite ignoramuses intent on attacking others' contributions and ignoring patients' observations. Sociologist Owen Whooley has, for example, argued that homeopaths intentionally portrayed their medical system as more flexible and amenable to change through empirical observation: "To regulars' opacity and elitism, homeopaths invited the public to assess competing knowledge claims. They also offered a sophisticated system of medical knowledge and articulated an epistemological program that claimed the scientific mantle through an appeal to empiricism."[40] Irregular physicians' recourse to personal experience also manifested itself in the clinical relationship. Historian Roberta Bivins has, for example, argued that homeopaths viewed their patients as partners in treatment. Whereas regular physicians looked with suspicion on patient descriptions of symptoms, homeopathic physicians would sometimes spend hours on an initial consultation, using their patients' experiences as a metric for calibrating treatment. Indeed, homeopathy's founder Samuel Hahnemann himself observed that the patient's "own account of his sensations is the most to be trusted."[41]

That homeopathy was able to claim the mantle of an empirically grounded therapeutic system is remarkable, because Hahnemann's entire therapeutic model was premised upon a theoretical explication of disease. He even referred to his guiding principles as laws. Again, what mattered was not whether a system was rational or empirical but how it was perceived, and irregular medical practitioners—most notably homeopaths—were gifted at presenting their sects as open-minded and progressive and regular medicine as outdated and dogmatic. It was, after all, Hahnemann who introduced the term "allopath" to counterpoise regular medicine in relation to homeopathy, while neatly identifying the sectarian theory upon which regular medical practice was premised. It was a brilliant move, and one that infuriated many regular physicians, such as the editor of the *Maryland Medical Journal* who, in 1885, wrote, "There is no word which so grates on the ears of a cultivated and scientific practitioner of the regular school of medicine as the designation, sometimes given to this school of Allopath." Expressing a keen understanding of Hahnemann's move, he summarized the situation: "It has come to be a fact . . . that the regular profession has allowed the homeopathic school to apply this term to all who differ with their peculiar dogma without resenting the absurdity of its application. It may be asked, what differences does it make what term is applied to the regular school? The answer appears in fact that the idea expressed by the term is deceptive, and classes those thus designated as followers of an exclusive dogma."[42]

Homeopaths successfully straddled rationalism and empiricism while appearing learned and sensitive to individual observation. The sect's openness to the observations of others was joined by its allowance of women to practice. It also sanctioned home health kits, allowing people to become their own doctors (a later incarnation of Thomson's approach to healing). In truth, homeopaths needed to do little to appear open-minded, for the attacks regular physicians waged on their healing system worked wonders to victimize them and make allopaths, helmed by the powerful American Medical Association, come across as bullies.

Thus, at the turn of the century, the Eclectic *American Medical Journal of St. Louis* could publish an editorial lamenting that, "Regular medicine to-day has more dogma, more prejudice, more intolerance, more irregularity, more empiricism, and more bigotry than any other of the schools."[43]

While one might presume that the rise of European laboratory science and the codification of germ theory would have settled allegations of dogmatic rationalism, the situation was not so straightforward. As regular physicians incorporated germ theory into their practice, some worried that the theory was, itself, becoming dogma. In an 1888 article, Dr. J. M. Taylor, former President of the Mississippi State Medical Association and Mississippi State Board of Health, expressed concern that germ theory threatened the contributions of the nation's rural physicians, an intrepid lot of healers who rode by day and night "on horseback, in buggies, and on railroad trains, in all seasons, over the hills and through the swamps, carrying, in a pair of saddle-bags or a little hand-bag, all the medicines, instruments and appliances used by them in the treatment of all diseases and injuries, medical, surgical and obstetrical."[44] While Taylor is careful to express his support for germ theory, calling it "one of the most beautiful and plausible theories that was ever launched on the sea of medical philosophy,"[45] he feared that acquiescence to it derogated the knowledge country physicians had gleaned through their practice:

> This beautiful theory supplies a desideratum in etiology long felt, and furnishes an easy solution to many problems which have greatly perplexed the profession for many generations. Immediately after its promulgation, the fertile mind of the discoverer, ever on the alert for something new, was set to work to find some means of killing these microbes, which like the giants that peopled Don Quixote's brain, cause all the miseries and all of the woes that afflict mankind. Antiseptic surgery, Minerva-like, sprang into existence in full panoply, and has carried the medical profession by storm, with all its boasted modern advancements. So strongly is it endorsed, that it is almost as much as any ordinary man's professional scalp is worth to express any doubts of its entire correctness.[46]

In a particularly pointed indictment, Taylor laments the dogmatic application of germ theory across wide domains of medical practice: "we are not yet freed from the superstition and credulity which have always prevailed in our profession."[47] Germ theory may be true, he submits, but it does not mean that its various applications were appropriate. The profession, in other words, was sacrificing not only experience but practicality for a theory that, while elegant, remained largely untested.[48]

Still, one might question the relevance of this current to late-twentieth-century health activism. After all, through the mid-to-late twentieth century, scientific empiricism was ascendant. The older distinctions between rationalism and empiricism, difficult to maintain even in their heyday, were relegated to the pages of dusty medical treatises. Yet in several important ways, we find that 1980s and 1990s–era unorthodox AIDS activism featured arguments remarkably similar in tone and content to those waged centuries earlier between regular and irregular medical leaders.

As I argue in chapter 4, many early-to-mid 1980s–era AIDS activists alleged that mainstream physicians were guilty of dogmatic thinking. Joseph Sonnabend, a community physician who played a significant role in the history of AIDS activism, complained that following the initial 1984 press conference wherein the viral cause of AIDS was announced, "the theory became a fact."[49] His patient, the prolific and influential Michael Callen, echoed his concerns: "In the weeks surrounding Gallo's announcement, press accounts would cautiously refer to [human T-cell lymphotropic virus type III] HTLV-III[50] as the 'putative' AIDS virus. Reporters were generally careful to remind readers that the assertion that HTLV-III was 'the cause' of AIDS was a hypothesis which was yet to be proven. Then, suddenly, the qualifiers disappeared and the caution evaporated. HIV was decreed to be the cause of AIDS. Wait? Did we miss something?"[51] Through the 1980s, Callen spoke out against mainstream medicine's rapid endorsement of the viral etiological model of AIDS, going as far as to say that it was a product of "scientific nationalism" and fit "nicely with most Americans' unsophisticated notion of germ theory."[52] The parallels between Callen's concern with the rapid acceptance of this model and Taylor's trepidation with germ theory are fascinating. In both cases, the authors based their criticism not on the validity of a given theory, but rather on the speed with which it was codified and operationalized.

CURRENT III: ANTI-AUTHORITARIAN SENTIMENT

The third current considered here is broader still, centering upon popular misgivings with the authority educated healers claimed over the lives and experiences of laypeople. Historically, it was, perhaps, best articulated by practitioners of Thomsonian medicine, which urged patients to eschew elite physicians and "become their own doctors." A century before bioethicists would speak of patient autonomy, Thomson, no doubt inspired by pecuniary interests in drumming up support for his proprietary healing system, spoke of patient empowerment: "[T]he common people have been found capable of examining, judging, and deciding correctly. Give them the facts, the whole facts, and nothing but the facts. By them, we conquer!"[53] This battle cry is best understood within the broader context of the Jacksonian era, a period wherein suspicion of centralized power was high. It was in this setting that Thomsonian medicine thrived, buoyed by what historian Michael Flannery terms a "pervasive anti-intellectualism that belittled both learning and the learned."[54]

While Thomsonian medicine represented a radical rejection of the authority of learned professionals, anti-authoritarianism sentiment could be found across other nineteenth-century healing sects such as hydropathy, homeopathy, and Eclectic medicine. Most commonly, anti-authoritarianism expressed itself through opposition to the monopolization of medicine. Here we find that regular medicine's efforts to respond to the success of sectarian practice fueled anti-authoritarian sentiment. As Nadav Davidovitch has noted, by the turn of the century, journals such as *Medical Talk for the Home, Homeopathic Envoy, Medical Liberty News, Journal of Zoophily,* and *The Arena* fiercely criticized the authoritarianism of regular medicine, invoking the language of monopolies to describe its behavior.[55] Mark Twain even weighed in on the issue in the final decade of his life. Appearing before the New York State Assembly, he defended osteopaths from the efforts of regular physicians to outlaw their practice. Twain testified, "I don't know as I cared much about these osteopaths until I heard you were going to drive them out of the state, but since I heard that I haven't been able to sleep. Now what I contend is that my body is my own, at least, I have always so regarded it. If I do harm through my experimenting with it, it is I who suffer, not the State."[56]

Twain's statements, echoed by many advocates of irregular medicine, do not turn upon the right of practitioners to choose their healing craft but rather that of patients to do with their bodies as they see fit. This popular expression of anti-authoritarianism expanded the anti-intellectual focus of Thomsonian medicine in a way that was compatible with multiple healing systems. It also tied alternative medicine with other early twentieth-century activist movements, most notably the women's health movement. For example, Mary Ware Dennett, birth control advocate and social reformer, served as a Special Lay Representative to the American Foundation for Homeopathy. In this position, she openly resented the "growing medical monopoly" demanded by regular physicians, arguing that people's freedom to choose health practitioners was related to their freedom to make sexual and reproductive decisions.[57]

The 1960s and 1970s witnessed a broad anti-authoritarianism on the macro level, exhibited in large-scale protests against governmental policies, and the micro level, exhibited in challenges to interpersonal and sexual norms. This anti-authoritarianism, coupled with the fear that physicians could cause great harm to patients, contributed to the professionalization of biomedical ethics as an adjunct discipline.[58] By the 1980s and 1990s, bioethical discourse had underscored the importance of informed consent and patient autonomy, challenging older paternalistic models of care.

Given this history, one might question any argument that turns to anti-authoritarianism to explain the origins of unorthodox AIDS activism. For if medicine had shifted from the baldly paternalistic practices of the nineteenth and early twentieth centuries to a more patient-centered model, it seems reasonable to conclude that it ceded some of the authority against which anti-authoritarian activism had organized. Yet a close examination of clinical care through the late twentieth century reveals important institutional and structural expressions of rigidity despite affirmations of patient autonomy. To appreciate the anti-authoritarian impulse of unorthodox AIDS activism, we must, therefore, understand these expressions.

As Barron Lerner has argued, during the 1960s and 1970s—pivotal years in the crystallization of American biomedical ethics and the codification of informed consent and autonomy as key principles of care—biomedicine continued to debate how to respond to patients who disagreed with or disregarded clinical instructions. For mainstream physicians, these patients were "noncompliant," an interpretation that defined them by their variance from an accepted standard of care. That this categorization was in direct tension with the tenets of patient autonomy and informed consent largely escaped critical analysis. Lerner, however, identifies it, arguing that "calling patients 'recalcitrant' and 'noncompliant' reinforced the widely held cultural belief that patients who did not follow physicians' advice were deviant and deserving of aggressive remedial interventions."[59]

Lerner's arguments suggest that it would be incorrect to assume that the rise of bioethics heralded a wholesale transformation in how physicians conceived of patients. A recent search of the National Institutes of Health PubMed database further supports this point. Polling the number of research articles mentioning the term "autonomy," it found an increase from approximately ten per year in the 1960s to 210 per year in the first half of the 1980s. A similar search of the term "noncompliance" reveals an increase from two per year in the 1960s to 730 per year at the start of the 1980s.[60]

Through the 1980s and 1990s, unorthodox AIDS activists articulated anti-authoritarian perspectives in their refusal to comply with biomedical efforts to order and treat their bodies. They argued that, not only did they have the right to be their own doctors, but their own researchers and regulators as well. This anti-authoritarianism was further fueled by fears and frustrations with the pain and damage biomedicine had perpetrated against queer communities in the mid-twentieth century in its medicalization of their sexual identities.

Thus, anti-authoritarian sentiment played an important role in inciting and inspiring nineteenth and twentieth-century unorthodox health activism, including activism organized in response to AIDS. Yet, interestingly, it ultimately would fail to sustain these movements. In the case of Thomsonian medicine, homeopathy, and osteopathy, we find the eventual establishment of medical schools and scholarly journals, directly contradicting the democratic, anti-elitist goals of its founder. And in the case of AIDS, as Steven Epstein has argued, activists who once derided the authority of biomedical researchers and physicians would, in time, transform themselves into lay experts who sought to influence the power structures of biomedicine.[61] Thus, in critiquing authority, the proponents of unorthodox healing systems cultivated their own expertism, demonstrating Foucault's observation that truth is linked "by a circular relation to systems of power which produce it and sustain it, and to effects of power which it induces and which redirect it."[62]

CURRENT IV: ANTIMODERN SENTIMENT

Antimodern campaigns have been launched from multiple berths throughout history. In each case, critics have argued that social, cultural, or economic changes had caused society to lose its bearings. For these individuals, the only remedy was to look backward to a time that was simpler in meaning and aligned with a moral compass that deepened our connections with ourselves, one another, or a higher power. As Jackson Lears has argued, antimodernism pulsed through society in the late nineteenth and early twentieth centuries, tied to apprehension with the changes wrought through industrialization, urbanization, and commercialization.[63] It would come to sustain and animate several unorthodox health movements.

Early-to-mid nineteenth-century concerns with social change were registered on the macro level, in the shifting patterns of commerce as the population expanded, and the micro level, in the transformations occurring in the structure and function of the American family. One representative—and fascinating—critic of these changes was a curmudgeonly preacher named Sylvester Graham. Born in the Connecticut River Valley during George Washington's presidency, Graham's antimodern fears prompted the creation of an influential popular health movement. His health activism, most notably antimodern critiques of U.S. nutritional habits, bear remarkable resemblance to later health movements, including the macrobiotic health initiatives advocated by HEAL. For these reasons, it is instructive to indulge in a brief exhumation of the cantankerous minister sometimes referred to as the father of U.S. vegetarianism.

Graham was deeply unsettled by the social changes taking place in the early nineteenth century, particularly those concerning the family. In response, he introduced a health system that critiqued intemperance in alcohol consumption, sexual behaviors, and dietary habits.[64] However, his beliefs became most associated with his campaign to forestall the fragmentation of systems of production. In it, he channeled his fury into a commercial product that epitomized processes of economic, communal, and familial fragmentation: white bread.

At the time of the nation's founding, bread was produced by families using wheat they had grown or procured from local farmers. However, by the mid-nineteenth century, families had begun purchasing flour prepared hundreds of miles away by faceless farmers and adulterated with additives and preservatives. No single product borne out of modern industrialization attracted greater scorn from Graham than white bread. For him, it not only heralded the disintegration of the family, but it posed direct harm to human health. In its place, he celebrated the virtues of his own "Graham bread," produced using what he called "family flour."[65] Students of history will struggle to find any nostrum in U.S. history possessing greater symbolic meaning than Graham's whole wheat bread. Folded into its grains were fears regarding the family's place in society, the effects of industrialization and commercialization on the family structure, and the underlying identity—we may even use the word "soul"—of the American populace.[66]

While it is easy to categorize Graham's health movement as an adjunct system that avoided commenting on core etiological aspects of regular medicine—a nineteenth-century version of "complementary" medicine—such a formulation would be inaccurate. Graham saw in his system a new framework for understanding all of health and disease. In his view, disease itself was a symptom of widespread, ingrained processes associated with marketplace capitalism, urbanization, and industrialization. Thus, even a disease such as cholera was symbolic of these larger problems. As historian Stephen Nissenbaum notes in his treatment of Graham's contributions to the history of healing: "The disease itself was nothing; what made it lethal and epidemic were the 'customs and circumstances of artificial life' that had reached so deep as to subvert the most basic structure of human need and behavior."[67]

By the late nineteenth century, apprehension with shifting social and economic arrangements reached a zenith. As Lears argues, this period witnessed the decline of Protestant dominance and a rise in secularism. As the nation embraced a culture defined by consumption, it lost its ties to the moral systems that once ordered and gave meaning to day-to-day activities. Furthermore, the explanatory frameworks ascendant during the period—vague, liberal Protestantism and sterile positivism—failed to fill the void left by the retreat of religious experience. As a result, society was afflicted by a "hovering soul sickness."[68]

In late nineteenth-century antimodernism, we find efforts to reclaim a religious or spiritual meaning to day-to-day life, expressed through a recourse to Christian principles and other faiths (e.g., Eastern religious practices). In the 1860s, for example, reformer James Caleb Jackson operated a well-known hydropathic institute in New York State that utilized Graham's system. The institute attracted many of the era's leading figures, including Susan B. Anthony, Frederick Douglass, and Clara Barton, as well as Ellen White, the cofounder of the Seventh Day Adventist religious group. White incorporated the alternative healing methodologies she learned at the institute into her own religious philosophy.[69]

The visitation of one of America's more colorful religious luminaries to Jackson's institute was more than quirk or coincidence—it speaks to the values shared between alternative health movements and religious practice. Closely allied with impositions for a return to a pastoral past and celebration of a simpler, more intimate existence were efforts to situate Americans in relation to a greater power. Many healthcare movements of the time shared this interest, invoking conceptions of a "vital force," a medium that bound body and spirit. Such was the case with American homeopathy, as historian Anne Taylor Kirschmann notes: "Viewing the cause of illness as the result of a disturbed vital force—affecting mind, body, and spirit—advocates counteracted the fragmentation of individual identity by reinforcing traditional notions of the integral relationship of mind, body, and spirit in healing."[70]

The links between irregular medical sects and spiritualism were also registered in the reflections of lay individuals. Recall, for example, Mark Twain's vocal support of irregular healing systems in New York State. In the same testimony before the state legislature wherein he invoked anti-authoritarian sentiments, he included personal reflections interpreting his childhood experience with hydropathy through a spiritual lens:

> I can remember well when the cold-water cure was first talked about. I was then about 9 years old, and I remember how my mother used to stand me up naked in the back yard every morning and throw buckets of cold water on me, just to see what effect it would have. Personally, I had no curiosity upon the subject. And then, when the dousing was over, she would wrap me up in a sheet and then wrap blankets around that and put me into bed. I never realized that the treatment was doing me any particular good physically. But it purified me spiritually. For pretty soon after I was put into bed I would get up a perspiration that was something worth seeing. . . . And when finally she let me out and unwound the sheet, I remember how it was all covered with yellow color, but that was only the outpourings of my conscience, just spiritual outpourings.[71]

At roughly the same time Twain offered these reminiscences, groups such as Boston's Emmanuel Movement and Mary Baker Eddy's Church of Christ, Scientist unambiguously preached the power of spirituality to cure disease.[72] These movements were extraordinary for their popular appeal during the years wherein germ theory was most clearly articulated and defended. Indeed, between 1900 and 1925, the same quarter century that witnessed Robert Koch earn the Nobel Prize for his work on *Mycobacterium tuberculosis* (1905) and Paul Ehrlich discover Salvarsan to treat syphilis (1909), Christian Science was the fastest growing religious denomination in the country. The rise of these spiritual approaches to treating disease, coupled with the broad antimodern turn in conceptualizing health, suggest that historians would do well to interrogate the intersections between religious beliefs and healing practices in the modern era. Historian Roy Porter has suggested as much, arguing, "The religious inputs in medical practice need much further study. Historians have been so concerned with questions such as the secularization of the medical-world view that they have neglected to study the continuing religious motivations for medical practice."[73]

What, then, is the vital spirit? A force that united the physical world with the spiritual, it served as a bridge between modernity's focus on materiality and premodernity's celebration of spirituality. The concept's history is extensive and beyond the scope of this analysis. Still, its manifestations are found throughout the history of medicine in the United States, with one of the most instructive articulations found in the writings of an eighteenth-century leader in both religion and medicine: Cotton Mather.

Mather enjoys passing reference in the history of eighteenth-century medicine, remembered as a Puritan minister who issued recommendations for smallpox inoculation in Boston. His efforts to wade into matters of medicine were often met with the opprobrium of leading physicians.[74] He deeply resented these critiques, viewing them as a sign of the fragmentation of body and spirit borne out of the Enlightenment rationalism of Thomas Hobbes and René Descartes. In response, he drafted a 1724 piece titled *Angel of Bethesda,* wherein he conceptualized a mediator between material and spiritual realms. Referred to as the "nishmath-chajim," a Hebrew phrase meaning "breath of life," this force has been described by historian Margaret Humphreys Warner as a vital spirit.

In Mather's view, the nishmath-chajim is present in every person, is acted upon by both material and nonmaterial forces, and mediates disease. Correspondingly, it is susceptible to the ministrations of both physicians and preachers. Using this concept, Mather devised a taxonomy of three physical explanations for disease (the particulate model, the animalcular theory, and intemperate living), and two nonmaterial explanations (sin and mental unrest). Demonstrating a command of history, theology, and philosophy and responding to the fear that medicine derogated spirit for flesh, Mather articulated a disease model that acknowledged the authority of scientific practitioners while demanding a seat at the table for the preacher.

While few later authors directly invoked Mather's nishmath-chajim in their analyses, the perseverance of the vital spirit in discussions of sectarian medicine is striking.[75] A century after Mather published his theory, Samuel Hahnemann cited a similar concept to explain the function of homeopathic dilutions. Hahnemann invoked the existence of a vital spirit that governed the physiological functioning of the body, upon which his dilutions acted.[76] For historian Robert Fuller, Hahnemann's description "caught the imagination of many intellectuals seeking innovative answers to the perennial question of the relationship of the world of matter to the world of spirit."[77]

Unorthodox health movements such as homeopathy have thus provided nexuses wherein the physical and spiritual worlds could coincide: antimodern spaces that sought to remedy Lears's hovering soul sickness. As such, they played an important role in facilitating what religious historians refer to as "awakenings," or phases in social life wherein communities reshape their identities and thought patterns.[78] For these reasons, they may have filled a void left by mainstream medicine's secularization. This possibility is intriguing, because some scholars have argued that medicine's secularization has contributed to the decline in the public's trust in physicians.[79]

In unorthodox AIDS activism, we see powerful recourse to antimodern sentiment, including efforts to revert to simpler living and reconcile spiritual and material conceptions of disease. This perspective expressed itself in diverse ways, spanning the political spectrum. For example, in explaining the origins of AIDS, we find invocations of divine retribution exacted against those who had, in the eyes of religious fundamentals, countermanded religious law.[80] However, such integrations of the material and spiritual were, by no means, limited to Christian fundamentalists. Among some AIDS activists, both the cause and purported treatment for AIDS were located in the spiritual and mental approach each individual adopted for understanding disease.[81] The leader of one unorthodox AIDS group even referred to himself using the honorific Reverend.[82] Others would turn to Eastern explanatory models, embracing Ayurvedic medicine, Chinese medicine, and other healing systems to conceptualize and respond to AIDS.

If ever there were a period rife for an awakening, it was the 1980s. After all, AIDS demanded a wholesale reconceptualization of identity, as individuals' most intimate behaviors—the fabric of identity itself—became exposed for the world to see. Just as individuals with AIDS struggled with their public association with a stigmatized group, society endured a crisis of identity as it was forced to respond to the fear racking its major metropolises. Out of these crises arose an awakening marked by the reshaping of social patterns and ways of conceptualizing identity and disease.

One final word on antimodern impulses is warranted. Readers may be surprised that I would link antimodern sentiment, epitomized by Grahamian entreaties to return to the traditional family structure, with a modern activist movement promulgated by individuals who faced untold attacks by those wielding these values as weapons against queerness. However, entreaties to antimodernism are not necessarily efforts to recreate the past but to place the present in dialogue with the past. Whereas Graham hoped to preserve the family as the primary organizational unit providing love, affection, safety, and well-being to society, unorthodox AIDS activists sought to redefine and recreate the family. This perspective was, perhaps, best articulated in 1988 by an anonymous author living with AIDS: "The AIDS crisis has shown us that we all have FAMILY. No, not the screwball ideas of family that Jesse Helms et al. promulgate to cheat us out of social benefits—like the right to have decent medical care or the right to live in decent housing. Each and every person who cares for a PWA, each and every cluster of human beings who huddle together in love but who are united by instinct to survive—that is family. There are more binding ties than the antiquated concept of blood relationships, or the horrible legal concoction, 'related by marriage.'"[83] In this passionate articulation of the modern family, we find sentiments that would have seemed familiar to health activists like Graham, who sought, first and foremost, to preserve the intimacy of social connection. In short, even in the modern, we find echoes of the antimodern.

In this chapter, I introduced an approach to conceptualizing the history of medicine and used it to identify several themes attending the rise of unorthodox health activism in the United States. In the following two chapters, I turn my attention to the precise ways in which these themes manifested in the decades preceding the first diagnosed cases of AIDS. In chapter 2, I examine changing popular conceptions of disease through the twentieth century, identifying how anti-authoritarian currents shaped laypeople's perspectives. In chapter 3, I focus on changing public perceptions of the character of medicine and eroding trust in the clinical encounter witnessed in the years immediately preceding AIDS.

2 ▸ A BROKEN MODEL

Twentieth-Century Transformations in the Social Constructions of Health and Disease

AIDS HAS AMASSED an impressive coterie of experts and authorities who have interrogated its every detail, mapped its epidemiologic and genomic profiles, and investigated its clinical, social, and moral sequelae. Virologists have conferenced with public health professionals, infectious disease physicians have lectured internists, policy analysts have advised government officials, and political science, sociology, psychology, bioethics, and gender studies scholars have all endeavored to shed light on the late twentieth century's most famed and feared disease. Analyses and expositions date back to the earliest days of the pandemic, before it was named, when seemingly healthy young people in U.S. metropolises perished from a poorly understood disease.

It was a time of innumerable questions, when neither the medical nor the scientific gaze seemed capable of taming the disease or identifying its most fundamental methods of action. Its natural history, to appropriate the language of clinical medicine, remained trenchantly and tragically unknown. Yet even as questions regarding its causative agent, its method of gaining access to and destroying cells, and its means of dissemination were raised by scholars and lay individuals alike, deeper fears reverberated throughout society. They reached beyond mechanistic diagrams, immunologic cell counts, and genomic guesswork and spoke to growing uncertainties regarding the state of health and disease in the modern world. How was it, many wondered, that we were staring through the haze at a disease lifted from the codices of the Middle Ages? What had happened to the progress and promise of yesterday and to the security society had been bequeathed by the forefathers of modern biomedicine?

These questions, intimated in the hushed whispers and uneasy stares greeting those suspected of harboring the unknown causative agent of AIDS, are the substance of historical inquiry. That this is the case is unsurprising, for societies have long turned to history for guidance when faced with existential threats, be they from the invisible waves of incurable disease or the armored legions of unstoppable aggressors. When the future appears in flux, society turns to the past to find islands of stability, reference points whereupon it may construct a compass for navigating the stormy waters of the present. Yet despite our age-old propensity for seeking guidance in the past, the precise ways in which people learn from, appropriate, and arrogate history to inform the present remain poorly understood.[1] Indeed, while we grant that individuals turn to historical memory and example to navigate treacherous times, much like sailors turned to constellations born out of history and myth to steer their ships, we do not always understand why people summon particular historical memories or what they mean to them.

I maintain that this deficiency in our understanding of the popular use and interpretation of historical memory is particularly acute in the case of AIDS. In the four decades since early cases of *Pneumocystis carinii*[2] and Kaposi's sarcoma were diagnosed in otherwise healthy gay men in New York and California, we have amassed a remarkable body of evidence exploring how AIDS has changed the way we think about and respond to disease, how we conceive of privacy in the context of illness, how we investigate and approve drugs, and how we mobilize as a lay society to influence health policy. In short, it has caused us to reflect critically upon what AIDS has meant to the history of medicine. Yet we know relatively little about what the history of medicine meant for people living in the early era of AIDS or how this history was invoked and interpreted. I suggest that to fully appreciate the history of AIDS—including the history of unorthodox AIDS activism—we must answer two questions: First, which strands of historical understanding did individuals in the 1980s and 1990s graft onto AIDS? Second, how did these historical narratives intersect and interact with their lived experiences and interpretations of recent history?

In this chapter, I explore each of these questions in sequence. First, I identify the dominant historical narratives into which AIDS was assimilated and through which it was explained. To address the second question, I argue that individuals confronted by AIDS interpreted the dominant historical narrative from a perspective shaped by disease discourse developed through the 1960s and 1970s. These interpretations challenged the dominant narrative, producing unsanctioned histories of the epidemic. It is in these unsanctioned pages of the AIDS historiography that we identify the underlying principles and perspectives that anchored unorthodox AIDS activism.

SANCTIONED MEANING: LOCATING AIDS WITHIN HISTORY

In the earliest days of the AIDS pandemic, as social commentators, politicians, and public leaders struggled to make sense of the sudden suffering and death visited upon countless communities across America, they turned to the metaphors and images born out of past events. The past to which they turned was a distant, discontinuous one that reached beyond recent memory. This trend was, perhaps, best exemplified by journalists' frequent use of the term "plague" to describe early cases of AIDS. In the developed world, the term was little more than an historical artifact, exhumed from time to time by newspaper columnists intent on regaling readers with harrowing accounts of the black death, cholera, and other monsters of bygone eras. During the 1980s and 1990s, however, the term enjoyed a resurgence in the popular press. In 1985, journalist David Black published "The Plague Years," a popular two-part article in *Rolling Stone*, the title of which summoned Daniel Defoe's 1722 account of the bubonic plague.[3] Columnists writing in the *New York Times* openly discussed "the plague of AIDS" and contemplated the existence of a "pre-plague" and "post-plague" gay culture.[4] Furthermore, the trend was, by no means, limited to New York papers. The term "gay plague" was used to describe AIDS in periodicals as far ranging as the *Washington Post*; *Minneapolis Star Tribune*; *Charlotte Observer*; *Irish Times*; *Times of India*; Toronto's *Globe and Mail*; and London's *Daily Mirror*, *Daily Telegraph*, and *Observer*.[5] Given its ubiquity, it is no wonder that medievalist Steven F. Kruger would lament, "The association of HIV/AIDS with the medieval has been most persistent in the intractable appellation 'plague,' assigned to AIDS even before its current name had been settled."[6]

While some authors located AIDS within the narrative of premodern disease through their choice of language, others reinforced this association through images. Consider, for example, the legacy of editorial cartoonists, who in ways both subtle and bold buttressed the notion that AIDS was best interpreted as a reconstituted horror of a bygone past. In some cases, cartoonists yoked AIDS to disease narratives recorded in modern civilization's origin texts, summoning fears of biblical scourges from Christian eschatology. This brand of symbolism was on display in early cartoons published in Los Angeles and London personifying AIDS as the four horsemen of the apocalypse.[7] A San Diego cartoon depicted a student with AIDS shunned by his peers, all of whom wore masks and bore crosses like those used in the seventeenth century to ward off bubonic plague. One cartoon published in London's *Daily Mirror* depicted a robed figure, presumably Moses, descending upon an orgy of naked men and women with a stone tablet emblazoned with the term "AIDS."[8] Furthermore, these images cut across social and cultural borders, appearing in countries with different experiences of AIDS. Consider, for example, the image of the scythe-wielding skeleton harassing the sick. Once popularly associated with American and British depictions of cholera, by the 1990s it appeared as part of the AIDS canon in newspapers from cities as wide ranging as Cincinnati, Ohio; Dallas, Texas; Miami, Florida; Minneapolis, Minnesota; Victoria, Canada; Madrid, Spain; Bonn, Germany; Zagreb, Croatia; San Pedro, Honduras; Lagos, Nigeria; Amsterdam in the Netherlands and Manila in the Philippines.[9]

At roughly the same time journalists and cartoonists analogized AIDS with historical and biblical scourges, conservative critics deepened the association by interpreting the condition as an expression of divine retribution. Using the suffering wrought by the disease as an opportunity to rail against the perceived excesses of the sexual revolution, they rained fire and brimstone on the "homosexual lifestyle." Ed Rowe, who had directed Anita Bryant's ministries in the late 1970s, famously condemned gays as, "anti-God, anti-Christ, anti-Bible, anti-moral, anti-life, anti-constitutional and anti-American."[10] Meanwhile, conservative pastors such as Jerry Falwell maintained that AIDS was "God's punishment . . . for the society that tolerates homosexuals."[11] These attacks, born out of what Robert Fogel terms the "Fourth Great Awakening" of religiosity in America,[12] yoked AIDS to 3,000 year old biblical narratives while simultaneously subverting a biomedical discourse that left little room for spontaneous acts of celestial wrath.[13] Indeed, for many public health professionals, religious leaders' efforts to present AIDS as an extension of ancient scourges meted out by a vengeful god crossed a line. Even Surgeon General C. Everett Koop, credited by some conservatives as a key force in the crystallization of the American evangelical movement,[14] challenged the association of AIDS with the plagues of the distant past, arguing, "Not since the days when people did not understand leprosy and put its victims in chains have we seen such outrageous behavior."[15]

As journalists, religious leaders, and others linked AIDS to historic plagues spanning recorded history and counseled the resurrection of nineteenth-century public health measures to combat its spread, historians went to work explaining the origins of these measures. It was in this tradition that Allan Brandt penned an early article—"AIDS in Historical Perspective: Four Lessons from the History of Sexually Transmitted Disease"—conveying the nuanced histories of late nineteenth and early twentieth-century venereal disease campaigns.[16] The same year, historians Elizabeth Fee and Daniel Fox released the edited volume *AIDS: The Burdens of History*, exploring the historical origin of infectious disease policies. While these authors set out to demonstrate the need for nuanced historical analysis that eschewed interpretations born out of presentism and Whiggish historiography, they also reinforced connections between AIDS and the distant past. The volume's epigraph, which immediately follows a 1930s-era syphilis awareness poster depicting a couple menaced by a skull silhouette, conveys this sentiment. Quoting the admonition of an early twentieth-century physician responding to polio, the editors avow, "We have learned very little that is new about the disease, but much that is old about ourselves."[17] Given the extraordinary degree to which individuals across multiple institutions and professions located AIDS within pre-twentieth-century plague narratives, we might regard this historical framing as the sanctioned history of AIDS, a mapping of the modern disease that was at once descriptive and normative.[18]

As the 1980s progressed, scholars continued framing AIDS in terms of past responses to turn-of-the-century epidemics, virtually all of which had been conquered through the interventions of modern biomedicine. In moving from premodern eschatology through nineteenth-century plague narratives to the clinical and public health lessons of the early twentieth century, the sanctioned historical framing of AIDS recapitulated earlier histories of disease leading up to the golden era of biomedicine. In the very language individuals used, in the narratives they appropriated, and in the metaphors they invoked, authors recreated the rough equivalent of a biomedical passion play, culminating in the miraculous taming of AIDS through the identification of its microbial cause and marshaling of the instruments of clinical medicine. So powerful was this progress narrative that, for some, society needed only identify the germ cause of AIDS and its eradication was but a fait accompli.[19] Margaret Heckler, Secretary of Health and Human Services under Ronald Reagan, fell victim to such reasoning. In 1984, with the announcement of the discovery of HTLV–III/LAV (later renamed HIV) as the cause of AIDS, she predicted the testing of a vaccine within two years, triumphantly declaring, "Yet another terrible disease is about to yield to patience, persistence and outright genius."[20]

But alas, this was not to be, for HIV would prove itself impervious to the best efforts of physicians and researchers. The vaccine Heckler had pontificated failed to materialize, even with the intercession of biomedical royalty such as Jonas Salk.[21] For half a decade, the mills of biomedical innovation seemed to grind to a halt. Fields lay fallow from either a lack of material resources or, some maintained, a drought of ingenuity. Moreover, even those tools available for use—the traditional measures of public health—had lost their purchase among many segments of the public. As Ronald Bayer has argued, society had entered an era of AIDS exceptionalism when past strategies—name reporting, routine testing, and partner notification—no longer seemed appropriate for combating AIDS.[22]

In this perceived incongruity, we register the distinction between the two questions that organize this chapter. Having identified the historical narratives through which AIDS was explained by journalists, cartoonists, religious leaders, and scholars, we addressed the first of these questions. We now turn to the second, more nebulous query, asking what these narratives meant for individuals living with and responding to AIDS in the 1980s and 1990s. In short, how was the light of historical plague refracted as it passed through lenses hewn by personal experiences, memories, and interpretations of the more recent past?[23]

UNSANCTIONED INTERPRETATIONS: THE MEANINGS OF HISTORY

For centuries, poets have reminded us of the kaleidoscopic nature of the past and how its meanings and lessons are obfuscated by the perspectives, opinions, experiences, and memories of the beholder. Yesterday does not sit idle and inert, waiting to be mined by the historian. It is, instead, mercurial, transforming based upon the historically and culturally mediated experiences and perspectives of individuals. William Wordsworth captured the sentiment nicely when, at the dawn of the Victorian Era, he argued that those wishing to ponder the noble promises of the past toiled in vain, for they would ever find themselves thwarted by "impediments from day to day renewed."[24] Nearly a century and a half later, another writer expressed a similar sentiment when he wrote, "'So my past is homeless now too,' I thought, / And slammed the window on the glimpse I'd caught." A young Charles Barber penned these words while attending an AIDS support group in the early 1980s. Within three years of having written them, on the anniversary of the nation's birth, he would die of AIDS-related complications.

Armed with Barber's chilling conjuration of a history bereft of meaning, we turn our attention once more to AIDS exceptionalism. As I have argued, through the earliest days of the AIDS pandemic, society demonstrated an eagerness to disinter the plagues of the past to graft meaning onto the new disease. Despite this, the public proved largely unwilling to consummate the allusion by responding to AIDS with the policies and approaches it had successfully employed for these older diseases. Indeed, we might say that society's response to AIDS was exceptional, not just because it differed from responses to prior infectious illnesses, but because it did so even as the sanctioned history of AIDS dramatically described it in relation to them.

One explanation for AIDS exceptionalism holds that the public's response to AIDS differed because of fundamental changes in social conceptualizations of individual rights through the mid-to-late twentieth century.[25] This approach weds analyses of AIDS with the historical rise of gay rights and patient activist groups such as ACT UP.[26] In describing society's failure to enforce traditional public health measures, the narrative implicitly explains suffering and death as a byproduct of the nation's embrace of individual rights. This broad historiographic approach explains tragedy as the cost of progress.[27]

Yet this rationalization masks other potential explanations for the changing meaning of historical experience in the early years of the AIDS epidemic. We should, for example, consider the possibility that exceptionalism resulted, at least in part, from fundamental transformations in the social construction of disease itself. For, if popular conceptualizations of disease had changed significantly through the early-to-mid twentieth century, then invocations of nineteenth-century public health measures would lack appeal. To invoke them would be to invoke a past that, in effect, had been rendered homeless.

As I shall argue, through the 1950s, 1960s, and 1970s, individuals embraced models of disease etiology that challenged the reductionism attending biomedicine's ascent during the golden era of biomedicine. Inspired by broad changes in the national health burden and the rise of social activism criticizing fundamental social arrangements, this discursive tradition sought to redefine health as a function of irreducible interrelations between physical, emotional, social, and environmental spheres. These perspectives would persist through the earliest days of the AIDS pandemic, challenging dominant AIDS narratives and efforts to respond to it. As I shall demonstrate, they shaped the lenses through which the light of AIDS would refract.

A CHANGING PAST: TRANSFORMATIONS IN CONSTRUCTIONS OF DISEASE AND HEALTH

> [W]e are, in a sense, at the end of the great era of the battle against infectious disease. We are entering the great era of cold war against chronic diseases for which we do not have biologic cures.
>
> —New York City Department of Health, 1961[28]

To understand the aims of unorthodox activists responding to AIDS in 1980s and 1990s–era New York City, it is important that we examine the transformations in the social discourse surrounding health in the first half of the twentieth century. Jeff Goldsmith has argued that this period ushered in a paradigm shift in society's response to disease.[29] By the 1920s, cardiovascular disease and cancer had supplanted the contagious illnesses of the previous generation as the leading cause of death in the United States.[30] As the century progressed, each decade reinforced the notion that, while infectious diseases remained an issue in segments of the population, their significance to the nation's overall health paled in comparison to chronic conditions. The antibiotic revolution of the 1930s seemed to sound the death knell for the once formidable germ.[31] In the 1950s, the National Tuberculosis Association had become the National Lung Association. By the 1970s, the nation's Communicable Disease Center, which had played an important role in the national response to malaria, venereal disease, and tuberculosis, was rechristened the Centers for Disease Control (CDC) to reflect a mission expanded beyond the parameters of infectious disease.[32] At roughly the same time, Richard Nixon signed the National Cancer Act, viewed by many as initiating the war on cancer, with funding for cancer research increasing from $377 million to $815 million between 1972 and 1976.[33] Furthermore, in 1979, just months before the CDC's *Morbidity and Mortality Report* disseminated word of a strange new disease visited upon the nation's cities, researchers who had assembled in Washington for a conference dedicated to developing disease strategies for the 1980s focused the vast majority of their attention on chronic conditions. In fact, the conference organizers made explicit their hope that those assembled would replicate the ingenuity of the "glorious age" of infectious disease as they tackled the chronic conditions that would surely define the decade.[34]

What of the lay public? May we assume that, as those located in the nation's intellectual and political nexus focused on chronic conditions, the same trend was exhibited in discussions had by families across the dining room table? Public opinion polls conducted in the 1960s and 1970s offer some insight into popular ideas. In 1973, G. Ray Funkhouser reported in *Public Opinion Quarterly* that of the top ten issues dominating the concerns of Americans, nearly half were related to chronic disease.[35] Preliminary evidence from newspaper sources further suggests that journalistic coverage of health issues changed in important ways through the twentieth century. In news outlets such as the *New York Times, Los Angeles Times, Amsterdam News,* and *Time Magazine,* coverage of chronic conditions such as cancer increased through the 1950s, surpassing articles examining infectious disease.

Thus, by the 1970s, by both professional and popular measures, national discourse surrounding disease had transformed, with discussions of chronic maladies supplanting earlier campaigns aimed at eradicating the pestiferous germ.[36] We might, therefore, conclude that Goldsmith's paradigm shift accurately captured changes in political, intellectual, and social discourse. Yet his chosen metaphor has limitations. For the term "shift" suggests that society moved from one system of conceptualizing disease (the infectious model) to another (the chronic) like shifting gears in a car.[37] However, disease paradigms are not instruments society exploits when the terrain becomes rough. They are historically contingent, culturally constructed languages for thinking about, ordering, discussing, and responding to the world. While they change over time, they do so for complex reasons that reach beyond a society's epidemiological profile. It is more appropriate to say that, over the course of the mid-to-late twentieth century, society developed an approach for conceiving of and discussing disease that harmonized with changing discourses regarding larger political, social, and economic issues.

That we would witness a fundamental change in the language used to define and respond to disease in post–World War II society is unsurprising, for the period brought great apprehension regarding social arrangements. Feminist critiques of systems and practices inimical to women's health harmonized with exposés of the dangers lurking in the interstices of a society overridden with industrial pollution, occupational abuses, and commercialized negligence. In 1962, Rachel Carson's widely influential *Silent Spring* exposed the latent toxicities of pesticides and other chemicals used to enhance food production in the industrialized world.[38] The same year, Michael Harrington's *The Other America* exposed the tragic reality of poverty in the nation.[39] Debates surrounding the detrimental effects of industrial excess and structural discrimination continued through the 1970s, with the publication of *Our Bodies, Ourselves* in 1970–1971 (re-released in 1973, 1976 and 1979) and extensive reporting on environmental disasters such as the Love Canal tragedy of 1978.[40]

During this period, authors who challenged the continued relevance of infectious disease and plague narratives premised their arguments upon a deep apprehension with these greater social and environmental issues. One of the most vocal and influential authors writing in this tradition was the French-born René Dubos, a microbiologist who had found fame in the discovery of gramicidin, the first clinically manufactured antibiotic.[41] While Dubos cut his teeth investigating cures for germs, he would go on to spend much of his career arguing that humanity's problems were of an order and scale far greater than the domain of the bacillus. For Dubos, one could not simply magnify and resolve health and disease to its base cellular or molecular dimensions, for it flowed from the complex relationship between the individual and the environment. It was born in the social and environmental arrangements that many uncritically accepted as the necessary conditions of modern progress.

If Thomas Hobbes argued that the individual required society to liberate him from a life that was "solitary, poor, nasty, brutish, and short," Dubos maintained that he needed protection from a modern structure which entrapped him in a world of "noise, dirt, ugliness, and absurdity."[42] From 1968 through his death in 1982, Dubos argued that disease resulted from the stresses posed by modern industrialization and the codification of the modern myth which held that "progress means introducing into our lives everything we know how to produce."[43]

Dubos did more than indict social arrangements permitting inequity and disease. He also criticized a scientific community that, in his view, had failed to adequately address the problem. Modern biomedicine had become fixated on what he termed "the doctrine of specific etiology," causing researchers to neglect interactions between individuals and their environment.[44] So enraged was Dubos at his colleagues' failures to address this complex relationship that he began his 1968 Pulitzer Prize–winning treatise *So Human an Animal* by asserting his "indignation at the failure of the scientific community to organize a systematic effort against the desecration of life and nature."[45] Throughout his work, Dubos—a self-described humanist who had coined the term "humanistic biology"—echoed the views of many that the reductionism of Western science was poorly suited to address the diseases of modern life.

Historian Charles Rosenberg would note that the reductionist turn in biomedicine began with the popularization of specificity—the notion that diseases were properly thought of as entities existing outside their unique manifestations in a given person. However, it was the adoption of germ theory, Rosenberg argued, that provided the "powerful argument for a reductionist, mechanism-oriented way of thinking about the body and its felt malfunctions."[46] While this reductionist approach would make extraordinary advances in medicine possible,[47] many authors began to echo Dubos's concerns with its unanticipated effects. Vijay Kumar Yadavendu, for example, has argued, "The process of individuation, biologism and reductionism started with germ theory. Through the shifts in epidemiology, the population dimension was reduced first to the individual dimension and finally to the molecular dimension. This effectively obviated the dynamics of interaction between the individual and his/her environment . . . In the final victory of molecular medicine over public health, the individual is completely robbed of his/her collective identity."[48]

Thus, to appropriate a term popularized by Michel Foucault, postwar critics argued that the "clinical gaze" was dehumanizing and myopic, reducing individuals to physiochemical reactions while systematically failing to consider their dynamic relationship with their environment. Many individuals wrote of biomedicine's myopia, arguing that its practices ignored the lessons laid bare by recent history. As biomedicine suffered, they argued, so did its patients. In 1954, example, New York Academy of Medicine spokesperson Iago Galdston published an edited volume titled *Beyond the Germ Theory* wherein he argued that traditional infectious disease models were insufficient for responding to the era's chronic diseases. In their place, he advocated etiological models prioritizing the importance of environmental stress, nutrition, and emotions.[49] These ideas were further developed by George L. Engel in his famous biopsychosocial model of illness.[50] For some readers, such arguments for a more socially and environmentally rooted clinical practice may call to mind the public health model of illness. Indeed, as Allan Brandt and Martha Gardner have argued, modern medicine's professionalization was marked, in part, by the erecting of boundaries between itself and public health.[51] In the developed world's twentieth-century transition to chronic disease, we thus find critiques of these boundaries.

Some of these critiques were quite direct. In 1978, John Ehrenreich lambasted the funds bequeathed to the stewards of biomedicine in the name of the nation's war on cancer. Ehrenreich maintained that society's investment amounted to little more than "devastating courses of radiation or drug therapy or debilitating radical surgery" despite the fact that the vast majority of cancers were caused by avoidable environmental hazards such as pollution, smoking, food additives, pesticides, and radiation.[52] For Ehrenreich, the unchecked pursuit of technology had led medicine down a path that promised little in the way of succor or amelioration of disease.[53] "Scientific medicine," he wrote, "for all its insights into the molecular mechanisms of carcinogenesis, has simply become unhinged from any fundamentally effective approach to the disease."[54] Other authors would question whether biomedicine had ever contributed significantly to decreases in mortality rates. For scholars such as Thomas McKeown, much of the credit went instead to changes in broad standards of living through the industrial age—an interpretation that complemented the environmental and structural focus of Dubos, Engel, and Ehrenreich.[55]

Thus, far from a mechanistic shift in paradigms, society's transition from germ theory-based infectious disease models to socially and environmentally mediated chronic disease models was, itself, an expression of more widespread critiques of underlying social, political, and economic arrangements. The transformation in health discourse parallels similar transformations in broader geopolitical discourse. During the same years that Koch and Pasteur conquered the germ, nations such as the United States and Great Britain openly pursued imperialist agendas. Successes in one domain strengthened the other, with both sharing a common language that yoked scientific progress to nationalist agendas.[56]

However, by the late twentieth century, as the New York City Department of Health declared, society had reached the "end of the battle against infectious disease" and entered the "great era of cold war against chronic disease." This word choice is telling, for in an environment of simmering hostility between former allies, the germ theory had lost its luster. The anti-authoritarianism of the 1960s and 1970s, fomented by widespread dissatisfaction with the nation's failed foray into the Vietnam War, buttressed fears that the policies and practices effected in an effort to make the United States stronger were, in fact, causing irreparable harm to its people.[57]

A reader may ask what strategies for decreasing morbidity and mortality are to be gleaned from the soaring idealism of René Dubos or the acerbic criticisms of John Ehrenreich. How precisely was society to address chronic disease if it did indeed spring from the relationship between people and their increasingly complex environment? Several avenues of intervention presented themselves. The first counseled a fundamental restructuring of social arrangements to address the inimical byproducts of industrialization, urbanization, and market capitalism. However, while we find several efforts to effect structural social change through the 1960s, it should come as little surprise that neither the U.S. Congress nor the American Medical Association's House of Delegates exhibited a hankering to codify wholesale anticapitalist critiques into law. Instead, through the 1960s and 1970s, we find the promulgation of less radical strategies for increasing health that would ultimately refract concerns with socially embedded and environmentally mediated sources of illness through the individual lens. Two such strategies bear mentioning here, as they would go on to play important roles in the social response to AIDS through the 1980s and 1990s.

The first of these avenues is considered the more conservative. For, while it granted that chronic disease resulted from individuals' interactions with their environment, it located its cause in the unhealthy decisions individuals made in those interactions. To the chagrin of many authors, this approach largely ignored deeper structural inequalities and inescapable sources of harm woven through society and instead focused on the inability of individuals to manage their own behaviors.[58] It was perhaps most influentially expressed in the writings of John Knowles, President of the Rockefeller Foundation,[59] in addition to state-sponsored documents such as Canada's 1974 "A New Perspective on the Health of Canadians" (commonly referred to as the Lalonde Report) and the 1979 U.S. Surgeon General Report *Healthy People*. For their authors, society could not depend upon biomedicine to cure the ailments of the modern age, because it had become hopelessly wedded to a paradigm that had run its course. Knowles himself underscored this point in radioactive rhetoric apropos to the Cold War era:

> The medical profession hitched its wagon to the rising star of science and technology. The results have been spectacular for some individuals in terms of cure, containment of disease, and alleviation of suffering; as spectacular in terms of the horrendous costs compounding now at a rate of 15 per cent annually. And even more spectacular to some because allocation of more and more men and women, money, and machines has affected mortality and morbidity rates only marginally. The problem of diminishing returns, if current trends continue, will look as large and pregnant to the American people in the future as the mushrooming atomic cloud does today.[60]

Underpinning Knowles's arguments were deep economic insecurities regarding the growing expense of healthcare in the context of an increasingly specialized clinical model. In many ways, Knowles extended the notion of the deviant sick role first introduced by Talcott Parsons in 1951. However, where Parsons's model focused on sick individuals' responsibility to become healthy so they could once more contribute meaningfully to society, Knowles and his enthusiasts generalized these arguments to the preventive domain, demanding that individuals actively work to remain healthy for the same reason. This extension of Parsons's model exhibits the characteristics of what Michel Foucault termed the "somatocracy"—"a regime that sees the care of the body, corporal health, the relation between illness and health, etc. as appropriate areas of state intervention."[61] We recognize the legacy of this approach in public health campaigns that convey a moralistic imperative for people to quit smoking, hold the sugar, cut the fat, and abstain from sex. In the years immediately preceding the first diagnosed cases of AIDS, and in an article in the same volume wherein Rosner and Reverby advocated a social historical approach to the history of medicine,

Robert Crawford critiqued this tradition's tendency to respond to structurally and societally mediated inequities through changes in individual behavior.[62]

This first avenue for conceiving of and responding to chronic disease would attract significant support through the late twentieth century, particularly with those allied with the right wing of American politics. However, another avenue warrants mention, as it would go on to influence the history of unorthodox AIDS activism in important ways. Like the Knowlesian perspective, this model granted the complex interplay between the individual and the environment in mediating disease, challenged the wisdom of clinical medicine's reductionism, and located responses to illness in the individual's actions. However, while Knowles's argument was premised upon a motivating morality, the second model was predicated upon what we might call a radical ontology. It counseled a metaphysical approach to re-mystify the human body, underscoring the complex interrelationships between the physical, emotional, environmental, and social spheres of life.[63] As advocates of this re-mystification professed, these interrelationships were difficult, if not impossible, to reduce.[64] Correspondingly, neither the highly technologized gadgetry of a reductionist biomedicine nor a rigid moralism would secure health. Individuals would have to grant the deep connections between these spheres of existence and implement changes in their lives that acknowledged and acted upon these interrelations.

For some readers, bubbling beneath this talk of irreducible dynamic interrelationships is a term associated with leftist radicalism: "health holism." This is no coincidence, for each of the authors whose work I discussed above advocated an approach to health and disease broadly consistent with holistic ideologies. Ehrenreich, for example, explicitly endorsed a "reexploration of more holistic approaches to health and disease" to understanding how the "body, mind, and environment . . . *interact* to produce disease or cure it."[65] Dubos, meanwhile, imbued holism with an air of historic legitimacy in his call for more universal models of health and disease: "Clinical and epidemiological studies show that the inextricably interrelated body, mind, and environment must be considered together in any medical situation whether it involves a single patient or a whole community. In a long, roundabout way, scientific medicine is thus returning to the Unitarian concept of disease intuitively perceived by the Hippocratic physicians 2,500 years ago."[66]

The full array of practices that fit this description is vast and defies straightforward characterization. However, despite this diversity, we may identify several common themes. In many of its iterations, health holism challenges Cartesian models of mind-body dualism, rejecting reductionism while embracing premodern conceptions of bridged physical and spiritual worlds, like the historic antimodern discourse discussed in chapter 1. For holistic health practitioners, health and happiness stem from a state of balance and harmony between the many domains of life. It was governed, as one *Chicago Tribune* reporter wrote in

1976, by "the search for the Certain Something, that elusive state of contentment and inner well-being."[67]

Furthermore, in challenging the technologism of modern medicine, health holism frequently glorified nature—yet another expression of antimodernism. While Hobbes had argued that mankind required society to improve its lot, holistic health reified the individual unpolluted by modern society, at times directly (and insensitively) invoking the image of a "noble savage" who found health through a connection with a primal mode of life.[68] In holism, we furthermore find a move away from Western modes of treatment in favor of methodologies developed in other nations—many of which invoked spiritual reasoning. Finally, practitioners of health holism often frame their movement using anti-authoritarian language that directly challenges the expertise of biomedical professionals. In some cases, these challenges also invoke the perceived toxicities of biomedical treatments, thereby invoking antiheroic currents.

Through the 1960s, 1970s, and 1980s, myriad health movements sharing one or more of these characteristics spread through the nation, each in its own way attempting to demonstrate how individuals could attain better health through an understanding and operationalization of the dynamic health model. The list of such movements is legion, running the gamut from herbalism, Chinese medicine, acupuncture, and macrobiotic diets to positive psychology, spiritual health, and visualization.[69] While these healing systems differed in their precepts and the degree to which they emphasized the dynamic interaction between the physical, emotional, and environmental, they all claimed to provide individuals with a means to achieve order, balance and stability in their health.[70] Holistic health models enjoyed success through the mid-to-late twentieth century.[71] In 1982, a mere month before the CDC introduced the term AIDS, James S. Gordon—who would go on to chair President Clinton's White House Commission on Complementary and Alternative Medicine Policy—marveled that holistic medicine had "rapidly emerged as a visible and controversial force in American medicine."[72]

Some readers may grant the proliferation of holistic health movements through the mid-to-late twentieth century and acknowledge the influence of Knowlesian arguments while nonetheless objecting to my decision to present them together. Surely, they would maintain, I have engaged in sloppy reasoning by categorizing Knowles's moralistic calls for responsible living alongside radical holistic health movements helmed by individuals some derided as left-leaning, crystal-wielding, "masters of doubletalk and weasel wording" quacks.[73]

To be clear, I do not mean to argue that the two avenues were identical or that their proponents frequented the same academic conferences. Yet they shared much in common. Both approaches were fundamentally conservative in empowering the individual to demand and achieve a healthier life. In the case of the moral injunctions found in *Healthy People*, the Lalonde Report, and John Knowles's writing, this empowerment flowed from the oft-cited injunction "ought implies can." In maintaining that people had an ethical obligation to maintain their health and overcome illness, these texts implied that individuals were indeed capable of proactively taking charge of their health. Meanwhile, for proponents of health holism, empowerment flowed from an understanding of the deep connections between the physical, emotional, and environmental spheres and the corresponding belief that action in one could effect change in others. In short, in both approaches, individuals were nominally empowered to participate actively in their care.

For readers still skeptical of the overlaps between Knowlesian and holistic approaches, a brief exercise may prove helpful. In 1976, a *Chicago Tribune* reporter penned an article wherein she quipped, "Of course, curing our own illness just may be the flip side of causing our own illness."[74] Without consulting the text of the article, one might ask whether the author here invokes Knowles, arguing that individuals must assume responsibility for the ills they had visited upon themselves by their own actions. Or, alternatively, is she advocating the direct empowerment of the individual through an operationalization of the interrelationships between behavior and environment, as well as emotional and physical health? Is she intimating that individuals are responsible for health as agents liable for its loss, or are they responsible as agents capable of commanding and creating it?

The title of the article—"Mind-Body Link and 'Heal Thyself' are New Medicine 'Miracle Drugs'"—solves the mystery. However, the ambiguity is more than a semantic parlor trick. Discussions of health frequently move between the primary and secondary connotation of responsibility, and in so doing transition between holistic and Knowlesian perspectives. In 1978, for example, Lewis Thomas, President of the Sloan-Kettering Cancer Center, bemoaned that individuals were resorting to "magical" thinking, assuming they could regain health by magically deciding to become healthy.[75] "Laetrile cures cancer," Thomas complained, "acupuncture is useful for deafness and low-back pain, vitamins are good for anything, and meditation, yoga, dancing, biofeedback . . . are specifics for the human condition."[76] In an article published in the magazine of the *University of California, San Francisco,* Joel Gurin examined the source of this magical reasoning, concluding, "The most prominent source for this view is probably John Knowles, president of the Rockefeller Foundation . . . [who] has written that, 'The next major advances in the health of the American people will be determined by what the individual is willing to do for himself.'"[77] The polysemy we register in Western conceptualizations of responsibility underscores the absence of clear borders between seemingly disparate health and disease paradigms—even when the practitioners of such ideas occupy diametrically opposed positions along the nation's left-right divide.[78]

Somewhere between Knowles and holistic health practitioners, we draw a line and the similarities between movements recede. We see only differences: the conventional versus the radical, the passionate versus the pathological. The history that subtends them erodes, leaving behind a narrative that presents one as an extension of orthodoxy and the other as a discontinuous break in historic progress. In drawing lines and erecting walls, we blind ourselves to the forces that cause individuals to position themselves within borderlands between systems, borrowing ideas and merging beliefs to construct meaning.

CONCLUSION: A PAST RENDERED HOMELESS

By the late 1970s, we identify a clear criticism of a reductionist biomedical system. In the context of growing disillusionment with biomedicine's ability to address chronic diseases and inspired by broad social movements underscoring unfair and destructive social arrangements, we witness a transformation in health paradigms. However, we must remember that these changes did not happen overnight, nor did they flow naturally or mechanically from changes in disease demographics. They were, instead, the result of gradual transformations in sociopolitical discourse.

Just as I have argued that society did not spontaneously shift health paradigms in the face of rising tides of chronic disease, it follows that it did not shift back to infectious models in the era of AIDS. As communities considered the visitation of a plague upon cities in the early 1980s, they processed infectious disease narratives through a perspective shaped by the discourse of the 1960s and 1970s. Even as journalists wrote of unchecked plague, cartoonists depicted medieval horrors, evangelicals preached of cataclysmal fury, and scholars mined the histories of syphilis and cholera, individuals interpreted the disease through behavioral, emotional, social, and environmental lenses, challenging the reductionism of biomedicine. This enduring lay discursive tradition never fully disappeared, even following the identification of the virus that causes AIDS. It persisted in the everyday forms of resistance and overt campaigns subsumed under the rubric of unorthodox AIDS activism.

Older models for ordering health and disease die neither noble nor ignoble deaths, but instead persist, resonating at various times with different segments of society. Unlike Kuhnian models of revolutions within scientific paradigms or Foucauldian conceptualizations of discontinuous ruptures between historical eras, old models coexist with the new, attracting and repelling individuals who move between them. We find, in other words, that individuals locate themselves in the borderlands of intersecting paradigms, their worldviews shaped by their positions within this broad network of models, systems, and traditions. Within such a complex network, binary oppositions of orthodox versus unorthodox, regular versus irregular, and traditional versus alternative lack clear meaning, and instead blind us to the rich interconnections between multiple systems for explaining health and disease.

3 ▸ A BROKEN TRUST

The Changing Character of Health Care

> What we call Man's power over Nature turns out to be a power exercised by some men over other men with Nature as its instrument.
>
> —C. S. LEWIS

IN THE PREVIOUS chapter, I focused my attention on fundamental changes in mid-to-late twentieth-century conceptualizations of disease. As chronic diseases rose in prominence, authors and commentators advocated models of etiology that factored in the dynamic interrelationship between physical, emotional, social, and environmental domains. The technologized and reductionist approach that had served biomedicine during an era of acute infectious epidemics appeared poorly suited to address illnesses that, many argued, flowed from the physical and emotional stresses of modern society. Critics alleged that it was necessary to reassess preventive and therapeutic health strategies and move away from narrow reductionism to empower individuals to take charge of their health.

Implicit in these broad health campaigns were appraisals of the social costs of an approach increasingly painted as dogmatic and provincial. For some, the biomedical system was guilty of dehumanizing its patients through its rigid attachment to reductionist responses to disease. However, even those less disposed to such sweeping allegations cast disapproving glances at a medical system resistant to change. In "The Responsibility of the Individual," John Knowles—himself a physician—spared his colleagues outright censure, arguing that their rigid attachment to a broken model flowed, in part, from society's historic fascination with science and technology. Yet in the same breath, he delivered a backhanded rebuke of their motives, arguing that they failed to consider new disease models because the "financial rewards of the present system are too great and because there is no incentive and very little demand to change."[1]

Thus, in mid-century evaluations of the biomedical model, we recognize a nascent criticism of the professionals Americans entrusted with their health. These reproaches would ultimately fuel a more widespread culture of distrust captured in outwardly critical attacks on the perceived failures of physicians, drug manufacturers, and governmental regulators to act in the best interest of patients. Launched by individuals in the medical community in addition to those outside its institutional and professional circles, these analyses accused biomedicine and its agents of squandering the public's trust through acts of incompetence, arrogance, and avarice. Some critics would allege that these sins had been institutionalized in the very structure of biomedicine, as physicians, drug manufacturers, and allied professionals placed personal interests over the needs of patients.

During the same period, biomedicine would witness the institutionalization of a professional discipline tasked with surveying its behavior and ensuring that it recognized patients' inviolable rights. Indeed, biomedical ethics arose to address the sins of the medical system by developing procedures to adjudicate ethically complex medical questions and institutionalizing oversight to prevent miscarriages in healing. It was, in effect, a professional response to distrust, aimed at shining a bright light into the corners and crevices of biomedical practice. Yet, as I shall argue, bioethics would largely ignore a broad category of concerns, which it dismissed as radical. Spurned in professional discourse, these unsanctioned expressions of distrust flourished in the darkness, ultimately provoking contentious debate regarding what some considered the unfulfilled promise of bioethical inquiry. To better understand the historic processes whereby some scholars dismissed these critiques as illicit, we must first consider the institutional routes and avenues through which some apprehensions were sanctioned as worthy of study.

A SANCTIONED DISTRUST: THE RISE OF BIOMEDICAL ETHICS

As many scholars have argued, bioethics as a formal discipline coalesced in a crucible suffused by the simmering anti-authoritarianism of the 1960s. It was catalyzed, in part, by startling allegations of abuse by research scientists and atomic-age insecurities regarding the dangers of unchecked scientific progress.[2] Fears that biomedicine had committed egregious sins against patients and research participants led to a reevaluation of patient protections and a critical analysis of how matters of ethics were adjudicated by clinicians and researchers.

As a result of these transgressions, the same clinicians who had once held quasi-mythical status among the public were deemed in need of oversight.[3] In the deputization of biomedical ethics as a formal discipline, an entire profession arose to provide this oversight.

By locating bioethics within the anti-authoritarianism of the 1960s and underscoring the prominent role it played in ushering in a power realignment in American medicine, scholars present the discipline as an exponent of the larger patient rights movement. In *Strangers at the Bedside,* the first history of the bioethics movement, David Rothman constructs a doublet of interlocking analogies comparing bioethicists to civil rights advocates. He begins by analogizing patients to groups of minorities bound in a common fight against authority. In their mutual powerlessness, he argues, patients were "at one with women, inmates, homosexuals, tenants in public housing, welfare recipients, and students." Furthermore, because bioethicists defended patients, they were like the "rights agitators" who fought on behalf of vulnerable parties. It was through such reasoning that Rothman could argue that bioethicists, a group largely comprised of career philosophers, were exponents of civil rights.[4] For they, like the leaders of interest-based advocacy groups, "looked at the world from the vantage point of the objects of authority, not the wielders of authority."[5]

Rothman's framing of bioethics suggests that it was dedicated to examining the expressions of distrust relevant to this analysis: critiques of the behaviors of a clinical system perceived to have amassed too much power. Yet, while the discipline has facilitated significant change in medical practice,[6] it largely ignored a class of objections that ran deep—one author would call them marrow deep—impugning the agents of biomedicine and the larger structures that facilitated its amassment of power.[7]

Indeed, by most measures, bioethics is a conservative endeavor. A branch of applied ethics, it is practical in its methodology, positioning itself within the biomedical model and working to modify physician practices to respect patient autonomy. In its scope and aim, it focuses almost exclusively upon what philosopher Anthony Weston refers to as "downstream" problems in healthcare, ignoring the upstream phenomena giving rise to them.[8] As Hastings Center Cofounder Daniel Callahan has admitted, in the practice of professional bioethics, "the larger and more fundamental human questions that should be engaged are put aside, and the focus is mainly on those issues that lend themselves to some concrete legal or legislative outcomes acceptable in a pluralistic society."[9] Hewing to this disciplinary approach, bioethics achieved tremendous success. In 2005, Arthur Caplan quipped that the field had grown "from a cottage industry of intellectually lonely misfits and malcontents . . . to a real field that whispers in the ears of Presidents, issues rules to bind the inquiries of Nobel Prize winners and is consulted by CEOs and media lights for advice and analysis."[10]

As bioethics amassed power through the second half of the twentieth century, critics contended that the field had gone astray. They argued that in transforming itself into an expression of the power of biomedicine, it had lost the ability to understand how that power operated. Feminist scholars were among the first to voice their dissent, arguing that in focusing on the promulgation of universal concepts of individual agency and informed consent, bioethics turned a blind eye to structural abuses that dictated and defined the patient experience. What good was informed consent, they asked, if individuals' social circumstances rendered them unable to exercise it? Furthermore, critics argued that in focusing on enhancing the clinical experience, bioethicists failed to consider the structural causes of health and disease in addition to the ways in which the clinical experience itself could be harmful. Feminist Christine Overall gave voice to these concerns in a rebuke of bioethical practice wherein she invoked the work of Ivan Illich, whose legacy I shall revisit later. Writing in 1996, Overall commented, "What Ivan Illich calls the 'ethical status of medicalization'—that is, the gradual incursion of medicine into, for example, sexuality, reproduction, disability, the emotions, nutrition, childhood, old age, and dying—is seldom recognized as an issue within bioethics. Nor are the marketing of infant formula and bottle feeding, the effects of environmental degradation on health, the drugging of athletes, or physicians' widespread participation in the certification of defiance, incompetence, and insanity recognized as such."[11]

In ignoring the structural correlates of health, bioethics failed to consider the rich discourse developed through the 1960s and 1970s interrogating the construction and operation of power in society. Interestingly, while the writings of Michel Foucault went on to profoundly influence academic disciplines such as history, anthropology, and sociology, they had relatively little effect on the practice of bioethics. In 2003, scholars Arthur W. Frank and Therese Jones analyzed American bioethics from a Foucauldian perspective, concluding that the French theorist would have adjudged it "yet another practice of power" which located individuals in a rigid hierarchy despite purporting to empower them.[12] By the late 2000s, bioethicists had begun to recognize their failure to adequately problematize power in their disciplinary approach. Writing in the *Hastings Center Report* in 2010, Bruce Jennings admitted, "Bioethics lives in the shadow of great structures and practices of power, and yet, it has not been notable for its contributions to an understanding of power. Indeed, the narrative that bioethics has fashioned for itself has been mainly a liberationist romance: a quest narrative in which the individual, seeking autonomy, struggled against limitations, constraints, and inhibitions imposed by forces from the outside."[13]

As Rothman's framing of the discipline underscores, many bioethicists presumed that by granting individuals autonomy, they were empowering them. Yet, as Foucauldians had long noted, giving individuals a voice in their care does little to change structural deficiencies, biases, and prejudices in the biomedical system, nor does it address the systematic abuses arising from the fundamental arrangement of clinical care.[14] The discipline similarly fielded critiques from those who argued that it ignored gender, race, and class-specific disparities in health care and the effects of broad power disparities on individuals' engagement with the system.[15]

As bioethics' proponents fielded criticism from feminist and Foucauldian scholars, they were faced with reinterpretation of their disciplinary history. In 2000, historian M. L. Tina Stevens challenged the canonical narrative of bioethics, arguing that it had sacrificed its radical origins in 1960s-era anti-authoritarianism and anti-technologism for an accommodationist posture that served the interests of physicians and researchers while furthering a reductionist, technologized care model.[16] Her work provoked the ire of Albert Jonsen, who in a review published in the *Hastings Center Report* argued that her interpretations were "driven less by the context and evidence than by her fundamental ideology as a historian, namely, that all historical analysis is nothing more than the record of power seeking to perpetuate itself."[17] Stevens's response, also published in the *Report,* disputed the bioethicist's claims while simultaneously delivering a backhanded rebuke, congratulating Jonsen on his 1998 work *The Birth of Bioethics* by calling it "informative history from a Whig perspective."[18]

While the points of disagreement between Jonsen and Stevens are fascinating, I am more interested in the topics on which the scholars agreed. Consider the broad structural critique Stevens levels at bioethics, which is like Overall's argument that bioethics excluded radical appraisals of the healthcare system from its analysis. In his review of Stevens's work, Jonsen agrees that bioethicists had engaged in the systematic elision of radical positions from their analysis. Moreover, he defends the practice, also invoking Ivan Illich: "I cannot imagine how the radical critics whom [Stevens] idolizes could ever have participated in this sort of public discourse. They could verbally demolish the social institutions that they accused of domination, but they had no means of actually revising or rebuilding them. They stood outside and shouted. Illich's slashing dissection of modern medicine and health care offered no alternative except the exhortation that people should take care of themselves."[19]

Thus, Jonsen, paints authors such as Illich as polemicists intent on destroying what biomedicine had built while offering little of value in return.[20] In his refutation, he demonstrates that bioethics declared no dominion over the vast arena of health care defined by self-care. Thus, ironically, a discipline of applied ethics that had constructed its authority upon the bedrock of patient autonomy would, in fact, recognize limits to that autonomy. Those who questioned the biomedical system's legitimacy writ large, or who advocated unorthodox approaches to healing that rejected its authority, simply went too far.[21]

The rabblerousing agitator who becomes too free for his own good is an old trope, exhumed from time to time by critics intent on branding those whose freedom offends their sensibilities as dangerous. Consider, for example, framings of the immigrant poor arriving on the shores of the nation in the early twentieth century. Addressing the Carnegie Institute in 1919, banker Otto H. Kahn argued, "They have become drunk with the strong wine of freedom. Brooding in the gloom of age-long oppression, they have evolved a fantastic and distorted image of free government. In fatuous effrontery they seek to graft the growth of their stunted vision upon the splendid and ancient tree of American institutions."[22]

My goal for the remainder of this chapter is to shine a light on those who had become drunk with the strong wine of freedom, identifying popular expressions of apprehension and ambivalence with the orthodox biomedical system in the years preceding AIDS. As I shall argue, radicalism of the sort articulated by Ivan Illich grew from and was expressive of concerns common through society in the mid-to-late twentieth century. Furthermore, Illich's theories, like the unorthodox AIDS activism they later fueled, had roots in earlier social movements that were not all deemed radical. Just as I have argued elsewhere in this analysis, if we hope to understand the radical firebrand, we must strive to apprehend the discourses that anchored and fueled him.

In the following two sections, I examine expressions of distrust shared by the public concerning the content and character of mid-to-late twentieth-century biomedicine. The first section examines concerns that the biomedical orthodoxy was, itself, directly injurious to the public's health due to its reliance on an armamentarium of potentially dangerous drugs. In it, I explore fears, widespread through the 1960s and 1970s, that the nation was overmedicated. Following this analysis, I turn my attention to changes in social perceptions of the competence and character of physicians during these years. I ultimately argue that the period witnessed a proliferation of criticism of the nation's healers not seen since the sectarian battles of the late nineteenth and early twentieth centuries.

Only after establishing this greater context of distrust and apprehension shall I turn my attention to the structural critique Illich launched, examining his analyses of clinical, social, and cultural iatrogenesis (physician-induced harm). I also consider the similarities between his critique and those of Foucault. In the final component of the chapter, I discuss the popular extensions of Illich's analysis, demonstrating the impact it exhibited on the growth of the self-help movement and unorthodox healing approaches. I reconsider the failure of professional bioethicists to address his critiques, arguing that in dismissing them as destructive expressions of radicalism, they failed to appreciate the distrust he articulated and the culture of self-help he inspired.

The Overmedicated Society

In 1980, Louis Lasagna, a clinical pharmacologist known for penning a modern adaptation of the Hippocratic Oath, edited a 600-page volume dedicated to examining controversies in clinical care. In the opening line of his introduction,

Lasagna identifies overmedication as one of the great fears of the era. "Few topics in medicine elicit such passions in the hearts of physicians," he writes, "as the question, 'Are we an overmedicated society?'"[23] The first two essays focused exclusively on the topic, with subsequent chapters directly and indirectly contributing to the discussion. In a piece titled "The Politics of Medication," John P. Morgan attests to the popular media's enthrallment with the issue, noting that everyone from high school groups to alcohol use counselors to reporters from *Time Magazine* and *Gentlemen's Quarterly* had approached him to discuss the nation's epidemic of overmedication.[24] "Everyone seems to know that we are an overmedicated society," Morgan observes, "and one imagines editors of publications small and large, common and arcane, swallowing benzodiazepines while rushing to meet a deadline with an article on the overmedicated society."[25]

Criticism of society's overreliance upon prescription drugs saturated both lay and professional publications in the years preceding AIDS. In 1980, Philip R. Lee—a former assistant secretary for health and scientific affairs under Lyndon Johnson who would later serve as the first president of San Francisco's health commission during the AIDS epidemic—noted with alarm that, since 1950, the number of prescriptions dispensed by community pharmacies, discount stores, and physicians tripled.[26] For many authors, the biomedical industry and, by extension, society in general had become dependent upon pharmacological solutions to everyday problems, seeking "a pill for every ill."[27] Lee's comments echoed research conducted by John M. Firestone who, in 1970, argued that in the United States, the volume of the drug business had grown by a factor of 100 through the twentieth century.[28] A startling report issued by The Consumers Union furthermore held that 20,000 tons of aspirin were consumed per year (almost 225 tablets per person) while, in England, every tenth night of sleep was induced by a hypnotic drug.[29]

It is impossible to locate a single overmedication discourse operative through the 1960s and 1970s, for the topic intersected numerous common anxieties, harmonizing with concerns voiced by individuals on both sides of the political spectrum. To say that society was overmedicated was to indict a vast array of social institutions and professionals, ranging from pharmaceutical corporations and governmental regulators to physicians. Correspondingly, throughout the 1960s and 1970s, we identify several overlapping discourses, each questioning the nation's growing reliance upon a biomedical industry painted as broken. In some cases, these discourses centered upon sensational revelations of new drugs with demonstrably debilitating side effects. In others, they focused opprobrium on more commonly prescribed medications believed to pose their own risks to the population. I maintain that each discursive tradition utilized its own conceptualizations of risk and harm; to appreciate the full measure of overmedication fears, we must consider each of them.

The first category of drugs I shall discuss here is, in many ways, the most recognizable, its story inscribed in the history of drug regulation. Through the 1960s and 1970s, authors published exposés arguing that the biomedical system produced an armamentarium of drugs whose toxic side effects far outweighed their utility. One of the most vocal and influential critics in this tradition was Morton Mintz, a *Washington Post* investigative journalist who, in 1967, published a volume critical of drug development and regulation in the United States. What its title sacrificed in brevity it gained in brass: *By Prescription Only—A Report on the Roles of the United States Food and Drug Administration, the American Medical Association, Pharmaceutical Manufacturers, and Others in Connection with the Irrational and Massive Use of Prescription Drugs that May be Worthless, Injurious, or Even Lethal.*[30] In it, Mintz provides an encyclopedic breakdown of the toxic drugs for which the pharmaceutical industry had sought, and in some cases received, approval. In addition to thalidomide (Thalomid), the archetypical drug whose history is closely associated with drug regulation reform, Mintz tells the tales of chloramphenicol (chloramphenicol sodium succinate; an antibiotic associated with aplastic anemia), zoxazolamine (Flexin; a muscle spasm remedy associated with liver damage), ethynerone (code-named MK-665; an oral contraceptive associated with breast cancer), dimethyl sulfoxide (an industrial solvent touted as a wonder drug and later associated with ocular conditions), and many others. A decade after its publication, Illich extolled Mintz's analysis as a masterpiece that had "done more than any other book to change the focus of the U.S. discussion of medicine."[31]

Surveying statements made by biomedical leaders, including testimony given before Estes Kefauver's 1957–1963 Senate Committee investigating the nation's health industry, Mintz paints a picture of widespread neglect. The reader encounters, for example, a concerned pathologist whose years of experience conducting autopsies led him to conclude that pharmaceuticals were killing patients, contributing to what he called "a sort of involuntary euthanasia."[32] We learn of analyses conducted by a well-respected statistician holding that three-quarters of published biomedical studies drew conclusions unsupported by their data. We read an FDA commissioner's concession that "the hand of the amateur" was evident far too often in drug testing data submitted to his office for review.[33] Furthermore, for those readers unimpressed with concerns voiced by biomedical researchers and regulators, Mintz invokes the memory of one of the era's most beloved champions of the public's health. His project, he made clear, was an extension of the mission undertaken by the late Rachel Carson, the conservationist whose name had become synonymous with efforts to protect the public from toxicities wrought through modern industrialization. On the second page of his preface, Mintz prints comments Carson made roughly a year before her death:

> The problem I dealt with in *Silent Spring* is not an isolated one. The excessive and ill-advised use of chemical pesticides is merely one part of a sorry whole—the reckless pollution of our living world with harmful and dangerous substances. Until very recently, the average citizen assumed that 'Someone' was looking after these matters and that some little understood but confidently relied upon safeguards stood like shields between his person and any harm. Now he has experienced, from several different directions, a rather rude shattering of these beliefs. Almost simultaneously with the publication of *Silent Spring*, the problem of drug safety and drug control, which had been simmering in the press for many months, reached its shocking culmination in the thalidomide tragedy.[34]

Narratives invoking the specter of substances such as thalidomide focused on the establishment of more comprehensive regulatory mechanisms to protect the public. The goal, they argued, was to catch the bad apples before they slipped through the regulatory net and into consumers' hands. These narratives deflected attention from larger social arrangements permitting an overreliance upon medication. For this reason, some maintained that they lost the forest for the trees. Furthermore, inherent in them was an optimism in society's ability to make biomedical practice better through more scientific knowledge. What society needed was someone to protect it from those who, out of negligence or malice, would cause it harm. In some iterations, that someone was constituted by the consumer rights movement—indeed, Ralph Nader penned a glowing review of *By Prescription Only*, which its publisher printed on its back cover. In others, they were embodied in heroized professionals—sentries in the mold of Frances Oldham Kelsey.[35]

Through the 1970s, leaders in the feminist and women's health movement would also engage in discourse regarding the safety of pharmaceuticals. Their contribution is best seen in their discussions of psychotropic medications, the third class of drugs to be considered in this chapter. However, they also contributed analyses of other classes believed to carry risks to women. Consider the case, for example, of high-dose estrogen birth control pills. In the late 1960s, journalist Barbara Seaman received letters from the readers of women's magazines documenting side effects they attributed to the pills. In 1969, she published *The Doctor's Case Against the Pill*, which underscored "the dark side of the pill, a sometimes lethal side . . . [which] seems to have been deliberately concealed."[36] Despite the medications' potential for empowering women, fears regarding their side effects inspired a widespread social movement complete with U.S. Senate hearings. Planned Parenthood described the debates as tantamount to "information wars between Congress, the FDA, the AMA [American Medical Association], and the women," underscoring public fears regarding the toxicities of pharmaceuticals, distrust in the biomedical industry, and the belief that people ought to have the right to protect themselves against harm.[37]

In these 1960s and 1970s–era protests, we locate the birth of a vibrant grassroots activist movement. Founded in 1967, the Health Policy Advisory Center became an important exponent in this movement, defining and critiquing the medical empire and the medical industrial complex.[38] In a similar vein, the National Women's Health Network published nine resource guides on an array of women's health issues, with one focused on health concerns with the contraceptive diethylstilbestrol (Apstil).[39] In these initiatives we register critiques of health structures, concerns with the dangers of medical interventions, and efforts to help people derive power through knowledge of their own bodies.[40] The movement was further informed by the work of Loretta Ross, who influenced women's health activism in her articulation of reproductive justice and her focus on the vulnerabilities of communities lacking institutionalized power.[41]

It is in moving from "bad drugs" to those of lesser toxicity that we better appreciate 1960s–1980s era social discourse surrounding the dangers of overmedication. Take, for example, a second category of drugs constituted by medications of questionable clinical efficacy that lacked the discernible toxicities of the first class. It is easy to dismiss this second class of useless medications as a minor concern in comparison with drugs of demonstrable toxicity. Alternatively, it is easy to conflate the two categories into one, noting, for example, that legislators addressed the second category of drugs in the same hallmark legislation—the Kefauver-Harris Amendment of 1962—that addressed the first.

However, focusing narrowly on legislative fixes blinds us to the effects pharmacologic duds would have on popular discourse surrounding medication. For through the 1960s and 1970s, as people contemplated useless drugs already on the market, we identify expressions of far more diffuse conceptualizations of risk. Perhaps, critics wondered, all drugs posed some level of harm. Unlike the dangers of thalidomide—discernible through more transparent testing standards and rigorous regulatory oversight—these other harms were unknowable, exacting their effects through complex pathways and facilitated through the dynamic interaction of multiple agents in each person.[42] In short, while many had granted that ineffective drugs posed harm to the purse, some began to question their effects on the person as well. Mintz expressed this concern in the opening line of his chapter dedicated to ineffective pharmacologic products. "Ineffective drugs can be dangerous drugs," he wrote. "There is no fact more crucial to an understanding of why we have wasted our money and our health."[43] This expansion of the notion of risk to include unknowable offenses also corresponds with an extension of interpretations of risk in tort law in the early-to-mid 1960s.[44]

The consumer rights movement would, similarly, focus attention on the theoretical risks of useless medications. Through the 1970s, critics accused the FDA of failing to adequately implement the provisions mandated by the Kefauver-Harris Amendment, arguing that many ineffective and potentially dangerous drugs remained on the market. In 1980, Sidney M. Wolfe, Christopher M. Coley, and Ralph Nader's Health Research Group published an influential volume chronicling these failures, titled *Pills That Don't Work: A Consumers' and Doctors' Guide to Over 600 Prescription Drugs that Lack Evidence of Effectiveness.* The authors' opening argument forewarned, "Neither you nor, in some instances, even your doctor realizes that one out of every eight prescriptions filled—169 million prescriptions costing over $1.1 billion in 1979—is for a drug not considered effective by the government's own standards."[45] The book lists 607 drug products deemed ineffective or unsafe, counseling patients to refuse doctors' advice if they should be prescribed one of them.[46] It also lists what it considers the "Top 30 Less-than-Effective Prescription Drugs," which had been among the top 200 drugs prescribed in the United States.

The authors fashioned the book as a self-help manual of sorts, aimed at decreasing the degree to which patients turned to physicians for the treatment of minor ailments and at "lessen[ing] the very dangerous gap between what the doctor knows and what the patient knows."[47] Despite its occasionally dry review of FDA policies and judicial pronouncements, the book was a phenomenal success. After Phil Donahue aired an hour-long conversation with one of its authors, sales skyrocketed. In November of 1981, Ray Walters of the *New York Times* observed, "To date, the book has sold 280,000 copies and the end isn't in sight." All said, it remained on the *Times*' trade-paperback bestseller list for six weeks and inspired the publication of a sequel investigating over-the-counter medications. Maintaining the self-help format of its predecessor, this volume told individuals which drugs to avoid and directed them to alternative, low-toxicity treatments.[48]

These volumes sparked debate regarding the appropriate response to failures in governmental regulation. Some authors, such as Peter Temin, argued that the correct response to the broken healthcare system was the empowerment of patients and corresponding dissolution of regulations concerning the purchase of potentially dangerous substances.[49] Historian Charles O. Jackson, on the other hand, criticized such free market positions, arguing for increased oversight for the good of the public.[50] These debates persisted through the late twentieth and early twenty-first centuries as society contemplated the regulation of agents purported to treat AIDS and COVID-19.

The refraction of health issues through the consumer rights movement relocated the nexus of power in health decisions from the physician's office to the individual's home. The best consumer, Nader intoned, was the educated consumer. Correspondingly, the healthiest patient was she who judiciously assessed the costs and benefits of taking any given medication. As physicians lacked the time or capacity to navigate patients through the minefield that was the modern healthcare system, patients would have to take the lead, making health decisions in the absence of clear information. Thus, in the tale of ineffective drugs, we uncover a social phenomenon bearing resemblance to the precautionary principle operationalized in population-level environmental policy debates through the 1970s and 1980s.

The final category of drugs I shall consider here comprises controversial psychotropic agents marketed and administered in large numbers through the 1960s and 1970s. Unlike the drugs in the first category, biomedical professionals conceived of the benefits offered by psychotropic agents as largely outweighing the harms they posed. Furthermore, unlike the other drugs thus considered, these agents effected clear biophysiological changes in the body. Thus, psychotropic agents provoked a rich public debate unique from discussions of the other two drug categories.[51]

As Nicolas Rasmussen has noted, through the 1960s, physicians readily prescribed amphetamines to patients presenting with symptoms of emotional disquietude. In short order, the drugs had become first-line treatment options, with one estimate holding that in 1969, enough pharmacologic amphetamine was produced to supply each American with fifty ten-milligram doses.[52] What amphetamines had done for low energy and depression, benzodiazepines would do for anxiety. In 1960, Hoffman-La Roche introduced chlordiazepoxide (Librium), the first benzodiazepine, which was later supplemented by diazepam (Valium) in 1963. Both replaced the anxiolytic drugs that had been popular in the 1950s. A 1979 Institute of Medicine conference report declared Valium the single most prescribed drug in not only the United States, but the entire world. Rounding out the national list were dextropropoxyphene (Darvon), a powerful painkiller later removed from the market, and Librium, Valium's analog.[53] As several authors noted, given the remarkable degree to which individuals sought recourse in psychotropic agents, it appeared that the nation had descended into an age of anxiety, a period famously articulated by poet W. H. Auden in his Pulitzer Prize winning eclogue of the same name.

It was, perhaps, only a matter of time before a nation ensnared in an age of anxiety would express anxiety with the skyrocketing national prescription rates of amphetamines and benzodiazepines. Growing realizations that medicinal psychotropics could become habit forming transformed national discourse; the same drugs once depicted in saccharine pharmaceutical advertisements as promising to transform overworked housewives into cheerful self-starters were soon associated with social unrest. During this time, we find tension between discourses celebrating the drugs as panaceas and those indicting them as poisons. In 1984, for example, a text on adult psychopathology noted that the drugs were widely considered safe by physicians and lay persons alike despite reports from the Addiction Research Foundation—cited in the same text—arguing that minor tranquilizers had become a major cause of drug-related toxicity.[54]

The popular press also registered disquiet with psychotropic drugs. The 1966 novel *Valley of the Dolls*, for example, presented characters whose lives had been destroyed by barbiturates and sleeping pills. A phenomenal success, it sold 17 million copies by 1974 and was recognized by the *Guinness Book of World Records* as the best-selling novel in publishing history. Meanwhile, the author of a 1975 *Los Angeles Times* article investigating the perils of Valium compared the drug to "soma," the dystopian cure introduced by Aldous Huxley in his 1932 novel *Brave New World*: "euphoric, narcotic, pleasantly hallucinant, [possessing] all the advantages of Christianity and alcohol and none of their defects."[55] Lest one assume that histrionic assessments of psychotropics were limited to popular fiction and newspaper articles, consider the following claim made in *Lancet* in 1973: "Sales of benzodiazepines are increasing in geometrical rather than arithmetic progression, and if the trend continues total tranquillisation of the population will soon be achieved."[56]

Some critics maintained that mood-altering drugs presented a harm that transcended discussions of individual side effects. For they appeared to threaten the fabric of social relations, robbing individuals of community-building experiences wrought through struggle and perseverance. The nation, many feared, had lost its nerve, flocking to the medicine cabinet at the slightest sign of disquiet.[57] Arthur Gordon, editor of *Good Housekeeping, Cosmopolitan,* and *Guidepost* magazines, epitomized this perspective when he implored individuals to reject mood-altering pills and "return to values of duty, obligation, and responsibility."[58] For such critics, psychotropic drugs represented a failure of collective will and the traditions they believed were foundational to the nation's values. Leslie Farber succinctly conveyed this sentiment in a 1966 *New York Times Magazine* article wherein he bemoaned, "It was only a question of time before man, in his desperation, would locate a divinity in drugs and on that artificial rock build his church."[59]

Interestingly, while in some analyses psychotropic medications provided individuals an opportunity to cede control over their lives and engagement with society, for others they represented tools of oppression used to subjugate segments of the population. Feminist authors, for example, argued that pharmaceutical corporations aggressively marketed psychotropic drugs to women. In 1979, then Representative Barbara Mikulski, speaking on behalf of the Congresswomen's Caucus, noted that 60 percent of psychotropic drugs, 70 percent of antidepressants, and 80 percent of amphetamines were prescribed to women.[60] In 1963, Betty Friedan famously described the use of medications to address "the problem that has no name": the lingering dissatisfaction many women experienced with the sharply delineated social roles they were expected to accept in the postwar years. For Friedan, in taking "tranquilizers like cough drops," housewives interpreted broad social problems through a narrow clinical lens, accepting personal responsibility for their own oppression.[61] Feminist concerns also found expression in the popular press, with articles exploring psychotropic use among women appearing in the *New York Times, Newsweek, Good Housekeeping,* and

Time. Further, in 1966, an obscure group of traveling troubadours spread Friedan's message to the masses in a piece of popular faire. Invoking the dangers of Valium use, they intoned, "Mother needs something today to calm her down. / And though she's not really ill, / there's a little yellow pill. / She goes running for the shelter of a mother's little helper."[62]

Thus, through the 1960s and 1970s, we locate a rich discursive tradition questioning biomedicine's reliance upon pharmacological treatments. In highlighting the harms posed by highly toxic drugs such as thalidomide, the theoretical harms posed by drugs of low efficacy, and the social harms posed by powerful psychotropics, authors expressed reservation with biomedicine's methods of treatment. Within a remarkably short period of time, we find the articulation of discourses questioning the magic bullets Paul Ehrlich had prophesied at the turn of the century. This reconceptualization of biomedical treatment would contribute to a gradual loosening of some patients' ties to the biomedical system and a resultant embrace of self-help and unorthodox healing strategies, much as nineteenth-century fears of heroic medicine led individuals to embrace alternative healing systems.

Also contributing to this loosening of ties were transformations in perceptions of the modern physician, with many authors questioning the competence and character of the nation's once venerated healers. It is to this transformation that I now turn.

A FALL FROM GRACE: POST-WAR CRITIQUES OF THE PHYSICIAN

As Susan Lynn Speaker has argued, through the 1950s and 1960s, overmedication discourse centered opprobrium on the sins of the pharmaceutical industry, with congressional hearings investigating the monopolistic practices and lax testing standards of the nation's drug-producing behemoths. By the 1970s, however, the public's reproach expanded to include other professionals and institutions within the larger biomedical system including, most significantly, the venerated physician. The link between patient and physician was far stronger than that which bound individuals to drug manufacturers; after all, the doctor-patient bond had been celebrated as a core component of Western medicine. From the omnipotent and sacerdotal physicians portrayed in the 1950s television series *Medic*, to the humane and compassionate *Dr. Kildare*, to the dependable, morally grounded *Ben Casey*, physicians were lionized figures expected to connect with patients, know what was right for them, and fight for it.[63] However, by the late 1960s and 1970s, many authors began to question both the ability and the resolve of physicians to achieve these ends. As Speaker argues, the period witnessed a fundamental transformation in the social perception of orthodox healers. Examining popular literature articles published in the 1970s, with a particular focus on articles concerning the prescription of psychotropic medications, she concluded that a minority presented physicians as competent authorities.[64]

Critiques of physicians' competence abounded in popular discussions through the 1970s, with authors arguing that doctors had lost the ability to shepherd patients through an increasingly bureaucratic biomedical system. The tone of attacks would, at times, slide into mudslinging, with some critics labeling physicians the "dupes of pharmaceutical companies' marketing departments."[65] Few possessed an aptitude for mud slinging surpassing that of Edgar Berman, surgeon and personal physician to Hubert Humphrey, who turned his acerbic wit on his own profession in 1976.[66] His volume—the cover of which includes a bolded disclaimer warning "Your Doctor May be Hazardous to Your Health"—portrays physicians as incapable of recognizing the absurdities of their craft.[67] In his sardonic and incendiary style,[68] Berman asks, "[I]s it the doctor's fault when he gives a patient MER 29 to lower cholesterol (by the same wonderful people that gave us thalidomide) and it causes cataracts? Was it not on the best advice of a detail man who has a college education with an A.B. degree in Urban Studies? If you can't trust a multibillion-dollar industry like pharmaceutical firms, whom can you trust?"[69]

Berman was not alone in his suspicion that physicians had become locked into a detrimental system of care controlled by corporate interests. Revisiting the chapter Philip R. Lee penned on overmedication, we find a review of clinical practice that, while less incendiary than Berman's, was no less insightful. In a brief discussion involving what he terms the "symbolism" of prescription practices, Lee suggests that physicians overprescribed drugs because they had been conditioned to believe they were necessary components of clinical care. If this were true, then doctors were incapable of challenging overprescription because the body of knowledge and practices they brought to bear upon human illness, and by extension their legitimacy as professional healers, were premised upon the provision of pharmacologic agents.[70] In discussing the symbolic meaning of prescription, Lee cites a claim Edmund Pellegrino made in a 1976 speech before the American Association for the Advancement of Science. "[I]t is prescribing which makes a clinical situation legitimately medical," Pellegrino deduced. "In its absence, [the physician] may regard the patient's problem as a personal or social matter outside the domain of medicine entirely."[71] Lee and Pellegrino's fears echo arguments made by health economist Charlotte Muller who, in 1971, argued that physicians relied upon prescriptions to designate the end of a clinical encounter and to express compassion and concern to patients.[72] For some authors, these concerns reverberated in the context of overmedication fears, with one 1960 *Science Newsletter* writer maintaining, "It is the doctors who need those tranquilizers, not the patient. Perhaps general practitioners are doling out the calming pills to relieve their own anxieties which develop when they do not know what to do for a patient."[73]

Several authors would go further still, suggesting that physicians' tendency to overmedicate extended beyond the prescription of drugs to include other clinical interventions as well. The problem, it appeared, was a cultural one—professional practice favored activist physicians who were inclined to intervene forcefully even when intervention was not indicated. One of the most well-respected authors to engage this topic was sociologist Eliot Freidson, who famously wrote on what he termed the "bias toward illness in everyday practice."[74] Physicians, he argued, were inclined to a certain degree of clinical interventionism, causing them to recommend treatments or procedures even when none were indicated. To support his claims, he recounted the results of a 1934 study investigating pediatricians' tendency to recommend tonsillectomies. The study began with 1,000 children, 611 of whom previously had their tonsils removed. A group of physicians was asked to review the 389 children with intact tonsils, and they deemed 174 (45%) of the group in need of tonsillectomies. The researchers then took the remaining 215 children with presumably healthy tonsils and presented them to a new group of physicians, at which point 99 (46%) were selected for the same procedure. The remaining 116 children were presented to a third group of physicians and, once more, roughly the same percentage (44%) was identified as needing surgery. Freidson concluded that, "Like the teacher who gives a certain proportion of failing grades no matter what the over-all quality of his class, so the physicians studied were inclined to remove a certain proportion of tonsils no matter what the range of signs observed."[75] Not all critics would share the same measured detachment from the issue. Three years after the publication of Freidson's *Profession of Medicine*, Louise Lerner, affiliated with the Health Policy Advisory Center, argued, "the doctor is trained and expected to be an activist, to engage in active intervention rather than passive observation. And what we get is Rambo, M.D."[76]

Some authors argued that physicians' propensity for resorting to aggressive surgical or pharmacologic interventions stemmed from their fundamental inability to understand an increasingly complex, technologized pharmacopeia. As Michael G. Michaelson argued in a sweeping 1971 *New York Review of Books* piece, physicians were ill-equipped to evaluate new medical devices and treatments and were thus inclined to buy almost anything, "the flashier it looks and sounds, the better." Citing Harry F. Dowling's damning 1970 work *Medicines for Man*, Michaelson suggested that physicians were incapable of challenging the pharmaceutical industry's hegemony.[77] For philosopher and religious scholar Jacob Needleman, the problem ran deeper still. Physicians, he maintained, had glorified science to the point that they were no longer capable of or willing to question it. In a passage printed in his 1985 epistolary volume *The Way of the Physician*, Needleman addresses an unseen doctor:

> [In the past,] it was not science you believed in, it was man. But today it is science you believe in and science, great as it is when it is good, is less than man, far less. When science was new to you, you believed in using it—but you were so very careful about it. You were always watching, looking, never taking anything for granted when you used the methods and the instruments of science. You were an observer and your eyes were in your heart as well as your head. But now science is no longer new for you. You no longer put it to the test when you act. More important, it no longer puts you to the test. It has swallowed your mind.[78]

In these analyses, we identify a movement toward victimizing the physician. Doctors may make poor decisions, overmedicate their patients, employ methodologies for recommending surgical procedures reminiscent of elementary school rubrics, but the moral outrage one might expect to find directed at them is tempered. Indeed, many discussions of clinical incapacity and inability suggested that physicians made poor decisions because they had become entangled in the same broken system as patients. In such framings, they were susceptible to the avarice of a pharmaceutical system bloated with power. In other cases, their errors are explained as the consequence of an entrenched reasoning system that taught them to believe that what they were doing was, in fact, good medicine.

However, in time, victimization narratives came under fire for two reasons. First, in defending physicians by assailing the professional institutions and practices that gave them meaning, the narratives conceded the very structural problems that motivated radical critiques in the first place. Second, by the 1970s, many critics directly challenged the notion that physicians were innocent bystanders in a broken system, arguing that they had directly and intentionally contributed to the problem. The issue, they maintained, was not merely one of competence, but of character. An exhaustive review of the factors attending transformations in social constructions of the character of physicians is beyond the scope of this analysis. However, three contributing factors deserve mention because they would anchor late-twentieth century unorthodox health movements: (a) the proliferation of critiques associating physicians with self-interested businesspeople who systematically prioritized profit over patient care, (b) the perception that professional organizations such as the AMA had squandered society's trust through self-serving political campaigns, and (c) allegations that medicine systematically harmed disempowered subpopulations through the selective provisioning of excessive or injurious care.[79] I shall briefly consider each of these issues in turn.

In mid-twentieth-century interrogations of clinical medicine's failings, many authors invoked the metaphor of the assembly line. To them, medicine had engaged in a Faustian bargain, sacrificing its connection with patients for efficient service defined by an increasingly specialized and fragmented clinical model.

The problems with clinical medicine were so well known that, in 1957, an attorney writing in the *Journal of the American Bar Association* urged his colleagues to resist making the same mistakes physicians had made in embracing a model defined by rampant specialization. "Today's patients often feel like a piece of machinery on an assembly line," he wrote, "with one man to put the rivets in the head and another to tighten the screws in the elbow. The doctor frequently doesn't even know their names."[80]

One might be tempted to argue that, here, the physician is conceived of as a victim in a bureaucratic system, analogous to the immigrant cogs in the industrial machine. However, the attorney's admonishment belies such an interpretation, for he wrote to implore his colleagues to resist making the same decisions physicians made. Indeed, the notion that physicians were complicit in the rise of assembly-line medicine appeared in popular literature through the 1950s and 1960s. A 1954 *American Magazine* article, for example, laid bare the irony of a clinical profession that demanded that patients recognize the "high priesthood of medicine" even as they processed bodies "on an assembly-line or chain-store basis, as if they were running a mass-production manufacturing or retail business."[81]

By all accounts, specialization was in vogue by the mid-twentieth century. Of the 271,000 physicians working in the United States in 1969, all but 58,000 limited their practice to specialties.[82] This was a transformation from the 1930s, when general practitioners outnumbered specialists five to one.[83] Furthermore, far from a phenomenon that swept up unwilling physicians in its wake, specialization seemed driven by financial interests. By assigning physicians to specialized domains of expertise, biomedicine granted healers dominion over a narrow range of increasingly complex technological and pharmacological innovations. As wielders of such nuanced knowledge, specialists watched their salaries rise, with a 1951 report issued by the U.S. Department of Commerce suggesting that the growth of specialization had been a key factor in the transformation of physician income through the twentieth century.[84] For historian Rosemary Stevens, the most concerning aspect of such specialization lay in specialists' failure to work collaboratively with one another, recognizing the complex ways in which disease and health were constituted. The illustrious specialists, she bemoaned, opted to "take the stand of isolationism, surveying with jaundiced eyes and outraged complacency the social facts of medicine in the second half of the twentieth century."[85]

By the 1970s, critiques of physicians' complicity in producing and sustaining the nation's broken healthcare system became more explicit, as testified in the writings of Edgar Berman. While it is possible to locate in his argument a critique of the underlying culture of medicine, Berman pulled few punches in his discussion of the role physicians played in creating that culture. Indeed, the volume's title alone—*The Solid Gold Stethoscope*—conveyed his belief that physicians debased patient care for financial gain. As he explained, the once sacrosanct doctor-patient relationship had been sacrificed on the altar of industrial efficiency:

> It happened the moment the computer found out that any time over nine minutes and thirty-three seconds spent with a patient is a bad investment. Every minute over that figure costs the average M.D. a minimum of 9 percent on the bank loan for his wife's new mink and the wall-to-wall carpet yet to be installed. How much rapport can be built up in a ten-minute contact in a cold cubicle, with a patient who's waited for four hours with no lunch and a doctor who has twenty more bodies to probe before dinner? Even to remember what each looked like last time around is a triumph in this revolving-door routine.[86]

Berman was not alone in his appraisals. In 1979, the esteemed Yale psychologist Seymour Sarason recounted a survey he had conducted among premedical students. In it, he asked them what satisfaction they expected to receive from their careers in medicine. While he thought nothing of their answers at the time, he was later struck with the realization that, in their discussions of the allure of high income, travel, interesting work, and high social status, none of them spoke of an interest in helping patients:

> [I]t dawned on me one day that I could not recall a single interview during which the student had said—spontaneously or in regard to any question or discussion in the hour or more long interview—that he or she had chosen medicine to help people, to contribute in some selfless or idealistic way to the betterment of society, to put any form of personal aggrandizement secondary to service to others and to the improvement of a larger scheme of things . . . there was a subliminal part of my thinking that did expect that some of these students, at least one or two, would describe themselves in relation to a medical career in idealistic terms. None had, although there had been ample opportunity for them to do so.[87]

For some, this naked self-interest merely confirmed an observation made by the sharp-witted George Bernard Shaw half a century earlier. Writing in the preface to his 1907 play *The Doctor's Dilemma*, the polemicist quipped, "That any sane nation, having observed that you could provide for the supply of bread by giving bakers a pecuniary interest in baking for you, should go on to give a surgeon a pecuniary interest in cutting off your leg, is enough to make one despair of political humanity."[88]

The transformation of the image of the American physician from a priest-like healer into a self-interested businessperson was facilitated by a controversial 1975 Federal Trade Commission (FTC) ruling requiring that the AMA lift the ban on advertising it had implemented in the mid-nineteenth century. The issue provoked profound disagreement within the medical profession, with many fearful that such an act would further tarnish the clinician's reputation. In a 1976 article in the *New England Journal of Medicine*, editor Franz J. Ingelfinger argued that in differentiating mainstream physicians from hucksters and quacks, the ban had preserved patients' trust in regular medicine. Noting that medicine had endured a decline in public confidence, Ingelfinger argued that for clinical medicine to survive, its leaders had to fight open advertising among physicians. "If the FTC has its way, and doctors succumb to hucksterism," he wrote, "no one need worry any longer about deprofessionalization. The process will have run its full course, for what better way than advertising to annihilate trust and confidence, what more effective means to convert medical practice into a purely commercial enterprise?"[89] Writing thirty years later, Nestor D. Tomycz confirmed Ingelfinger's fears, revealing that in demanding the lift of the ban, FTC Chairman Michael B. Pertschuk admitted his intent to treat medicine as a business that responded to the same marketplace influences as other industries.[90] The effort appears to have succeeded. For, as Tomycz argues, "If American medicine has lost some of its prestige in the last few decades, perhaps it is because the best advertisement for physicians was the original decision not to advertise."[91]

While the increasingly specialized, fragmentary, and impersonal nature of clinical care threatened to undermine the physician-patient relationship, another critique arose through the 1950s, 1960s, and 1970s holding that physicians sought to trade on this sacred bond to sway public opinion on key pieces of national health legislation. Through the mid-to-late twentieth century, the AMA was a central player in debates surrounding this topic, launching campaigns opposing universal health care. These campaigns attracted heated criticism, such as one 1943 column decrying the AMA's social outlook as "scarcely distinguishable from that of a plumber's union."[92]

One of the most dramatic critiques of professional medicine's meddling in universal healthcare debates is found in a 1951 *Harper's Magazine* article by historian Bernard DeVoto.[93] In it, DeVoto describes AMA literature he had received in the mail urging him to voice his opposition to the compulsory health insurance plan being debated in Congress. He decried the propaganda for cheapening the image of the noble family doctor by suggesting that the nation needed his protection from not only infectious ills, but the perils of "political enslavement" as well.[94] The historian's attack is cutting, impugning everything from the AMA's antisocialist invective to the hubris of a profession feverishly grasping at the reins of power even as it failed to adequately treat the nation's chronic disease epidemics. Most of all, he argues that physicians had foolishly sullied the bond between healer and patient: "Your ad speaks of the trust between physician and patient, so noble it says here, so sacred, so certain to be destroyed by what the propaganda calls socialism. But I do not like any kind of solicitation that trades on prestige or on such fears and hopes as illness necessarily involves, and I will not tolerate political solicitation in a relationship of trust. Solicitors who call at my house must use the back door."[95]

The AMA's efforts to derail public health legislation persisted through the 1970s, with various authors decrying their campaigns. Richard Carter's *The Doctor Business*, published in 1958, presented a stinging attack on the AMA and was identified by one writer as a key exponent in changing public perceptions of physicians.[96] In the 1960s, Richard Harris meticulously chronicled the AMA's efforts to derail landmark Medicare legislation, published first as a series of articles in the *New Yorker* and later as a bounded volume.[97] Similarly, in 1971, Michael G. Michaelson published a review of nine volumes critical of medicine published between 1967 and 1971.[98] In many ways, the review constituted its own, tenth addition to the series, with Michaelson making clear his revulsion with the state of American health care.[99]

While the first two factors thus considered impugned the character of physicians by arguing that they were self-interested businessmen sacrificing the doctor-patient relationship for personal, professional, or political gain, critiques flowing from the final factor were, perhaps, more nefarious. For they maintained that contemporary medicine systematically harmed certain groups through the selective provisioning of injurious care. In these critiques, physicians were seen as possessing phenomenal power, wielded with bias to dictate and define their patients' lives. Exponents of this interpretation of clinical care would argue that, far from a benevolent institution, medicine exerted tremendous social control, assuming a power previously reserved for religious and legal institutions.[100]

As Susan Lynn Speaker has noted, social control theory had been cited in discussions of medicine, especially psychiatry, as early as the 1960s, most notably in the writings of R. D. Laing and Thomas Szasz. The antipsychiatry movement Laing and Szasz inspired maintained that medicine pathologized normal states of being, coercing individuals to accept care they did not want or need. In many ways, Szaszian critiques were an expression of the overmedication discourse introduced earlier. However, his ideas expanded the critique, arguing that biomedicine was pathologizing mental states society did not understand or like, including homosexuality, hysteria, depression, schizophrenia, sexual perversions, and drug addiction.[101] A controversial figure, Szasz maintained that psychiatrists wielded a phenomenal power to subjugate and suppress individuals, and he ultimately tasked Americans with "abolishing psychiatric slavery."[102]

The antipsychiatry movement was not alone in accusing medicine of policing the bodies of the marginalized and disempowered. As noted, the feminist movement would accuse mainstream physicians of practicing sexist care, registered in the overmedication of women with psychotropics, frequent recourse to unnecessary gynecologic procedures, and the medicalization of natural stages of women's lives. The first edition of *Our Bodies, Ourselves* cited Carter's *The Doctor Business* in arguing that one-third of all hysterectomies conducted in a leading hospital were performed on women who suffered no disease.[103] While the authors of the Boston Women's Health Collective granted that financial interest played a role in these unnecessary procedures, they argued that women were specifically targeted as a result of the operationalization of trenchant sexism in medical practice.[104]

In the face of such potent critiques, physicians would find little succor in victimization narratives. Invoking language that had appeared in *Fortune Magazine*, the Collective argued, "[T]he doctors created the system. They run it. And they are the most formidable obstacle to its improvement. It is the doctor who decides which patients will be treated, where, under what conditions, and for what fee; who will enter the hospital, for what therapy, and for how long; what drugs will be purchased and in what quantities."[105] The feminist framing of the character of mainstream physicians underscores the complex ways apologists and critics mobilized structural arguments to support their aims. Biomedical sympathizers, for example, cited structural factors to exonerate physicians from responsibility for harms wrought by biomedicine while ignoring the structural critiques of "radical" detractors. Similarly, feminists lamented biomedicine's failure to explore structural factors influencing health outcomes while sometimes disregarding the ways in which physicians were, themselves, subject to entrenched structural forces.[106]

For many critics, biomedicine's problems ran deep and would not yield to traditional responses such as the empanelment of bioethics committees. Extending autonomy to its logical conclusion, they counseled self-care and suspicion with biomedical orthodoxy, earning the opprobrium of an emerging professional discipline built upon the autonomous patient archetype. Impassioned and impolitic, stimulating and seditious, they were the radical rabble-rousers who endeavored to achieve Rothman's maxim of looking at the world from the vantage point of the objects of authority.

Of all the radical rabble-rousers of the 1970s, few were as prolific or polarizing as Ivan Illich.[107] One recognizes in Illich's analyses many of the objections to clinical medicine outlined above. However, Illich's work was especially controversial for his detailed explication of how medicine served as a form of social control that systematically and unavoidably harmed patients. His writings earned the opprobrium of many medical scholars, and it is not difficult to see why. For Illich's critique cut a rift that was, at once, broad and deep. In his review of medical failings, he anathematized the medical system for structurally disempowering patients and, in so doing, causing harm. He covered a vast array of topics, failing to articulate a consistent or easy-to-summarize position on many of them. He was, furthermore, prone to histrionics, penning statements destined to attract the condemnation of orthodox readers.[108] A consummate provocateur, he endeavored not only to shed light on the failings of an immensely powerful system but to offer recommendations for wresting from it individual freedom and autonomy.

In sum, he offered an important critique of the biomedical system—one that scholars, including bioethicists, would ignore at their own peril.

THE PROPHET OF CUERNAVACA: IVAN ILLICH'S RADICAL DISSENT

Referred to by one contemporary author as a "quasi-mythical being," Ivan Illich was one of the most fascinating critics of modern medicine.[109] The child of a German Jewish mother and Croatian father, he was a polymath and polyglot who spoke German, Italian, French, Serbo-Croatian, Greek, Latin, Spanish, and English. After earning graduate degrees in history, philosophy, and theology, he was ordained a Catholic priest. Although he was expected to move up the ranks in the Holy See, he instead requested an assignment at a parish in New York City's Washington Heights. As journalist Chase Madar has noted, his time in the Manhattan community influenced his anti-authoritarian outlook: "The experience of tending to immigrant parishioners as they got flashfried in urban modernity left a lasting impression of the grotesque inadequacy of large-scale, rationally administrated institutions in dealing with basic human needs."[110]

Recognized for his intellect, Illich was soon sent to Puerto Rico to serve as the vice rector of the Catholic University in Ponce.[111] Once there, he made waves among church leaders, refusing to accede to the indoctrination of missionaries and, under a pseudonym, espousing controversial views on topics such as contraception. He was summarily sent to Cuernavaca, Mexico to prepare North American Catholic church workers to serve in Latin America. However, true to form, he opted instead to establish an ecclesial community supporting grassroots lay initiatives and attracting independent-thinking priests and nuns expelled from other South American churches.[112] A career firebrand, Illich soon fell out of favor once more with church superiors; this time, however, as Harvard Professor of Divinity Harvey Cox has explained, "it appeared that Brer Rabbit had finally reached the briar patch." He was summoned and chastised by the Sacred Congregation for the Doctrine of the Faith in Rome and requested a release from his priestly vows in 1969.[113]

Through the 1970s and early 1980s, Illich penned several works critical of the systems and structures that had come to define modern society. He advocated a disestablishment philosophy, arguing that the very systems mankind had invented to enhance life—education, transportation, and medicine among them—disabled individuals from acting on their own. Through their pernicious and malignant spread, these systems became "radical monopolies," destroying individuals' abilities to act freely and independently. "Ordinary monopolies corner the market," he wrote, "radical monopolies disable people from doing or making things on their own . . . Intensive education turns autodidacts into unemployables, intensive agriculture destroys the subsistence farmer, and the deployment of police undermines the community's self-control."[114] For a period, the world was bewitched by Illich's ministrations. As Madar has noted, "His books were best-sellers, his lectures jammed auditoriums, his essays appeared in the *New York Review of Books* (back when it was radical, fun, and widely read) and even the square-john *Saturday Review*."[115]

In 1975, Illich turned his attention to the state of the modern medical system, penning the expansive and divisive *Medical Nemesis: The Expropriation of Health*. In it, he argued that the biomedical health care system was responsible for a great deal of human suffering, indicting it on three counts of iatrogenesis. His first category of harm, clinical iatrogenesis, is the most recognizable to a modern audience and subsumes many of the harms considered earlier in this chapter. Included within its purview were the dangers posed by exposure to toxic, useless, and addictive drugs, in addition to unnecessary and potentially dangerous medical procedures. Had Illich ended his argument here, his critique would have been like many of the works considered earlier. However, he believed that clinical iatrogenesis was a symptom of deeper harms. Demonstrating his penchant for allegorical imagery, he argued, "[A]ny charge against medicine for the clinical damage it causes constitutes only the first step in the indictment of pathogenic medicine. The trail beaten in the harvest is only a reminder of the greater damage done by the baron to the village that his hunt overruns."[116]

Illich's second and third categories of iatrogenesis together form his most damning critique of contemporary medical practice. In his formulation of social iatrogenesis, he rails against the medicalization of life, wherein much of everyday experience is subsumed under the physician's authority. As he wrote, "Once a society is so organized that medicine can transform people into patients because they are unborn, newborn, menopausal, or at some other 'age of risk,' the population inevitably loses some of its autonomy to its healers."[117] Social iatrogenesis constituted a category of harm that was, at once, deeper and more pernicious than clinical iatrogenesis, for it occurred invisibly, in the diffusion of the medical system into all areas of life.

In cultural iatrogenesis, Illich expanded upon the consequences of social iatrogenesis, arguing that, as a result of the proliferation of an increasingly hegemonic health system, individuals lost the ability to conceive of health and illness in a manner unique to their own lives and experiences.[118] Both it and social iatrogenesis, therefore, multiplied disabling dependence, allowing the physician to render individuals unable to process or order their lives and unwilling to independently endure states of being deemed abnormal, deviant, or disabled. In Illich's worldview, when this happened, individuals ceded control over their lives to professionals who, in turn, rendered them illiterate in the language used to describe their own bodies.[119]

For Illich, the fundamental problem with contemporary medicine was that it misused scientific achievement to strengthen the growth of industries and professions rather than facilitate personal growth.[120] While branded a Luddite by his contemporaries,[121] Illich's concern was not technology itself but its weaponization to suppress individuality and autonomy. In his view, the public had been taught to conceive of technologized orthodox systems for explaining health and disease as the only legitimate systems. They were, therefore, blinded to the harms wrought by inimical social arrangements and rendered incapable of perceiving the dangers posed by the medical system itself. Channeling 1960s-era feminist arguments, Illich maintained that in disempowering patients, biomedicine "exempt[ed] them from the scene of political struggle to reshape the society that has made them sick."[122]

Illich's indebtedness to feminist and consumer rights advocates is clear, for he freely cites their arguments throughout his volume. However, while he would write approvingly of their activist initiatives, he simultaneously made clear that many of their arguments were too accommodationist for his taste. This was particularly apparent in his discussion of Nader's work enhancing public awareness of the dangers posed by clinical medications. Praising the consumer rights movement, he nonetheless argued, "Unless it disabuses the client of his urge to demand and take more services, consumer protection only reinforces the collusion between giver and taker, and can play only a tactical and a transitory role in any political movement aimed at the health-oriented limitation of medicine."[123]

For Illich, the problems he unearthed would find no resolution in consumer reports or empaneled review boards. The only solution was to recapture a culture of self-care society had lost in the institutionalization of a powerful biomedical system. He made no effort to disguise his embrace of self-care—in the very opening of *Nemesis,* he called for the "laicization of the Aesculapian temple . . . leading to a delegitimizing of the basic religious tenets of modern medicine."[124] His arguments were difficult for many clinical professionals to endure. For, as he saw it, medicine could not fix the problem because it was the problem; only the layperson could effect a cure. By rejecting the excesses of the modern biomedical system and redistributing its powers into individuals' hands, Illich hoped to establish a community of self-care wherein individuals determined what constituted disease, reaffirmed their ability to identify structural and environmental health determinants, freed themselves from harms wrought through biomedicine's commandeering of science to eradicate suffering, and developed the capacity for embracing all stages of life and death.[125]

Despite his popularity during the early-to-mid 1970s, by the end of the twentieth century, Illich's works had faded from memory. In 1989, *New York Times* book reviewer Anatole Broyard commented that he took special delight in purging Illich's volumes from his library.[126] How was it that a man who had rattled and enraged the keepers of orthodoxy, filling auditoriums and penning popular columns, faded so precipitously from memory?

Several explanations present themselves. One might argue, for example, that by the 1980s, the anti-authoritarian and anti-institutional sentiment that had anchored and fueled Illich's work faded in the face of a new conservatism. However, it is too simplistic to paint Illich as the liberal agitator whose works soured in a conservative climate. In truth, Illich was a liberal to conservatives and a conservative to liberals; far more than an ecclesiastic nomad, he was an intellectual one, passionately expressing views that, in one way or another, estranged him from both poles of the political spectrum. In rejecting biomedical orthodoxy and advocating self-care, for example, he alienated himself from the bioethicists and clinical authorities who dismissed him as a radical firebrand intent on dismantling the modern healthcare system while offering little in its place. At the same time, to liberal audiences, he was viewed as a conservative advocate of the free market principles famously espoused by Milton Friedman. Writing in the *New York Times*, H. Jack Geiger expressed such misgivings, arguing that Illich's volume began with a socioeconomic bang but ended in a political whimper, valorizing free will and individual enlightenment while ignoring the need for more radically progressive economic redistribution.[127] "It is all the more disappointing," Geiger argued, "that from Illich's cocoon of apparent radical humanism there ultimately emerges no bright butterfly of revolutionary change but rather, in a curious inversion, a caterpillar of petty conservatism."[128]

In the final analysis, through his contrarian invective, Illich offered society a prism through which it might view, raw and naked, the dangers posed by the institutions that had come to dominate everyday life. His arguments concur, to a point, with the critiques of Michel Foucault. Indeed, Illich directly states his indebtedness to the French scholar in his chapter discussing the invention of disease. However, Illich would part ways with Foucault in his exposition of recommendations for responding to the institutional dangers. Surveying the individual and social ills wrought by modern medicine, he identified an antidote in the reclamation of individual autonomy. Interestingly, much like the bioethicists' perspective, his approach assumed a romanticized—and perhaps naïve—valorization of free will, a harkening to the past that, as Geiger noted, was roughly Rousseauian.[129] Ironically, the radical polemicist, dismissed by many as destructive, would ultimately express an abiding faith in the capacity of the enlightened individual, freed from his iron cage, to once more claim control over his health.[130]

Ultimately, Illich was a German Jewish Roman Catholic Priest deeply suspicious of institutions, a traditionalist harkening back to a purer and simpler past, and an optimist who saw in humankind the capacity to free itself from the servitude of pernicious institutions. He cited Foucault while embracing autonomy and valorized free will while alienating bioethicists. He was that rare individual who spoke myriad languages but was seldom understood, who was versed in innumerable traditions but who had no home.

Illich's theories may have faded from the literature. However, his memory renders itself apparent whenever healthcare discussions impugn institutional orthodoxies. In some cases, biomedical leaders acknowledge his historic influence. Such was the case when, in 2003, a former editor of the *British Medical Journal* observed that the closest he had ever come to a religious experience was listening to Illich.[131] Perhaps even more significant was Illich's impact on the development of a robust self-help and alternative medicine movement. Speaking at a 1980 conference dedicated to the rise of self-care, Yale University Professor of Public Health Lowell S. Levin credited Illich with challenging conventional beliefs and raising public awareness regarding the dangers of an ineffective and harmful biomedical model.[132] Many authors, including alternative medicine historian James C. Whorton and holistic medicine advocate David Kopacz, credit Illich with catalyzing the American holistic health movement.[133] Indeed, in his commemoration marking Illich's death, theologian Harvey Cox went so far as to declare him a prophet of alternative medicine.[134]

The synergy between Illich's work and the alternative and holistic health movements is easy to understand. Each, in its own way, embraced a model of self-care and resistance to orthodox healing methodologies. Even as leading columnists purged their libraries of Illich's texts, his beliefs resurfaced wherever unsanctioned expressions of distrust breached biomedical practice. When faced with apprehensions regarding the competence and character of their healers and healing system, the public would disinter the prophet of Cuernavaca and his radical critiques. So it was in the early 1980s, as gay men living in U.S. metropolises endeavored to process, respond to, and cope with a disease that cast intensely stigmatized facets of their private lives into the clinical gaze, while offering little in the way of salve. In this caldron of fear, suspicion, and distrust, we find individuals deriving inspiration and guidance from Illich's work.[135]

In dismissing Illich as a radical detractor, professional scholars, such as mainstream bioethicists, disregard the long history of distrust that anchored and fueled his analysis. Bioethics constructed a rigid border around orthodox biomedicine, claiming it as its sovereign domain while ignoring the wilderness that lay outside its walls. In so doing, its practitioners blinded themselves to the consequences of unsanctioned distrust and its potential to do more than destroy, but to produce. This distrust ultimately prompted individuals to explore unorthodox systems of healing, migrating between them irrespective of the borders bioethics policed. It is in this movement that we find self-care.

Interestingly, in ignoring Illich's analysis, bioethicists also deprived themselves of a critique of alternative and holistic health care movements. A decade after publishing *Medical Nemesis*, Illich once more exhibited his unparalleled ability to alienate the very communities who supported his ideas. In an interview, he lamented the health movements his work had inspired, arguing that health holism had replaced orthodox medicine with alternative systems of control that taught individuals how to conceive of their bodies, to strive for health, and to combat illness. Thus, he believed that they ultimately failed to effect fundamental change for the better.[136] An explication of his misgivings with health holism was not forthcoming, for while he agreed that *Nemesis* was properly seen as a popular rabble-rouser, he adjudged his later reflections on holism to be "very delicate, not necessarily for mass consumption."[137] Whether he feared that a detailed explanation of his concerns would be received as support for orthodox medicine is impossible to ascertain, for Illich died in 2002 without further expounding on the topic. His death was, in a word, Illichian: he died of cancer after refusing to excise a tumor that had appeared on his face, fearful that the surgery would interfere with his ability to speak.[138]

It is easy to dismiss Illich by labeling him radical. Yet when we do, we blind ourselves to a valuable perspective through which individuals perceive and interpret the world. Fears, anxieties, apprehensions, and distrust cut across political spectra and defy rigid binaries demarcating the appropriate from the inappropriate, the sanctioned from the unsanctioned, the left from the right, or the orthodox from the radical. Just as Illich himself defied such dichotomies, so did the movements inspired by his ideas. For whether it is in 1980s-era unorthodox AIDS activism or 2020s-era unorthodox COVID-19 activism, we find echoes of Illich and self-care—of individuals drunk on the strong wine of freedom.

PART 2

THE SEEDS OF UNORTHODOXY

The Emergence of Unorthodox AIDS Activism

As the previous two chapters demonstrate, while the late twentieth century witnessed the ascendance of a modern biomedical juggernaut exerting tremendous influence over daily life, interwoven between promises of pharmacological panaceas were lingering doubts regarding the nation's health-care system. Critics pointed to several factors that suggested the system had gone awry: the rise of a highly technologized, pharmaceutical-driven clinical model; the elaboration of an outsized role for the state as scientific entrepreneur; and the unfettered promulgation of a culture that glorified and heroized the search for cures. Some scholars would go further still, arguing that the nation's health-care system had become institutionalized as a massive, impersonal, profit-driven bureaucracy, a health-denying behemoth Barbara Ehrenreich, John Ehrenreich, and the Health Policy Advisory Center famously dubbed the "Medical Industrial Complex."[1]

This lingering distrust and disillusionment catalyzed the development of robust, poorly understood unorthodox health activist campaigns through the

1960s and 1970s. From the dissemination of alternative health advice by the Boston Women's Health Collective, to the resurgent interest in New Age therapeutics, to the polarizing popularity of nontraditional cancer therapies, a host of health activist movements arose in the postwar years to challenge what some deemed a biomedical hegemony. In advocating their contrarian perspectives, unorthodox activists tapped into the same currents of anti-authoritarianism, antidogmatism, antimodernism, and antiheroism that had attended the rise of irregular medical sects through the nineteenth and early twentieth centuries. These currents of resistance are among the few constants to be found in our nation's long experiment with healing, having endured eras of bloodletting heroics, antibacterial animus, and biotechnological breakthroughs.

So, too, would they persist in the age of AIDS. Yet few analyses of AIDS activism explore linkages with these enduring currents of resistance, even as authors frame AIDS as a regression to the plagues of yesteryears.[2] Instead, they interpret AIDS activism as a watershed moment in the postwar patient rights and gay rights movements.[3] We thus observe the effects of two contradictory biases—one that projects a very old narrative onto AIDS and another that interprets the social movements it engendered as modern. Such framings of the disease are attractive, for they pair the tragedy of regression narratives with the promise of progress narratives. Yet they are misleading, severing both the disease and the activist response it begat from their historical moorings.

In the next section, I identify several expressions of AIDS activism that directly and indirectly intersected the nation's long history of alternative healing practices. I focus my analysis on two New York City–based activist initiatives, with chapter 4 dedicated to the campaigns of the People with AIDS Coalition (PWAC) and chapter 5 to the works of the Health Education AIDS Liaison (HEAL). Often overshadowed in AIDS scholarship by organizations such as the Gay Men's Health Crisis (GMHC) and AIDS Coalition to Unleash Power (ACT UP), PWAC and HEAL strove to empower individuals living with AIDS to claim ownership over their disease and their bodies. Their activism was neither the loudest nor the most visible amongst AIDS organizations, yet by promoting unseen, everyday acts of resistance, they played a pivotal role in empowering those affected by AIDS. As I shall argue, each organization, in its own way, encouraged its members to challenge biomedical orthodoxies, thereby laying the foundation for an engagement with alternative healing systems.

In the archives of HEAL and PWAC, we find tales of heroism and heartbreak, of unalloyed courage and unallayed despair. The groups' apologists included among their ranks individuals who summoned tremendous personal energy to organize a robust activist response as their bodies collapsed under the burden of their illness. So, too, do they include individuals promoting useless and, at times, dangerous perspectives. For this reason, some may argue that an exhumation of unorthodox AIDS activism serves as little more than a cautionary tale against the credulous embrace of health quackery by desperate individuals. Yet were we, as historians, to dismiss these individuals' stories, we would commit an offense tantamount to that which mobilized their activism in the first place, treating them as victims twice disempowered—first by virtue of their disease, and then by virtue of their desperation. I present this historical project as an antidote to this bias—an attempt to locate expressions of agency in a setting of tremendous social, political, and clinical disempowerment.

4 ▸ EVERYDAY UNORTHODOXIES AND THE PEOPLE WITH AIDS COALITION (PWAC)

Out of the AIDS epidemic arose a powerful health activist movement many authors credit with fundamentally transforming the patient-healer relationship.[1] Echoes of this activism resonate in the public memory, coalescing around the riotous chants and impassioned pleas of protestors beseeching action by government researchers and pharmaceutical corporations. We may trace these echoes to precise loci of protest—the streets of Greenwich Village whereupon ralliers unfurled hand-painted banners demanding "drugs into bodies," the meeting halls of medical conferences wherein protestors interrupted biomedical leaders to demand the reframing of AIDS as a national priority, and the offices of FDA officials wherein people with AIDS staged die-ins.[2] In our shared reminiscences—transmitted through lived memory, oral history, journalistic reporting, and faded photographs—we recall AIDS activism as an exercise in overt resistance staged in the public arena. Whether demonstrators marched on Washington, besieged St. Patrick's Cathedral, or stopped traffic before federal office buildings, they expressed their impassioned views in fora chosen to maximize public exposure.

While popular protests echo loudest in our historical memory, to summarily reduce all AIDS activism to such vocal demonstrations ignores a vast array of resistance that remained largely hidden or shielded from the public sphere. The location of expression for this activism was neither the streets of New York City nor the fields of the National Mall, but the bodies of men and women living with and dying from AIDS.[3] Where public protestors would claim as tools a compendium of bolded banners and rancorous chants condemning federal bureaucracies, activism located on the scale of the body registered resistance through individuals' decisions to claim ownership over their disease, questioning the etiological and therapeutic paradigms of mainstream biomedicine. It was manifest in the actions of the young man who eschewed antiretrovirals and turned to soy lecithin solutions he religiously mixed in his East Village apartment, or the person who rejected pharmacological cures to pursue a treatment plan grounded in herbal nostrums. These individuals' acts of protest, effected before medicine cabinets each morning and facilitated by underground networks, are no less examples of everyday forms of resistance—namely to mainstream biomedicine—than the private protests of peasant farmers famously explicated by James C. Scott.[4]

Historians stand to learn a great deal by studying these hidden expressions of activism.[5] Consider, for example, the history of queer and gay individuals living in New York City through the twentieth century—a cohort of relevance to the history of AIDS activism. Popular conceptions of the queer rights movement identify demonstrations such as the Stonewall Riots as watershed moments in the expression of resistance and opposition to sexual norms. However, long before the first glass was shattered outside the Stonewall Inn, individuals who engaged in same-sex interactions—be they in private bedrooms, downtown bathhouses, or the dark of Central Park—expressed their opposition to gendered orthodoxies through their everyday actions effected at the level of the body.[6] Far from marking the end of these expressions, the AIDS epidemic catalyzed transformations in private acts of protest, with individuals claiming ownership over their bodies in an effort to quell a disease increasingly attributed to sexual liberation.

Although I have presented everyday expressions of resistance as private acts, they were, in fact, sustained and supported by an array of underground networks and communities. In the case of 1960s–1970s era sexual liberation, for example, we find the establishment of institutions (e.g., bathhouses) and cultural practices (e.g., nonverbal means of communicating interest) that enabled queer individuals' acts of resistance. During the first decade of the AIDS epidemic, we similarly recognize the development of underground groups that assembled to empower individuals to assert control over their treatment. Through anonymous publications and support groups, these organizations encourage individuals to reject the external ordering of their bodies, defy mainstream biomedical ministrations, and claim expertise over their own healing. Among the first and most successful of such organizations was New York's PWAC.

Scholars are torn in their descriptions of the PWAC's core mission. Some categorize it as a service organization in the mold of the Gay Men's Health Crisis (GMHC), while others argue that it was a direct-action protest group more like ACT UP.[7] In truth, it defied such rigid binaries, for it was not solely concerned with linking individuals to support services or taking to the streets to demand action. Instead, it sought to empower individuals by encouraging them to claim ownership and expertise over their bodies, transforming 1960s–1970s era cultures of bodily resistance into forms more appropriate for a decade defined by disease.[8] In a poem he penned while hospitalized with AIDS, poet and PWA Tony J. Giordano eloquently captured the linkages between 1960s and 1980s–era expressions of bodily activism. Reflecting upon his liberated past and gazing forward into a precarious future, Giordano discerned from both directions the harrowing "sounds of furious living"—the furor of individuals demanding and commanding lives of resistance and protest.[9]

This chapter tells the history of furious living in the era of AIDS and of the empowerment attained by impassioned and intrepid individuals who lived with and perished from AIDS in America's great metropolis. I begin with an examination of the foundational texts that motivated the PWAC's creation, arguing that these documents established the organization's allegiance to a culture of radical empowerment and articulation of unorthodox perspectives. I also argue that the movement embraced the unorthodox currents introduced earlier in this volume, and that those currents were propagated through 1970s-era activist initiatives such as the women's health movement. I then move on to an examination of the discourse the PWAC embraced in its critique of biomedicine, focusing on several organizational publications: the *PWAC Newsline* (1985–1993), the dual volume *Surviving and Thriving with AIDS* collection (1987 and 1988), and Michael Callen's *Surviving AIDS* (1990).[10] In the final section of the chapter, I examine how these critiques gave rise to PWAC contributors' direct engagement with unorthodox responses to AIDS.

As I shall discuss, despite launching several initiatives to expand outreach to the larger PWA community, the PWAC was an organization whose history and mission were defined in large part by gay White men. Thus, it offers just one view into expressions of unorthodox AIDS activism early in the pandemic. Furthermore, despite its relative homogeneity, the group was heterogeneous in terms of the positions, beliefs, and initiatives its members embraced. Some advocated unorthodox philosophies, while others allied more closely with biomedical orthodoxies. Perhaps even more importantly, many did both. The PWAC famously lacked internal consistency—but then, it was not its goal to establish homogeneity of thought or action beyond its shared interest in empowering individuals with AIDS.[11] In describing the *Newsline*, for example, one PWAC cofounder commented, "AIDS is full of non sequiturs and incomplete thoughts and so is the *Newsline*."[12] As I argue, we should view this heterogeneity not as a sign of diluted unorthodoxy but an example of the borderland model in action. Rather than claim citizenship in the kingdom of biomedicine or any of the myriad alternative sects dotting the landscape, individuals moved between them in overt and covert ways. The history of the PWA movement charts these migrations—of the ways people organized amidst tremendous fear and uncertainty to contest received wisdom, share hope, and reject the external ordering of their bodies—in short, to live furiously.

A BILL OF RIGHTS, A WAR BULLETIN, AND THE BIRTH OF THE PEOPLE WITH AIDS COALITION

As sociologist Susan Chambré has chronicled, by the early 1980s, myriad professional and lay groups had organized on both coasts to provide support services for those diagnosed with AIDS and to raise funds for biomedical research.[13] The earliest of these groups assembled informally in living rooms and kitchens, convened by individuals—mostly gay men—who had been diagnosed with AIDS.[14] In 1982, the city's first professional AIDS service group, the GMHC, was founded. While renowned for its support services, by 1983, GMHC would attract complaints by some who viewed its attitude toward patients as broadly patriarchal and patronizing. As two prominent AIDS activists later noted, "New York PWAs and PWArc [people with AIDS-related complex[15]] began to express frustration at attending GMHC forums where those of us with AIDS would sit silently in the audience and hear doctors, nurses, lawyers, insurance experts, and CSWs tell us what it was like to have AIDS . . . The 'real experts,' we realized, weren't up there."[16]

This concern with the health service community's victimization of AIDS patients dramatically came to a head in June of 1983 at a national Gay and Lesbian Health Conference in Denver.[17] In the midst of conference proceedings, a group of 14 men living with AIDS—many from California and New York—stormed the stage to read prepared comments asserting their right to participate in the national AIDS discourse.[18] Their opening statement eloquently and emotionally gave birth to the PWA movement: "We condemn attempts to label us as 'victims,' a term which implies defeat, and we are only occasionally 'patients,' a term which implies passivity, helplessness, and dependence upon the care of others. We are 'People with AIDS.'"[19] By the end of their protest, the group had enumerated 17 principles—remembered today as the Denver Principles—outlining the rights of those living with AIDS. Half a decade after the conference, activists Michael Callen and Dan Turner registered the moment's lasting effect on the PWA movement: "[I]t simply hadn't occurred to those of us in New York who were diagnosed that we could be anything more than the passive recipients of the genuine care and concern of those who hadn't (yet) been diagnosed. As soon as the concept of PWAs representing themselves was proposed, the idea caught on like wildfire."[20]

Given the prominent role they played in shaping the public response to the epidemic, it is unsurprising that scholars and activists remember the Denver Principles as a cornerstone of AIDS protest. It is also unsurprising that a leader of the AIDS movement would, in 2005, refer to them as "the Magna Carta of AIDS activism, our Declaration of Independence, Constitution and Bill of Rights rolled into one."[21] What is surprising, however, is how we choose to remember them. Consider, for example, the first six principles, intended to shape the behavior of healthcare professionals. The result of compromise between East and West Coast activists, this set of principles captured positions rightly viewed as unorthodox. Representatives of California, for example, successfully lobbied for a provision (Principle 5) advocating the holistic treatment of patients, while those from New York secured a plank (Principle 2) recognizing the diversity of opinion surrounding the etiology of AIDS.[22] Yet many contemporary discussions of this foundational PWA text ignore these intersections by literally eliding the first six principles from the historical register. In reproductions published by ACT UP New York and the Joint United Nations Programme on HIV/AIDS (UNAIDS), for example, both organizations redact, without comment, the first six principles. Where once there were seventeen, the groups list only eleven, even as they ensure readers that they remain "as relevant and powerful today" as when they were first drafted.[23] While it is difficult to ascertain the cause for this elision, its consequence is clear: it severs the PWA activist movement from the unorthodox principles that once formed its foundation.

Following the Denver Conference, the eight East Coast PWA attendees returned home to form "PWA—New York," the city's first PWA organization.[24] The group registered some success—producing, for example, the first safe sex posters to appear in New York bathhouses—but soon disbanded following internal dissension, the death of many founders, and perceived hostility from professional service organizations such as GMHC.[25] In its wake, several of its leaders formed the People with AIDS Coalition (PWAC), an organization that would persist for nearly a decade.[26] With a budget approaching one million dollars by the early 1990s, the PWAC differed from ACT UP, which it predated, in that its leaders relied less on public expressions of protest,[27] endeavoring instead to empower individuals to effect changes in their conceptualizations of and responses to their disease. It was well regarded for hosting discussions and support groups but exerted greatest influence through its print publications, including the two-volume collection of essays *Surviving and Thriving with AIDS* and, even more importantly, its monthly *PWAC Newsline* newsletter. First distributed in June of 1985, the *Newsline* began as a sixteen-page resource editor Michael Callen described as a "breathless war bulletin from the front lines"[28] and included essays, reflections, interviews, letters, poems, and cartoons written by and for PWAs. By the late 1980s, the publication had burgeoned into a forty-eight-page resource distributed monthly to 14,000 individuals in hospitals, private homes, offices, and incarceration facilities throughout the city, state, and nation.[29]

Both the *Newsline* and *Surviving and Thriving with AIDS* were living documents airing diverse, contradictory, and controversial perspectives aimed at helping PWAs find order and meaning amid profound uncertainty. The texts bore resemblance to publications produced by the feminist and women's health movement, particularly the Boston Women's Health Collective's popular text *Our Bodies, Ourselves*. Indeed, the broader PWA movement shared many characteristics with the women's health movement.[30] In his 1990 text *Good Intentions: How Big Business and the Medical Establishment are Corrupting the Fight Against AIDS*, Bruce Nussbaum describes how the feminist and women's health movements would come to inspire PWAC leaders such as Callen, who cofounded the group and edited its core publications:

> The feminists and lesbians in the AIDS Network had been talking to Callen about the women's health movement of the seventies, but he didn't quite understand it. He had been out playing in the seventies. Callen couldn't connect it to himself until that moment.[31] One of the key issues in the women's movement was the arrogance and condescension of male doctors toward female patients. Doctors saw themselves as deities and were treated as gods by the older generation. Women, however, wanted to take responsibility for their own health . . . *Our Bodies, Ourselves* was one of many books to come out reflecting this dramatic shift in the relationship between patient and doctor. The notion of self-empowerment, borrowed from the women's movement, began to play itself out in the gay community.[32]

Callen later recognized the degree to which the women's health movement would come to influence his philosophy. "We felt that we had a right to tell our own stories, to control to a greater extent who said what about us," he reflected. "Our experiences were a reaffirmation of the feminist principle that the personal is indeed political."[33]

It is difficult to overstate the feminist and women's health movements' impact on PWAC activism.[34] If, as I have argued in this volume, unorthodox health movements have been propagated by antiheroic, anti-authoritarian, antidogmatic, and antimodern currents, then feminist activism, in addition to Black liberationist activism, were the conduits through which many of these currents acted upon the early AIDS movement.[35] Yet as leaders pursued activism inspired by radical feminist ideas, they encountered resistance, as Callen described in a 1985 edition of the *Newsline*: "The concept of PWA activism was not well received

here in New York . . . Drawing on the feminist and black liberationist concept of self-empowerment, we demanded certain rights in an effort to retain some control over our lives. But heaven forbid that PWA should express an opinion about etiology, about organizational structure, about service delivery, about the politics of AIDS! No, we were only permitted to participate in forums as performing bears brought in at the end to make them cry before the hat got passed."[36]

In Callen's view, accommodationists advocated a conservative activism that used the PWA experience instrumentally, as exemplified by initiatives that presented ill PWAs for fundraising purposes. Instead, he advocated an approach that impugned systems of oppression he believed the gay community had internalized. He was not alone in his conviction. Jim Fouratt, a founding member of several gay rights and AIDS organizations, has suggested that debates between accommodationist and radical AIDS activists recapitulate the divide between visions of gay empowerment articulated by the Gay Activist Alliance and Gay Liberation Front.[37]

While the women's health movement served as an important conduit through which unorthodox currents propagated within the PWA movement, it was not the only activist tradition to exert influence. Callen, for example, identified Marxist principles as motivating his activism. In a recent biography, musicologist and cultural critic Michael J. Jones argues that Callen was particularly inspired by author-activist Gayle Rubin's 1975 essay, "The Traffic in Women: Notes on the Political Economy of Sex," which utilized a Marxist critique to interrogate social systems that oppressed women.[38] Furthermore, though seldom discussed, the Denver Principles and the larger PWA movement were informed by progressive philosophies in nursing practice. This link is explicit: one of the authors of the early PWA movement was a nurse named Bobbi Campbell. Joe Wright has argued that Campbell's nursing education influenced the drafting of the Principles, noting that some of the content, "reflects Campbell's own approach to how to be a clinician, and would have been the sort of instruction a progressive nursing educator might have given at the time."[39] This education would have included 1970s and 1980s-era engagement with feminist and postcolonial ideas, rejection of expertism and paternalism, and embrace of holistic ideologies.[40]

Inspired by these activist traditions, the PWAC sought to empower PWAs. Some of the most powerful tools it wielded in this pursuit were its publications. Many PWAs who remained painfully stigmatized and isolated by both their health status and sexuality viewed the *Newsline* as nothing short of a lifeline.[41] Through the early 1990s, it existed as one of few fora wherein individuals could engage their conditions as both anonymous readers and contributors, sharing strategies for survival and wresting control over their disease narrative from a medical industrial complex viewed as hegemonic, a government viewed as negligent, and a mainstream media viewed as sensationalist. PWAC leaders argued that this level of engagement was crucial to the long-term survival of PWAs, with one member observing, "You cannot underestimate the therapeutic value of feeling like a soldier in the war against AIDS."[42]

It is easy to interpret these calls for engagement as benign expressions of the patient rights movement—appeals for the education of individuals so they could participate in healthcare decisions as informed, autonomous agents. Such a framing, however, simplifies what was, in fact, a far more complex and contentious activist tradition. Many PWAs viewed biomedicine not as a symphony strengthened by the addition of patients' unique vocal registers, but as a cacophony that had fallen badly out of tune. This critique was one reason some GMHC leaders initially viewed PWAC activism as dangerously radical.[43] For in many regards, the group's activism bore less in common with the patient right movement's Kantian individualism than it did Illichian anti-institutionalism.[44] A radical repudiation of health bureaucracies, it located hope not in systems of ennobled expertise but in individuals' power to direct their own care. As Callen would write, borrowing the words of democratic socialist Michael Harrington, to support PWA activism was "to sense the seed beneath the snow; to see, beneath the veneer of corruption and meanness and the commercialization of human relationships, men and women capable of controlling their own destinies."[45]

Callen vigorously maintained this philosophy through his editorship of the *Newsline*, arguing that PWAs possessed the capacity and the right to engage therapeutic and etiological debates on their own terms. He evidenced his position most clearly in his support for the newsletter's *Medical Matters* section, wherein PWAs openly debated the wisdom of mainstream biomedical practice.[46] Throughout its run, the column attracted criticism from some readers who accused it of sanctioning almost guerilla-style attacks on mainstream biomedicine. Unflinchingly committed to PWA empowerment, Callen rejected their critiques, often invoking the language of the Denver Principles: "[R]equiring that articles by PWAs/PWArcs who happen not to be medical experts be censored or fact-checked by so-called medical experts runs contrary to the basic philosophy of the Newsline . . . The PWA self-empowerment movement was born out of a general distrust of expert-ism. One of the founding principles of our movement states that we PWAs are, in one sense, the *real* experts about AIDS; we demand to be included in all decision-making processes [with] full and equal credibility as other so-called experts."[47] Callen was so committed to this principle that, in a 1986 *Newsline* column, he recommended that PWAs speaking publicly about their condition first recount their medical histories, "much in the way that other experts list their credentials."[48] Other *Newsline* authors took this call for PWA engagement further still, transforming individuals' right to challenge experts into an obligation. In a 1986 *Newsline* column titled "How to Talk to Your Doctor," PWA Bob Herman, for example, suggested that patients who refused to challenge received wisdom and instead passively followed the advice of physicians were "choosing not to heal" themselves.[49]

Through the 1980s and 1990s, numerous *Newsline* and *Surviving and Thriving with AIDS* contributors heeded Callen's call for open engagement with their disease, penning articles critical of the experts entrusted with the nation's health. Their critiques betrayed a fundamental distrust and disillusionment with institutions and individuals who wielded power in AIDS research and policy, including the National Institutes of Health (NIH), the FDA, pharmaceutical corporations, mass media outlets, and political leaders. Ranging far and cutting deep, they impugned virtually all aspects of the mainstream response to the epidemic, including how biomedical leaders (a) discussed AIDS, (b) organized research efforts, (c) theorized about etiology and pathology, and (d) developed treatments. In short, they waged a full-scale offensive against the orthodox response to the epidemic.

In the second section of this chapter, I explore these four broad domains of dissent and protest in greater detail. As I shall argue, in articulating distrust of biomedicine, PWAC contributors tapped into and expressed the same core themes of anti-authoritarianism, antidogmatism, antiheroism, and antimodernism that have historically subtended alternative and irregular health activism throughout U.S. history.

Disputed Words: Challenges to Universal Fatality Narratives

Many scholarly analyses of AIDS activism focus on discussions of the anger and frustration pervading the gay community in the first decade of the epidemic. As sociologist Deborah Gould has argued, the most famous expressions of AIDS activism harnessed shared sentiments of anger and rage to mobilize highly public activist responses.[50] By the late 1980s, protestors had begun taking to the streets in record numbers, staging die-ins to remind the public that, absent active intervention by an apathetic government, they were fated to perish from their disease. One can craft near endless histories of AIDS focused upon such expressions of fury, bringing to bear compendiums of faded photographs capturing the bodies of protestors forcing the public to gaze upon the face of death and suffering.

Yet these histories would comprise but one part of the larger story of AIDS activism. To capture the full range of AIDS protest, we must consider other emotions that catalyzed acts of resistance. These emotions included hope—an abiding faith in the capacity of individuals to survive with their disease. As we shall see, PWAC leaders such as Michael Callen and Max Navarre argued that empowerment was predicated upon awakening within individuals a belief that they would survive. For these authors, hope was more than a cheerful or optimistic disposition; it was a prerequisite for survival. Furthermore, it was under siege.

Through the 1980s, Callen deemed the print media ground zero in an unrelenting assault on PWAs' capacity for hope. In one 1986 *Newsline* piece, for example, he complained, "Every time I pick up the paper, I choke on that boilerplate paragraph about AIDS being 'invariably 100% fatal.'"[51] In a column published a year later, he similarly condemned reporters' practice of framing AIDS as "uniformly, inevitably, ineluctably, always, without exception . . . fatal."[52] Callen committed himself to challenging these macabre characterizations, dedicating his 1990 text *Surviving AIDS* to finding and interviewing long-term survivors of AIDS to prove that it was indeed possible to persevere with the condition.[53] In his text, he surveys the ubiquity of universal fatality narratives, demonstrating that they reached beyond sensationalist headlines to influence visual representations of the condition as well. In one passage, for example, fellow PWAC cofounder and photographer Jane Rosett recalls submitting photos of PWAs for a spread in a major news magazine, only to have the editor reject them for being "too healthy looking." Dumbstruck by the editor's response, Rosett replied, "That was the point."[54]

It is easy to dismiss Callen's critiques as nothing more than semantic quibbles—the call for the use of politically correct designations to describe those suffering from illness. However, for both Callen and fellow PWAC editor Navarre, they were about much more. Less than a year before his death, for example, Navarre would write, "Does anyone consider the impact of [the] cult of the victim? Does anyone realize the power of the message, 'You are helpless. There is no hope for you?' I'm not immune to the reinforcement of hopelessness that surrounds me. That reinforcement causes despair, and I believe that despair kills people with AIDS as much as any of AIDS' physical manifestations."[55] Similarly, in his opening to *Surviving AIDS*, Callen observed, "A common thread that has run through my AIDS activism has been a passionate belief that hopelessness kills. This is why challenging the myth that everyone dies from AIDS has become an obsession."[56] Both Callen and Navarre argued that the purveyors of universal fatality narratives—including mainstream media and the biomedical leaders who influenced it—were fundamentally incapable of championing the survival of PWAs, for they forestalled its possibility. The activists' views of hope and hopelessness were not romantic but radical, blurring distinctions between physical and symbolic forms of violence. For this reason, their positions resonated with the supporters of attitudinal healing movements, as I argue later in this chapter.

While PWAs criticized news outlets for fomenting fatalism, they also challenged the authority of biomedical leaders for fueling the fire with unsophisticated assessments of the disease. In the second volume of *Surviving and Thriving with AIDS*, for example, Callen criticizes New York City Health Commissioner Stephen Joseph for stating that the proportion of long-term PWAs was greater than he "would have intuitively expected it to be." Callen's response was unequivocal: "What the hell does that mean? In New York City, 15% of us have survived five or more years. Shouldn't the City's own Health Commissioner have known that? And is it enough for him and others to now say, 'Oops! Guess we were wrong about 100% mortality?' Is there no one to hold accountable for the lie and its harmful effects on PWAs?"[57] In the same publication, Joseph Sonnabend, Callen's physician and a leader in the PWA movement, suggested that mainstream biomedicine's fatalism derived from its exaltation of laboratory science over the experiences of community physicians who were in the trenches working with PWAs.[58] Sonnabend railed against the power and influence afforded academic and research physicians, many of whom he viewed as distant professionals ensconced in their labs, lacking necessary clinical experience with patients.[59]

Just as Callen, Navarre, and Sonnabend accused the mainstream media and biomedicine of robbing PWAs of the hope requisite for survival, so, too, did they express frustration with the city's AIDS service organizations. In an essay appearing in the second volume of *Surviving and Thriving with AIDS* communicating frustration with the universal fatality narratives encountered at major AIDS service organizations, PWA Max Navarre includes a short poem: "What shall we do with Max? / He will not face the facts. / He insists he's alive. / And continues to thrive. / What shall we do with Max?"[60] Callen put an even finer point on the matter, arguing that GMHC actively promulgated universal fatality narratives to elicit greater public support and funding. In *Surviving AIDS*, for example, he recounts with horror an early encounter at a GMHC event:

> Once, after giving my "hope speech" during a public forum organized by the Gay Men's Health Crisis, I was angrily pulled aside by a gay man who worked in the GMHC Education Department. He begged me to stop saying that AIDS might not be 100 percent fatal. Shocked that a gay man would make such a request, I asked for reasons. He gave three: (1) efforts to persuade gay men to practice safer sex might be undermined because they would "take AIDS less seriously"; (2) it was bad for fund-raising; and (3) it would make lobbying for increased federal funding more difficult. "After all," he said, "if not everyone who gets it dies, then maybe AIDS isn't *really* the crisis we're being told it is."[61]

In *Surviving AIDS*, West Coast-based PWA Stephen Pieters reported receiving similar pushback when he announced to members of the AIDS Project Los Angeles that he had gone into remission. There, a group representative quietly asked him not to share his story, arguing, "[I]t'll be real bad for fund-raising that it gets out that people are doing well."[62]

For Callen and Navarre, such mainstream practices were health denying. Their positions were anti-authoritarian in nature, impugning mainstream society and biomedicine's ability to frame the disease and give voice to the epidemic.

Moreover, they represent a fascinating transformation of antiheroism discourse; for whereas nineteenth-century critics would argue that physicians were injuring people through heroized treatments, Callen and Navarre argued that late-twentieth-century clinicians were doing so through villainized disease narratives. Through their *Newsline* and *Surviving AIDS* commentaries, they encouraged PWAs to project their own voices, ideas, and perspectives onto AIDS discourse, supplanting a biomedical framing they viewed as not only misguided but dangerous.

Armed with this understanding of 1980s-era critiques of mainstream fatalism discourse, I move now into more familiar terrain, mapping PWA engagement with biomedical professionals' early efforts to research AIDS and develop drugs to treat its symptoms. As I shall argue, many PWAs expressed concern with virtually all aspects of the mainstream biomedical research response, betraying grave distrust and disenchantment with the commitment and competence of biomedical professionals.

Disputed Actions: PWAC Activism and Allegations of "Fourth or Fifth Rate" Science

Many scholars have recounted the history of PWA discontent with researchers' failure to develop treatments for the condition until half a decade into the epidemic. The history of PWA protests surrounding these issues is well known, because it inspired the most vocal public forms of AIDS protest. PWAC publications aired these complaints as well, with authors lamenting a research response that appeared woefully underfunded to address the suffering at hand.[63] However, by focusing exclusively on top-down research funding issues or the truancy of national leaders, we blind ourselves to an even more radical critique logged in the pages of PWAC publications, as authors expressed growing concerns that the biomedical research system was profoundly misaligned or broken.

Through the 1980s and early 1990s, many individuals writing in the *Newsline* expressed concern with the mainstream professionals tasked with researching and treating early cases of AIDS. Joseph Sonnabend made little secret of his feelings toward professional researchers, arguing that they lacked a real understanding of the needs of those living with AIDS and had badly fumbled early efforts to study the condition. In a 1991 *Newsline* interview, he told of the earliest days of the epidemic when researchers first realized that the disease was linked to T cells. As the field of T cell subtyping was still relatively new, Sonnabend tracked down a pioneer in the area, certain that many biomedical professionals would have called the researcher for counsel. He was shocked to learn that his was, in fact, the first AIDS-related call the man had received—even though, as a community physician, Sonnabend lacked the resources, prestige, or clout enjoyed by academic researchers. Experiences such as these shaped his opinion, causing him to conclude that, "the caliber of people who've gone into the field of AIDS research is abysmal."[64] Michael Callen, Sonnabend's long-time patient, echoed these concerns, arguing that a mixture of incompetence and complicity had forestalled the free expression and testing of ideas among researchers. In the second volume of *Surviving and Thriving with AIDS*, he declared, "[W]hat's going on in terms of AIDS research—or should I say, what's not going on in terms of research—is a form of passive genocide . . . I think that the caliber of science that has been brought to bear on the problem of AIDS is fourth or fifth rate at best."[65]

Attacks on biomedical researchers were joined by lingering doubts, consistent with the narratives of distrust chronicled in chapter 3, that self-serving pharmaceutical corporations had hijacked the nation's biomedical research apparatus. Many authors contributing to the *Newsline* underscored these fears, arguing that the federal research and drug testing bureaucracy was designed to profit pharmaceutical corporations, not heal patients. In 1987, for example, the *Newsline* published a statement from PWA activist Marty Robinson, who argued that the FDA had "hidden behind a guise of cautious scientific detachment" in failing to prevent the excessive profiteering and delay by big pharma.[66] A second *Newsline* piece cited reflections from a former NIH lab director, who stated that researchers structured their clinical trials primarily to benefit pharmaceutical manufacturers, not PWAs.[67]

Another *Newsline* piece invoked well-known West Coast AIDS activist John S. James. "The commercial forces driving AIDS treatment research favor high-tech, patentable options, the very ones which take the longest to develop," the article quotes James as saying. "Simple, available, off-the-shelf treatments, already well known in human use, could be applied much more quickly; but these kinds of treatments have little commercial potential."[68] The comment reinforced a fear expressed by many *Newsline* contributors—that no matter what evidence PWAs marshaled in support of potential remedies, if they derived from a plant, health food, or commonly available chemical, they had virtually no prospects of seeing the light of day due to the monopolistic hold big pharma exerted on research. Here, we recognize the echo of antimodernism, pitting the simple and the natural against the manmade and artificial.

The biomedical critique published in the pages of *Newsline* reached such a level that some readers felt compelled to pen letters to the editor defending its legitimacy. In one such defense, published the same month AZT was approved, a contributor urged other PWAs to accept on faith that mainstream researchers operated with a "certain degree of sophistication."[69] Callen, who regularly published pieces critical of his own perspectives, printed the letter while appending a rebuke. "It remains my view," he wrote, "that the gay community's (and the media's) unwillingness to demand the *best* science—it's 'willingness to assume on faith, at least provisionally, a certain degree of sophistication among AIDS researchers'—is costing us our lives."[70]

In addition to impugning the commitments and capacities of mainstream researchers, PWAs writing in the *Newsline* and *Surviving and Thriving with AIDS* took issue with biomedicine's insistence upon gathering "clean" or "pure" data, a topic Steven Epstein explores in his 1996 volume *Impure Science*.[71] Rigid entry requirements for clinical trials, such as rules forcing PWAs to forego the use of unapproved therapeutic treatments before or during trials and to submit to randomization, effectively forced individuals to choose between their regimens of self-care and the potential promise of new experimental agents. Both literally and figuratively, they demanded that PWAs submit to systems of control, while simultaneously asking that they prioritize statistical power over individual expressions of power. In their design and administration, they attempted to contain PWAs within neatly bounded and bordered domains, proscribing the movement between systems characteristic of the borderland model.

For many PWAs, the request was too bitter a pill to swallow. Callen, for example, counseled PWAs to avoid federally sponsored trials. "The federal government's track record of unethical, poorly designed trials speaks for itself," he wrote in the conclusion to *Surviving AIDS*. "Don't be willing to die for the supposed greater good of the greater numbers. Besides, a government trial is likely to be so poorly designed and executed that the data will end up being worthless anyway."[72] Navarre voiced similar concerns in the second volume of *Surviving and Thriving with AIDS*, noting, "I question the advisability and effectiveness of gay people sacrificing themselves on the altar of science in the hope of preventing the onset of symptoms. Is that really the responsibility of the gay community?"[73]

Perhaps the clearest articulations of resistance to systems of control were found in individuals who feigned deference to scientific authority while simultaneously working to undermine that authority. One remarkable 1989 *Newsline* article captures this dynamic, relaying in vivid detail the efforts an anonymous PWA undertook to gain entry into a clinical trial of the experimental drug ribavirin, which he had previously procured at great personal expense from Mexico. The trial had rigid entry requirements, accepting only PWAs with T4 cell counts below 600. Concerned that his high titer would prohibit his enrollment, the man took actions to effectively cheat his way into the study and then violated its protocol when accepted so that he could maintain his self-care regimen:

> In order to try to lower my T4s a little, I went out the night before [my pre-trial test], partying and barhopping with friends with little sleep. It didn't work. My T4s were 680. Another appointment was made for me to try again a few days later. This time, I stayed out the entire night before, and with NO sleep at all (I am not advising this!), my blood was taken again. The result was 630. I was accepted anyway . . . Then it dawned on me that although there was some difficulty in recruiting for this program, there are so many people with ARC who could

> benefit from free ribavirin. So I cheated to get into this study. Also on my mind was the fact that I could be fucking up the results which may or may not jeopardize (again?!) the approval of this beneficial and life-saving drug by the goddamn FDA. I felt very guilty and had very mixed emotions about what I was doing. But I would be saving myself and family a lot of money since the medication was costing a fortune . . . When I got in the study I cheated; I began to stockpile Ribavirin. I continued with my 5-days-on/5-days-off schedule even though the protocol required that I take it every day. I now have enough Ribavirin to last me through November. My doctor commented once that I seemed to have lower blood levels of Ribavirin than others and I laughed and denied selling it on the street . . . It's just a goddamn shame that one has to cheat, lie and who knows what else to obtain what you need to live. May God bless our government.[74]

As this brief analysis underscores, PWAs engaged in a rich, multilayered critique of biomedical research practice through the 1980s and 1990s, calling into question the competence and character of mainstream researchers and the broader biomedical research paradigm. Their arguments challenged the authority of not just individual researchers but entire systems and cultures of practice. Moreover, they exercised this resistance through both words and actions, fomenting distrust through emotionally charged opinion pieces while subverting clinical trial protocols to procure unapproved agents and pursue individualized systems of self-care. In some ways, by questioning the capacities of mainstream research paradigms and advising PWAs to pursue their own self-care programs, these individuals engaged in expressions of activism even more disruptive than protests staged in the public arena. For they robbed the biomedical system of the one resource it required to conduct its business: controlled bodies.

Disputed Thoughts: HIV, AIDS, and the "Unholy Holy War"

Of all the topics discussed in the pages of PWAC publications, few were as controversial as debates surrounding the etiological models biomedical leaders adopted to explain AIDS. In his authorship and editorship of the *Newsline, Surviving and Thriving with AIDS* and *Surviving AIDS*, Callen was well known for contesting the claim that HIV caused AIDS and for maintaining an editorial policy receptive to critiques of orthodox etiological theories.[75] Others also contributed their voices to the opposition of the so-called "killer virus" model, including members of HEAL, who wrote into the *Newsline* expressing their support for the editor. As a whole, this culture of opposition and resistance censured biomedicine for, in its view, uncritically accepting the HIV etiological model, replacing falsifiable knowledge with dogma, and failing to heed the concerns of those who questioned its legitimacy.

Despite this rich culture of engagement and protestation, many scholarly treatments of AIDS activism underemphasize the role PWAs played in so-called "dissident" or "denialist" etiological debates, focusing instead on the contributions made by rogue scientists such as University of California, Berkeley retrovirologist Peter Duesberg. It is difficult to determine the reasons for this elision, but several possibilities suggest themselves. Some scholars, for example, exhibit an almost paternalistic defensiveness toward the memory of PWAs, perhaps striving to protect them from the stigma now attached to HIV dissidence. Such expressions of benevolent paternalism may, for example, explain the characterization of Callen's activism found in some works.[76] Others may presume that scientists are the only legitimate experts to consult in scientific disputes, even when said experts have been denounced by their colleagues. Whatever the cause, the effect of this bias is clear: it has reduced a complex social movement into neat questions of scientific legitimacy. In one 2009 volume dedicated to unorthodox etiological AIDS debates, for example, the author diminishes the role PWAs played in contrarian etiological activism, arguing that, "HIV denialism starts and ends with Peter Duesberg."[77]

There is, of course, irony in scholarly analyses of unorthodox AIDS activism that recognize as legitimate only those expressions of resistance originating from within the halls of biomedicine. For it was precisely a discomfort with "expertism" that motivated the editorial policy of PWAC publications—and, more broadly, inspired the drafting of the Denver Principles in the first place. Suggesting that PWA expressions of dissidence depended upon Duesberg both misrepresents the chronology of etiological activism and recapitulates the systematic disempowerment of PWAs against which individuals like Callen protested.[78] Furthermore, equating HIV dissidence with Duesberg's theories reduces a multifaceted tradition of resistance to a purely scientific disagreement debated according to the traditions and standards of modern biomedicine. As I shall argue, PWA engagement with etiological disputes reached beyond questions of viral titers or statistical power analysis to interrogate the full measure of the power biomedicine wielded over the ill. Indeed, throughout the 1980s and early 1990s, authors writing in the *Newsline* and *Surviving and Thriving with AIDS* asked probing questions regarding the power of experts to dictate truth, the power of a theory to influence individuals' lived experience of their disease, and the power of PWAs to define and respond to their condition on their own terms.

For Callen, the HIV etiological model's rapid ascent from questionable hypothesis to received truth, a phenomenon Epstein chronicles in *Impure Science*,[79] smacked of that most pernicious exponent of expertism: dogma.[80] The situation was a perfect storm for controversy: a new theory promulgated by a controversial American researcher and announced with fanfare by an administration widely deemed negligent was rapidly codified by a media establishment viewed as sensationalist.[81] Callen argued that in condoning this process, biomedicine had branded itself into something far worse than fourth or fifth rate science—it had become, in effect, religion masquerading as science. Writing in the *Newsline* in

1986, he argued, "Regarding the virtual non-debate about the etiology of AIDS, HTLV-III[82] has become a matter of faith—almost a religion. To question its central role in AIDS is heresy."[83] He would carry his distrust in biomedicine's embrace of the killer virus etiological model for the remainder of his life. Seven years after the *Newsline* piece, in one of the last letters he penned before his death from AIDS-related complications, Callen reflected, "Naïve poor Midwestern boy that I was, I thought this battle would be fought according to the rules of science. It came as quite a shock to discover that the true discourse of AIDS is theological. There are received truths; papal bulls (papal bullshit, more like it), and various sects and denominations who launch jihads against one another. It's an unholy holy war."[84]

In addition to believing that viral etiological theory wrapped religion in the garb of science, Callen worried that the public would use the theory to further stigmatize and disempower PWAs. He disagreed fiercely with the leaders of mainstream AIDS organizations who argued that a narrative centered upon a specific germ would diffuse some of the spotlight that had remained sharply focused on gay men's sexual practices. He maintained that viral narratives merely made matters worse by allowing conservatives to cast gay men as vectors threatening to infect mainstream America with their malady. Writing as early as 1985, he identified new expressions of discrimination enabled by the virological model, with parents in Queens, New York protesting the admission of children with AIDS into classrooms and small towns in America passing ordinances requiring antibody testing for food handlers. "As many gay activists are only now beginning to realize," he wrote, "we've painted ourselves into a very dangerous corner by our uncritical acceptance of the simplistic and *unproven* hypothesis that LAV[85] 'causes' AIDS."[86]

Callen's critique of the HIV etiological model flowed from his support of an alternative etiological theory first proposed by Joseph Sonnabend in 1983. The multifactorial theory viewed AIDS as the consequence of repeated infections with known sexually transmitted pathogens coupled with other environmental factors that, over time, wore down individuals' immune systems.[87] The theory was never popular among AIDS service organizations or protest groups such as ACT UP, almost certainly because its focus on the sexual and recreational practices of gay men bore too close a resemblance to the condemnations of the religious right.[88] The mainstream viral etiological model was, in many ways, more palatable, as Raymond Keith Brown argued in *AIDS, Cancer and the Medical Establishment*. "A single disease agent that just happened to have emerged within the gay community," Brown explained, "absolves its members from individual or collective responsibilities for containing or controlling the spread of AIDS."[89] Despite this, Callen maintained that the multifactorial theory was the only etiological model that explained reality, arguing that he had failed to meet a single PWA who refuted his belief that AIDS resulted from the constant barrage of infections over time.[90]

Sonnabend's multifactorial model was a product of its time, expressive of significant shifts in the public experience of disease through the early-to-mid twentieth century. As discussed in previous chapters, in the decades preceding AIDS, the developed world witnessed a fundamental shift in the overall burden of disease, with chronic conditions replacing infectious diseases as the primary cause of morbidity and mortality. During this time, professionals and the lay public alike came to interpret intransigent chronic diseases such as cancer through multifactorial models. Indeed, early in the AIDS pandemic, researchers and journalists appropriated cancer language to describe the new condition: early reports labeled AIDS a "gay cancer," a much-feared AIDS-defining condition was a form of skin cancer, the NCI coordinated a great deal of AIDS research, and Robert Gallo initially theorized that AIDS was the product of a cancer-causing virus.

Perhaps most importantly, for PWAs the chronic disease lens suggested that they could persevere with their condition.[91] Interestingly, most histories of AIDS activism fail to recognize the empowerment engendered by the chronic disease model. In their impressive 1992 volume *AIDS: The Making of a Chronic Disease,* Elizabeth Fee and Daniel Fox paint chronicity as a failure of sorts. As they argue, "[T]he idea that AIDS would become another killer chronic disease, like heart disease, cancer, and stroke, has been unpalatable because it adds to the already overwhelming financial and organizational problems of health policy."[92] Yet for PWAs, chronicity meant one thing: survival.

Callen offered at least two additional arguments in support of the empowering potential of the multifactorial theory. For one, he maintained that, by forcing PWAs to examine high-risk behaviors, the theory made it easier for communities to identify the structural roots of discrimination that had ultimately led gay men to seek out risky sexual interactions in the first place.[93] Perhaps most importantly, however, Callen believed the theory empowered PWAs directly by suggesting they could reverse the course of their disease by making real and lasting behavioral changes. In rejecting the notion that an unlucky sexual encounter could transmit a killer virus, the model replaced chance with agency, preserving a role for individual action in both preventing and treating the disease. Reflecting upon his support of the model in *Surviving AIDS,* he admitted, "Whether or not Joe's multifactorial theory of AIDS ultimately proves to be correct, discovering a different way of thinking about AIDS at such a crucial turning point in my life provided a framework for me to justify believing that I might survive my disease. It was a life raft that kept me afloat in a sea of doom and gloom."[94] Even Rob Schick, a *Newsline* columnist famously critical of Callen's positions, admitted, "We'd like to believe that AIDS is caused by Michael's proposed 'fane lane' urban lifestyle because we could change that lifestyle ourselves. As Michael himself points out, belief in HIV is disempowering."[95]

Thus, some maintained that the HIV model was disempowering because it provided few opportunities for PWAs to engage their condition and effect their own cures, a topic to which I shall return in the final section of this chapter. The multifactorial model, in contrast, allowed PWAs to explain their disease as the consequence of long-term behaviors and to derive power by accepting responsibility for making changes to those behaviors. In so doing, it inverted the aphorism that great power brings with it great responsibility. For Callen, the power requisite to survive AIDS came from owning one's body and one's past, a point he underscored in the closing of *Surviving AIDS*. "[T]he survivors I interviewed took responsibility for their own healing, and this expressed itself in a number of ways," he noted. "Many voiced strong opinions about the need to acknowledge some personal responsibility for life-style choices, both in terms of getting sick in the first place and in terms of getting well."[96]

In 1983, Callen and Richard Berkowitz, in collaboration with Joseph Sonnabend, published *How to Have Sex in an Epidemic: One Approach*, seeking to utilize the principles of gay liberation to respond to AIDS. In addition to critiquing the single virus etiological model, it advocated a transformation in intimacy in the gay community to include a role for love, affection, and responsibility. In Callen and Berkowitz's view, the promise of gay liberation had been undone by the development of markets and cultural institutions that commodified and commercialized sex.[97] This critique of institutions is reminiscent of Ivan Illich, and indeed Callen was no stranger to Illich's work.[98] Callen and Berkowitz also borrowed from feminist critiques, particularly those of Cindy Patton, in interrogating the systems and structures that undergirded the politics of sex and intimacy.[99] The work generated significant debate among members of the gay community who feared it would further stigmatize their members, despite Callen and Berkowitz's structural analyses and fervent support for sex-positivity.[100]

In Callen's championing of unorthodox etiological models, he invoked a resistance to dogmatism reminiscent of nineteenth and early-twentieth-century defenses of nontraditional healing movements.[101] As I shall argue, the advocates of unorthodox AIDS healing systems found a home in the *Newsline*, though Callen's own views on unverified healing systems were far more complex. Ultimately, however, the multifactorial model failed to generate traction among the biomedical community, with mainstream research organized about the viral etiological model.[102] Correspondingly, most pharmaceutical research through the 1980s and 1990s focused upon developing antiretroviral agents to target HIV. The first agent to receive FDA approval, AZT, generated profound enthusiasm and concern among many in the PWA community. It is to these concerns that I now turn.

Disputed Treatments: Curses, Cures, and the "Promiscuous Use" of AZT

In the previous sections, I identified ways in which individuals contributing to PWAC publications expressed positions rooted in anti-authoritarianism, antidogmatism, and antimodernism, three of the themes identified in chapter 1 as common to historic expressions of unorthodox health activism. By the late

1980s, with the approval of AZT, these publications began featuring arguments more clearly evocative of the fourth theme: antiheroism. PWAs invoked themes of antiheroism in two distinct ways, first by focusing on AZT's toxicities and further by more broadly critiquing biomedicine's narrow pursuit of magic bullets targeting HIV.

Granted expedited review and FDA approval in 1987, AZT stoked remarkable controversy in the pages of the *Newsline* and the second volume of *Surviving and Thriving with AIDS*. Much of it centered upon the drug's toxicity and the fact that the NIH had ended the AZT clinical trial early after initial results suggested that it prolonged the lives of PWAs.[103] As early as 1986, a *Newsline* article planted seeds of doubt in discussions of the drug, warning readers that little was known about its toxicity beyond the two-week mark.[104] By 1987 and 1988, the tenor of criticism increased, with PWAC cofounder Paul Lande declaring it "morally negligent, if not criminally negligent, to push AZT without carefully explaining how little is known about it."[105] Meanwhile, *Newsline* editor Max Navarre bemoaned what he termed the "medical love affair with AZT," which led physicians to prescribe it even to those with few symptoms of AIDS.[106] Navarre linked his fears of the drug's toxicities with the historic marginalization of gay people. As he argued, the rush of PWAs to take potentially dangerous drugs such as AZT "sounds to me like more dyed-in-the-wool, gay community lack of self esteem: we don't count, so why not throw ourselves to the wolves? Why not sacrifice ourselves on the altar of 'progress.'"[107]

As early as 1986, several *Newsline* contributors had begun to air concerns with AZT's side effects. In fact, in the same article that announced the initial AZT clinical trial results, the editorial issued a warning: "Anecdotal reports of serious side effects—particularly bone marrow suppression—abound. The Coalition knows of several individuals who had to drop out of the trials due to side effect."[108] The drug's early history as an experimental anticancer agent, coupled with the fact that it inhibited DNA synthesis, did little to bolster its reputation among skeptical PWAs and their advocates. In 1989, Joseph Sonnabend declared the drug "incompatible with life."[109] However, it was Callen who would launch the most sustained critique of what he termed society's "promiscuous use of AZT."[110] In article after article, he indicted and imprecated the drug, referring to it as "Drano in pill form,"[111] and arguing that prescribing it to combat AIDS was like "swatting a fly with a thermonuclear warhead."[112] So vociferous was he that his detractors would, in fact, take to calling him an "AZT terrorist."[113]

To support his claims, Callen turned to the interviews he had conducted with long-term PWAs, arguing that the overwhelming majority of those who had beaten the odds to survive for longer than three years refused to take AZT.[114] He noted, for example, that well-known PWA John Lorenzini refused to take the drug and quoted a second PWA, A. J. Roosevelt Williams, who argued, "You can't cure anyone with a poison, and AZT is obviously a poison."[115] Many of these contributors pursued regimens of self-care featuring alternative therapeutic components—a topic I will explore in greater detail in the final unit of this chapter. Williams, for example, rejected the antiretroviral agent in favor of mainstream drugs such as sulfamethoxazole/trimethoprim (Bactrim) and aerosolized pentamidine (NebuPent), alongside nontraditional healing approaches including garlic pills, germanium, food grade hydrogen peroxide, egg lipids, and visualization.[116] Interviews such as these informed Callen's 1991 volume *Surviving AIDS* and generated controversy with the book's publisher. As Martin Duberman has described, HarperCollins begged Callen to exclude a chapter titled "The Case against AZT" from the final manuscript. Ever allergic to censorship, he refused their request.[117]

Concerns with AZT's toxicities were closely linked with trepidations regarding the methods and motives of pharmaceutical corporations. In 1987, former PWAC Executive Director Michael Hirsch penned a letter to Burroughs Wellcome, the manufacturer of AZT, requesting information regarding the drug's clinical trials. The pharmaceutical giant replied with a letter so nakedly paternalistic that an exasperated Hirsch submitted it for publication in the *Newsline*. "[I]t can be difficult, and in some cases ill-advised, to provide complex scientific information directly to the news media or the general public," the letter argued. "As a pharmaceutical company, we feel it is very important to preserve the integrity of the patient-physician relationship. This relationship is a critical one and a very important way for patients to get answers about their individual condition and experiences."[118] The response underscores the chasm dividing pharma's conceptualization of benevolent expertise and the PWA empowerment movement's celebration of radical engagement. Sonnabend would rail against such casual disempowerment of PWAs. "There is nothing worse than treating people like cattle," the community physician argued, "giving something which is presented with conviction only for the purposes of maintaining order or lack of confusion."[119]

For some PWAs, the biomedical fascination with AZT stemmed from a mainstream professional culture that had come to glorify the search for cures and, in the process, lost sight of the actual needs of PWAs. Callen, for example, argued that the biomedical research apparatus had become fixated on the "Nobel-prize winning prospect of curing" as opposed to engaging in the "unglamorous, labor intensive task of KEEPING PEOPLE ALIVE."[120] *Newsline* Editor Bree Scott-Hartland echoed similar sentiments in a 1992 interview wherein he rejected Paul Ehrlich's well-worn metaphor describing clinical therapeutics. "People are screaming for a magic bullet," Scott-Hartland lamented. "Their energy would be better spent learning to live with the disease. We don't all die within six months. There are people who have lived with AIDS for ten years and are still thriving."[121] In fact, for PWAs who were dying of unglamorous opportunistic infections, the word "cure" had become a curse. This point is underscored by a 1989 *Newsline* article penned by a representative of Boston's AIDS Watchdog Group. "While the old-boy researchers at Harvard play Star Wars with pie-in-the-sky antiviral strategies, people are dying from infections that need not kill them," its author argued. "'Looking for a cure' is a phrase that has little meaning in the here and now . . . 'Cure' is a useless word; in fact, it's a deadly word."[122]

Thus, the debate among PWAs regarding AZT was about much more than a single drug. In their critique of pharmaceutical corporations' practices, we find expressions of anti-authoritarianism and antidogmatism, particularly among authors who critiqued AZT out of a belief that research had not sufficiently demonstrated the HIV-AIDS relationship. Most noticeably, we recognize expressions of antiheroism centered upon the known and unknown toxicities of AZT, coupled with the fear that the search for cures was costing PWAs their lives. The problem, in short, was not just about AZT—it was about a mind frame that would soon echo through the streets of Greenwich Village: "Drugs into bodies." Callen deplored the term and deemed it the product of "the conveyer-belt conceptualization of AIDS" which held that because AIDS was universally fatal, any experimental drug was worth taking.[123] Thus, while in the mid-twentieth century critics alleged that clinical care was becoming defined by assembly-line efficiency, here we see an extension of the metaphor into the very conceptualization of disease.

Appeals to antiheroism provoked diverse responses in the *Newsline*. Callen, for example, used his critiques of AZT to encourage PWAs to engage in their own explorations of less toxic drugs and agents, both conventional and alternative.[124] Others, however, expressed even more radical positions. The *New York Native* reporter John Lauritsen, who coauthored a 1986 text explicating a multifactorial, toxin-based etiological model for AIDS,[125] argued in a September 1989 *Newsline* article that the only solution to AIDS was in foreswearing the use of all drugs, recreational and medicinal, in favor of a "healthy lifestyle."[126]

AZT provoked impassioned debate in the *Newsline*. In its January 1990 volume, for example, readers encountered an anti-AZT article followed immediately by a pro-AZT article, which was rebuffed by an anti-AZT article, only to be countered by another pro-AZT article.[127] It was, in no small part, a consequence of Callen's critiques of mainstream biomedical practices, coupled with his ardent support for PWAs' open contestation of received truths, that the *Newsline* would continue to air critiques of AZT years after the drug's approval. In fact, articles contesting the drug continued to appear even after he left the publication in September of 1989.

When a 1993 study questioned the efficacy of early AZT dosage regimens, Callen felt that his half-decade long activism had been vindicated. Yet in reflecting upon his years at PWAC, he expressed reservation with some of the principles he had espoused. In his support for PWA empowerment and his critique of authoritarianism, he worried that he had helped engender the very "drugs into bodies" activism he loathed. He feared, for example, that his "rabid anti-expertism" had allowed a small group of non-experts at ACT UP's Treatment and Data Committee to successfully advocate for the early approval of AZT.[128] Though Callen's later reflections do not change the history of the unorthodox AIDS movement he helped inspire, they are a fascinating coda to his activism. They furthermore call to mind another supporter of self-empowerment who would, at the end of his life, express misgivings about the effects of his activism: Ivan Illich.

In sum, the *Newsline* and *Surviving and Thriving with AIDS* volumes were safe harbors wherein PWAs could engage their condition on their own terms, sharing questions, theories, hopes, fears, strategies, ideas, and practices for defining and responding to their disease. Moreover, they were lively, contentious publications airing impassioned perspectives of contributors committed to questioning the practices, principles, and pronouncements of mainstream biomedical professionals. Much of this was the result of Callen's commitment to publishing diverse content, even that with which he disagreed.

For Jane Rosett—unique among PWAC cofounders in that she was the only woman and the only person who did not have AIDS—Callen's vigorous defense of editorial diversity was, in fact, the only factor that cohered the group. Early on, she had wondered whether the PWAC was indeed a true coalition, because it was founded almost entirely by gay White men who met weekly in the city's Gay and Lesbian Community Center. "[I]f, as a publication we are a coalition," Rosett observed, "it is all thanks to Michael Callen's commitment to create and maintain varied editorial content."[129]

Thus, despite being fairly homogenous in its leaders' identities, the PWAC expressed a wide array of perspectives and opinions. Among the topics that elicited the most impassioned debates were the four considered in this unit. They constituted loci of resistance around which individuals organized their own responses to the epidemic, rejecting the efforts by others to order their bodies. Through their engagement with these issues, PWAs expressed positions and opinions that invoked themes of resistance that have long attended alternative and nontraditional health activism, including anti-authoritarianism, antidogmatism, antimodernism, and antiheroism. They, in turn, established a forum conducive to PWAs' direct embrace of alternative and nontraditional healing systems. In the final section of this chapter, I turn my attention to these direct points of intersection, examining the healing practices and traditions whose tenets found expression on the pages of PWAC publications.

EMBRACING UNORTHODOXIES: PWAC CONTRIBUTORS' EMBRACE OF ALTERNATIVE HEALTH SYSTEMS

Both *Surviving and Thriving with AIDS* and the *Newsline* regularly featured columns, letters, and advertisements embracing a wide array of alternative health modalities, ranging from herbalism and homeopathy to macrobiotics, chiropractic medicine, acupuncture, yoga, biofeedback, Ayurvedic medicine, orthomolecular medicine, crystal curatives, and attitudinal healing. The very first edition of the *Newsline*, in fact, featured an article titled "Acupuncture as an Alternative" wherein PWAC cofounder David Summers explored the benefits of Chinese medicine while criticizing organizations such as GMHC for neglecting nontraditional healing systems.[130] Similar articles appeared through the close of the first decade of the epidemic, seemingly unfazed by advances in biomedical research and drug development. Indeed, if anything, PWA engagement with nontraditional healing systems increased in frequency and intensity following AZT's approval. This trend distinguishes the history of unorthodox AIDS activism from earlier alternative health movements such as homeopathy, which declined in influence following the development of antibiotics.[131]

A cursory review of the unorthodox healing modalities advocated in the pages of PWAC publications underscores many areas of overlap and synergy. For example, the advocates of guided visualization, yoga, hypnosis, biofeedback, and the teachings of Louise Hay shared concerns with the fatalistic narratives Callen railed against. One proponent of such systems, writing in a 1986 *Newsline* column, expressed concern with the "conspiracy of hopelessness" surrounding AIDS, facilitated by victim narratives promulgated by mainstream researchers and the popular press.[132] Similarly, in the second volume of *Surviving and Thriving with AIDS*, self-hypnosis instructor Gail Spindell argued, "If you imagine yourself with three months to live, how does that help? Instead, imagine yourself well. There is a blurry line between fantasy and reality . . . the body and the mind make little distinction between the real and the imagined."[133] Many authors writing in support of nontraditional health modalities would, furthermore, invoke antimodern and antiheroic arguments, eschewing pharmaceutical agents in favor of herbal and nutritional strategies they deemed more natural.[134]

However, perhaps the single most important link uniting diverse alternative health systems was their shared view of orthodox biomedicine as rigidly reductionist and dogmatic. The supporters of the alternative health system articulated a robust critique of the killer virus etiological model, and sometimes the germ theory writ large, painting both as simplistic and outmoded. In one 1989 *Newsline* column, for example, Tom Herman extolled the virtues of homeopathy while lambasting biomedicine's reliance on the germ theory of disease. "To a homeopath," Herman observed, "to say a sore throat is caused by a streptococcus germ is like saying that a murder is caused by a bullet—true in a way, but the most important part is left out. Our modern obsession with 'causative' agents may be the legacy of the so-called Pasteurian model of disease."[135] This tactic of acknowledging germ theory's legitimacy while denigrating it as one-dimensional has roots in the early twentieth century, when the supporters of irregular medical sects recognized that they could no longer paint germ theory as wholly fallacious.[136] These individuals, like those writing in the *Newsline* three generations later, argued that their chosen health systems enriched a germ theory-based clinical model by identifying and treating other dimensions of health and disease. Similarly, those writing in the 1980s and early 1990s would expand upon Sonnabend's multifactorial model, arguing that AIDS resulted from irreducibly complex interrelationships between stressors spanning environmental, behavioral, interpersonal, emotional, and spiritual domains.[137]

In short, contributors advocated models of health and disease that were holistic in design.[138] Consider, for example, Alex Idavoy's 1992 *Newsline* piece, "Holistics 101: An Alternative Beginning." In it, he dismisses mainstream biomedicine for relying upon reductionist pathological models and toxic cures and, instead, posits health holism as an enlightened etiological and therapeutic paradigm. "Since holistic medicine holds that the physical, emotional and spiritual are interconnected, there could be a myriad of explanations [for AIDS]," he writes. Included among these explanations were "chronic malnutrition, long-term abuse of over-the-counter as well as illegal drugs and alcohol, long-term exposure to environmental toxins, sexually transmitted diseases, exposure to immune-suppressive vaccines, even unresolved psychological trauma and/or long-term locked up emotions."[139] In his framing of AIDS, we register echoes of both Sonnabend's and Lauritsen's multifactorial models, augmented by psychological and emotional sources of illness. This holistic multifactoriality is particularly interesting when we recognize that it appeared ten years after Sonnabend introduced his multifactorial model, during a period in which two antiretrovirals, AZT and didanosine (ddI; Videx) had already secured FDA approval and a third, zalcitabine (ddC; Hivid) was looming on the horizon.

Readers may profess exasperation with Idavoy's conceptualization of health holism, for he lists a vast array of stressors underlying AIDS while making little effort to reconcile them into a unifying conception of etiology or pathology. For these readers, health holism may appear less panacea than pastiche, failing to offer a logical or coherent plan for responding to disease. However, such a reading misinterprets the goal of the holistic health construct. Many PWAC contributors treated holism not as a remedy for AIDS, but as an antidote for a broken biomedical system that had become too dogmatic and reductionist to adequately address their experiences. Consequently, the same features that befuddle and bewilder modern audiences in fact differentiated holism from the mainstream system it sought to undermine. Its expansive explication of nebulously interacting variables defied reduction, while its openness to near constant emendation by individuals positing ever more physical, emotional, or spiritual causes for AIDS protected it from allegations of dogmatism. It was, thus, a broadly philosophical rejoinder that capitalized on the uncertainties and ambiguities of AIDS, coupled with the distrust and disenchantment of those who questioned the wisdom of mainstream biomedical responses. The model was extraordinarily powerful, particularly because those who invoked it seldom incurred any real obligation to defend its many constituent healing systems. Instead, they merely carved out a subset of variables and elected their chosen alternative healing system—homeopathy, macrobiotics, attitudinal healing, and so on—in an effort to act upon these variables.

Health holism was, thus, a vessel of sorts, grouping alternative health practices bound by their distrust for the mainstream biomedical model. The term was sufficiently loose and open ended that authors could invoke it to refer to all manners of healing practices. Alan Burns, for example, construed holistic healthcare as including macrobiotics, vitamin therapy, herbology, Reiki, and the visualization therapies of Louise Hay and the AIDS Mastery;[140] Michael Hirsch used the term to refer to Reiki, Transcendental Meditation, and yoga;[141] Bob Lederer used it in conjunction with acupuncture, herbalism, nutritional supplements, and spiritual healing;[142] Peter Dvarackas invoked it while discussing Chinese medicine and acupuncture;[143] and Alex Idavoy argued that it subsumed homeopathic, Ayurvedic, traditional Chinese, and orthomolecular healing systems.[144]

In voicing their support for holistic health practices, these PWAC contributors echoed the organization's underlying mission, suggesting that PWAs were capable of self-organizing to challenge the dictates of a hegemonic biomedical orthodoxy, claiming ownership over their disease and responsibility for their healing.[145] Some supporters of alternative healing systems painted this reclamation of responsibility in a moral light, as when an executive director of the PWAC penned a *Newsline* letter defending the practitioners of one alternative healing system by arguing that they were "working hard at taking responsibility for their own well-being and quality of life."[146] Here, one recognizes the links between causal and moral responsibility of disease. Further, three months after publishing the letter, the *Newsline's* editorial staff renamed its monthly alternative health column "Holistic Approaches," arguing that the title conveyed a sense of PWA self-empowerment. In their announcement, they quoted the Holistic Medical Association's definition of holistic medicine as "a system of medical care which emphasizes personal responsibility, and fosters a cooperative relationship among all those involved, leading towards optimal attunement of body, mind, emotions and spirit."[147] Of note, this framing of holistic medicine as an avenue for personal responsibility and empowerment contrasts with common presentations of holistic healers as quacks preying on impressionable patients.[148]

While it is beyond the scope of this analysis to review the many alternative health movements PWAs embraced through the 1980s and 1990s, one in particular warrants mention. Referred to by PWAC leader Michael Hirsch as "the most popular and most simple holistic approach used by PWAs/PWArcs,"[149] it was epitomized by visualization and attitudinal health methodologies promoted by Louise Hay and AIDS support service Northern Lights Alternatives. The attitudinal health movement, inspired by the late 1970s to early 1980s volumes *Getting Well Again* and *Love, Medicine and Miracles,* suggested to PWAs that they could use their minds to influence their course of illness.[150] Hay, for example, argued that PWAs could secure their health by acknowledging and rejecting feelings of self-loathing and internalized rejection, while the Northern Lights Alternatives AIDS Mastery workshop taught participants to "find inner peace and come to understand the meaning of their lives" as a step in effecting their own cures.[151] The systems were far more radical than benign entreaties to optimism, for they argued that one could harness his or her mind—through, for example, visualization exercises—to influence the disease process.

Perhaps more than any other alternative healing system, attitudinal health modalities embodied a radical allegiance to the view that PWAs possessed the innate capacity to heal themselves. In one 1987 *Newsline* column, PWA Steven James summarized what he referred to as the "personal power" PWAs derived from visualization, arguing of his own treatment regimen that, "There was a satisfaction in knowing that I was using my *own* willpower to do something to further my own health."[152] Others focused on the attitudinal health movement's ability to develop within PWAs a capacity for self-control—a fascinating concept that further links notions of empowerment and morality.[153] Some authors also linked visualization practices with forgiveness, such as PWA Michael Hirsch who argued that visualization exercises "advocate that one take more control over one's life, that one re-examine one's self-image and attitudes about one's world, and that one forgive oneself and others for the past."[154]

The attitudinal health movement purported to help PWAs wrest control over the conceptualization of and response to their disease from a biomedical orthodoxy viewed as fatalistic, dogmatic, and heroic. It also provoked ardent debate among PWAC contributors, with some (including Callen) deriding leaders such as Louise Hay as charlatans and others praising them for empowering individuals to assume a direct role in their own healing.[155] Despite such critiques, many PWAs, including Callen, incorporated elements of attitudinal healing into their syncretic healing approaches.[156] In many cases, attitudinal healing systems endorsed such syncretism. The AIDS Mastery, for example, taught PWAs that visualization and meditation could help them better understand which complement of healing strategies would work best for them.[157] Even Louis Nassaney, an ardent proponent of Hay's methodology, revealed to Callen that he combined attitudinal health modalities with other unorthodox and orthodox healing systems.[158]

Thus, PWAs' approaches to conceiving of and responding to their health needs were complex and defied rigid categorization. This was the case for Callen, who called himself "rabidly [and] rigidly rational" and critiqued Hay's Church of Religious Science on several grounds, including his fear that it suggested PWAs who died had failed to embrace the right attitude. Yet he also tried her healing system, finding some value in its conceptualization of a "bi-directional mind-body connection." In many ways, he practiced the sort of impassioned open-mindedness he demanded from biomedicine: Someone who believed strongly in an idea but was open, through new experiences, to amending those ideas. Perhaps most importantly, he maintained an open editorial policy, publishing pieces—be they about AZT or attitudinal healing—whose claims he found questionable.

This underscores a point of great importance to understanding unorthodox AIDS activism: it was not the product of any one person's philosophy. I have invoked Callen's perspective many times in this chapter due to his role in cofounding the PWAC and editing group publications. Scholars also benefit from the fact that his archives have been preserved and reflections of his life rendered by those who knew him and his activism. However, Callen was by no means the most ardent proponent of alternative medicine; indeed, though he noted that he used several alternative strategies, he also strongly critiqued many holistic perspectives. That he was viewed as radical—and his contributions considered here as unorthodox—is more a testament to the biomedical system's resistance to his critiques than it was to his wish that biomedicine be burned to the ground. At times, he expressed views that were paradigmatic of unorthodox health activism. At others, he demonstrated an allegiance to scientific empiricism, a critique of alternative medicines, and a concern with anti-expertism. Perhaps most importantly, he nurtured unorthodox AIDS activism through his words and actions, helping to form the soil out of which it grew.[159]

Though PWAs disagreed with one another about the particular etiological and therapeutic models they endorsed in their engagement with AIDS, most likely would have agreed that no single model held all the answers. In the first volume of *Surviving and Thriving with AIDS*, Steven James reports utilizing unorthodox healing strategies to modulate his use of mainstream medications. As he explains, "I have used alternative methods such as Applied Kinesiology, or muscle-testing to determine the precise dosage of Bactrim [a mainstream antibiotic] which seems to be optimal for my body. I also take herbs and vitamins, and I follow a diet low in red meat, white flour, and sugars."[160] Many of the PWAs Callen interviewed for *Surviving AIDS* also reported pursuing hybrid approaches, with one swearing by Bactrim and macrobiotics,[161] another by egg lipids and AZT,[162] and Callen himself by high dose acyclovir, Itraconazole, egg lipids, and homeopathic doses of naltrexone.[163] Furthermore, in a 1988 *Newsline* article titled "My Doctor and My Chiropractor," PWA Larry Peck discusses his use of conventional therapies administered by his physician combined with alternative therapies—including body manipulation, kinesiology, herbal-flower remedies, homeopathic treatments, and natural nutritional supplements—prescribed by his chiropractor. Interestingly, while Peck credits his mainstream physician with helping him overcome an early bout of PCP, he portrays the orthodox therapeutic model's focus on fatal viruses as inherently disempowering compared with unorthodox approaches that identify a curative role for personal intervention.[164]

While this chapter has focused on how PWAC publications helped PWAs to pursue individualized, syncretic approaches to bolstering their health, I would be remiss if I did not mention several of the other initiatives organized by the group's leaders. In the late 1980s, for example, they would form the PWA Health Group, an independent organization committed to helping PWAs gain access to experimental treatments for AIDS.[165] "We do not speak of drugs," the group's Statement of Purpose read. "[W]e consider our products to be food substances and/or vitamins and enzymes . . . As frustrating as it sometimes seems, we never talk about dosages; we talk, instead, about recommended servings."[166] Among the substances discussed and distributed by the group were AL-721, an egg lipid mixture and dextran sulfate (Gentran, LMD), a polysaccharide that group leaders avowed was "a food, like broccoli or eggs."[167]

PWAC leaders also would work to establish the Community Research Initiative (CRI) to "act as the administrative coordinator of experimental drug trials."[168] The group was inspired by a critique of biomedical bureaucracy institutions and, for some, a desire to invest more funds and attention in treatment strategies, including alternative avenues, that they felt biomedicine was ignoring. Though the group would not make any breakthrough discoveries that changed the course of the pandemic, in its very incorporation it demonstrated the commitment of individuals seeking to wrest control over their lives from a biomedical bureaucracy they deemed negligent, if not inimical to their health.

For a relatively homogenous organization, the PWAC thus included a dizzying diversity of unorthodoxy. Some PWAs chose to invest their energy in avowedly holistic health models while others sought to create new systems that harnessed the scientific process in ways they felt biomedicine had failed to accomplish. Most importantly, many did both, demonstrating not only migration within the borderlands of healing systems but within the borderlands of unorthodoxy itself. These different expressions of resistance were not identical, but they shared a common roof—indeed, sometimes literally: among the subtenants the PWA Health Group considered for its offices were Northern Lights Alternatives, an initiative that embraced visualizations and spiritual responses to AIDS.[169]

The PWAC offers one lens through which we may understand unorthodox AIDS activism. However, as I have noted, we must recognize that the conclusions we may draw are limited by the group's membership. As longtime member Jane Rosette commented when describing the PWAC, "[C]oalition is quite a broad term to use to describe this predominantly gay white group."[170] Callen, too, would recognize the limits of their coalition, lamenting the underrepresentation of people of color in PWAC publications.[171]

In 1989, Callen resigned from the PWAC. In his letter of resignation, he reflected upon all that he had hoped, but failed, to achieve. He also expressed frustration with changes in the organization and its establishment of new bureaucracies that he felt failed to appreciate the diversity of perspective and experience he had brought to the PWA movement. Thus, once more we identify the complex ways in which grassroots anti-authoritarianism can give rise to bureaucracies that perpetuate dominant power structures. Yet Callen closed his tenure with a characteristic note of empowerment: "I'm a bit bruised, but I'll survive . . ."[172]

CONCLUSION: QUACKS, DUPES, AND PWA EMPOWERMENT

The PWAC's activism was neither the loudest nor the most visible form of protest organized in the 1980s and 1990s in response to AIDS. Rather than taking to the streets to demand changes in the federal research response, it sought to empower PWAs by encouraging them to claim ownership over their bodies and responsibility for their conditions. Through its print publications and allied initiatives, it fostered radical engagement among its members, fomenting deep distrust and disillusionment with the systems tasked with responding to the growing pandemic. In pursuing its aims, it cultivated a multilayered discourse that invoked and intersected many of the same themes that have historically subtended alternative health activist movements throughout U.S. history.

In addition to capturing links between PWA protest and historic expressions of alternative and nontraditional health activism, this analysis challenges commonly held perceptions regarding the workings of power within communities facing deadly diseases. For one, as noted above, it contests a persistent scholarly bias which summarily dismisses the practitioners of alternative therapeutic modalities as dupes. While it is certainly true that some of the advocates of nontraditional healing systems engaged in chicanery, there is no reason to suggest that their presence somehow negates the willful actions of individuals who eschewed orthodox biomedical practice. The "quack" and the "dupe" are tropes that, by their very nature, deny the possibility of empowerment for those who look beyond orthodox biomedicine for treatment. My analysis of PWAC activism suggests that many individuals who turned to alternative healing traditions through the 1980s and 1990s did so out of an avowed belief that these nontraditional systems were more empowering than orthodox biomedicine. Just as they refused to be construed by physicians and researchers as disempowered patients, they would, no doubt, reject historical framings painting them as victims of quackery.

My analysis furthermore suggests that, far from pledging allegiance to a particular bounded system of therapeutic practice, PWAs frequently moved between systems to craft responses that resonated most with their experiences and beliefs. Health holism facilitated this movement, as it grouped seemingly incompatible healing systems under a common rubric. Consequently, the history of AIDS-era engagement with alternative health modalities diverges from older historical framings focused on sectarian medical battles between bounded systems of healing. It demonstrates that, as scholars continue to examine alternative and unorthodox health activist movements, we should focus not on the philosophies that delineated thought systems but on the messy and muddled movement of individuals who passed between their permeable borders.

This chapter focuses primarily on written publications appearing between 1985 and 1993, because this was the zenith of PWAC activism. Beginning in the early 1990s, the PWAC endured financial difficulties owing to a decrease in contributions and increase in real estate prices in Chelsea. The group declared bankruptcy in 1993 and officially closed, only to be revived later under a different name. By the mid–1990s, much had changed in mainstream PWA care, with physicians and researchers generally acknowledging the missteps taken with AZT's early use. New classes of biomedical therapeutics—most importantly protease inhibitors, first introduced in 1995—drastically improved the lives of PWAs while avoiding the toxicities of high-dose AZT. It is difficult to assess the persistence of everyday expressions of activism or the importance of the borderland model of action during these years. However, I anticipate that future historians will find that, even in eras of biomedical triumph, individuals find ways to loose themselves from the moorings of orthodoxy and explore the borderlands between healing systems. In short, they will find that, in times of triumph and tribulation, people find ways to live furiously.

5 ▸ PATIENT, HEAL THYSELF

The History of Health Education AIDS Liaison (HEAL)

In the previous chapter, I examined the history of the People with AIDS Coalition (PWAC), chronicling its members' endorsement of unorthodox etiological and therapeutic paradigms for describing and responding to the AIDS epidemic. Inspired by the activism of leaders such as Michael Callen, the group questioned mainstream biomedical practice, arguing that PWA survival was predicated upon individuals' willingness to directly engage their disease. I also discussed the tendency for some scholars to elide from the historical record the group's most unorthodox, alternative, and radical activism, thus recapitulating uncontroversial formulations of the patient empowerment movement. This historiographic abridgement is most evident in recreations of the Denver Principles that omit references to unorthodox resistance and in scholarly discussions of Callen's activism that excise his more contrarian beliefs.

While this scholarly treatment of AIDS activism has resulted in a myopic picture of the PWAC, it has virtually blinded students of history to the initiatives of a second health activist group founded in the earliest days of the AIDS epidemic. Forged in the same crucible that gave birth to the Gay Men's Health Crisis (GMHC) and PWAC, Health Education AIDS Liaison (HEAL) pursued a much more open, avowed embrace of nontraditional health modalities, with its literature extolling "alternative, complementary, non-toxic, natural and holistic approaches to living with AIDS and staying healthy if at risk."[1] One of the earliest AIDS support groups of any kind organized in the city, HEAL predated ACT UP—which scholars have studied extensively—by five years. What's more, it would remain active for two decades, with its mission and reputation undergoing transformation as its leaders pursued an increasingly unorthodox activist agenda.

Given its remarkable history, one might expect HEAL to have earned a place within the late twentieth and early twenty-first-centuries' body of historical and sociological AIDS scholarship. Yet by nearly every measure, its story remains obscured, appearing today as little more than an anomalous aside or fringe curiosity relegated to the footnotes of scholarly works. On the rare occasion when one comes across reference to the group in the index of a scholarly piece, it generally points him or her to a slim paragraph listing HEAL as one of several early AIDS groups.[2] Others dismiss the grassroots organization as an exponent of a radically dissident fringe inspired by the perspectives of rogue retrovirologist Peter Duesberg.[3]

This chapter seeks to redress this dearth in scholarship, exhuming HEAL's history so that we may add its unique voice to the record of AIDS activism. Exhumation is indeed an apt descriptor for the methods brought to bear in my research process. For no central repository houses the group's collected ephemera. A grassroots organization through and through, by the early 2000s its leaders had consigned surviving group documents to whichever members' apartments could house them. My research took me far from the august archives of major academic institutions and into the dusty closets of East Harlem apartments and bedraggled berths of Long Island garages, where boxes of HEAL literature sat, in many cases untouched for the better part of a decade.

It is my hope that in analyzing the group's newsletters, news clippings and correspondence, the reader may share in the excitement I experienced upon first sifting through this forgotten archive. Yet a word of caution is warranted, for raw archives pose unique historiographic challenges affecting historians' ability to reconstruct the past. While I was fortunate to review thousands of pages of documents, countless pieces of correspondence and literature have, no doubt, been lost to time. Furthermore, many surviving documents lack authors or dates, often necessitating an approximation of their origins. In general, the group's later initiatives enjoy greater representation within the archive, likely a consequence of HEAL's increased focus on print publications post-1990 and the fact that those individuals who eventually housed the archives came into leadership positions at roughly this time. To redress gaps in the print archive, I have conducted supplementary oral history interviews with former group leader Michael Ellner,[4] and have additionally consulted independent interviews compiled as part of the New York Lesbian and Gay Experimental Film Festival's *ACT UP Oral History Project*.[5]

As I shall argue, the transformations witnessed in HEAL's membership and mission through the 1980s, 1990s, and 2000s reveal a dynamic organization in a near constant state of flux. From its earliest years, members explored and advocated a wide array of alternative health paradigms, ranging from macrobiotics and herbalism to chiropractic and positive psychology. Interestingly, despite its unorthodox philosophy and members' willingness to openly question the pronouncements of biomedical professionals, through the early 1990s, the group enjoyed the respect of the city's larger AIDS service organizations. Yet by the mid-1990s, the winds had changed. The same group once lauded as a nontraditional resource for individuals seeking to engage their disease on their own terms had become derided as a dissident organization spreading dangerous misinformation. In the first section of this chapter, I review HEAL's early history as an alternative and complementary health activist group, demonstrating its synergistic relations with more mainstream AIDS support groups. I then juxtapose this early history with the group's eventual embrace of contrarian and dissident perspectives, arguing that HEAL's turn toward dissidence resulted, in part, from the radicalization of two holistic health principles underlying its alternative health activism.

THE CONSONANT CONTRARIANS: HEAL'S EARLY YEARS

A quintessentially grassroots organization, HEAL's early history is the stuff of historical lore. Cofounded by a prominent gay rights activist just two weeks after GMHC opened its doors, HEAL was among the first groups to meet in New York's newly inaugurated Lesbian and Gay Community Center. Operating on the thinnest of budgets, it initially assembled weekly in one of the center's broken-down bathrooms, the toilets of which had been removed from the walls to create a makeshift discussion space.[6] Here, HEAL created a safe space wherein members—by and large gay men—could discuss alternative and unorthodox responses to the strange new disease that had racked their community. The group's earliest meeting space captures its relationship with the larger AIDS activist community—proponents of contrarian holistic health philosophies, HEAL members embraced a model of patient engagement that resonated with the larger PWA empowerment movement. Thus, they enjoyed a place—albeit one somewhat out of sight—in the larger network of AIDS service providers.

While HEAL would become known for its embrace of heath holism, its founding had less to do with promoting holistic health paradigms than it did with more broadly nurturing individuals' hope in their capacity to survive their condition. As noted in chapter 4, the earliest days of the AIDS epidemic were fraught with anxiety, uncertainty, and fear. As one longtime HEAL president would note, the period signified nothing less than the "Dark Ages" of gay society.[7] It was into this crucible that gay novelist Larry Kramer injected his famous

New York Native articles alerting gay men to the crisis that had arrived at their doorsteps. Intentionally incendiary, Kramer sounded a death knell that would reverberate throughout the gay community. "If this article doesn't scare the shit out of you, we're in real trouble," he wrote in March of 1983. "If this article doesn't rouse you to anger, fury, rage, and action, gay men may have no future on this earth. Our continued existence depends on just how angry you can get."[8]

For Jim Fouratt, a well-known gay rights activist who had served as an active member of the Gay Liberation Front (GLF) and participant in the Stonewall Riots, this type of fatalistic hyperbole exacted a toll. In his estimation, liberal media outlets had, in their efforts to cultivate a politically propitious fury amongst gay audiences, written off individuals diagnosed with AIDS as fated to die. "This was at the height of the AIDS hysteria," Fouratt later reflected. "Even the gay newspapers, all they could talk about was death, death, death. And I remember thinking it was just an awful environment in which to be diagnosed and in which to be concerned about being sick because it was so negative."[9] The situation was far worse amongst conservative media outlets, many of which had literally adopted apocalyptic language to argue that AIDS was the equivalent of a modern-day biblical plague.[10]

In 1982, less than a month after Kramer cofounded GMHC, Fouratt organized his own support group with a decidedly different focus. Originally named Wipe Out AIDS (WOA), the group strove to shift the tone and tenor—or "emotional habitus" of AIDS activism—from one of despair to one of hope.[11] Shortly after its inception, WOA changed its name to Health Education AIDS Liaison (HEAL), which more directly communicated its mission of engendering self-empowerment.[12] In its early years, it adopted holistic health paradigms as tools for helping PWAs claim ownership over their disease, turning first to the macrobiotic diet popularized by Michio Kushi in the 1970s and 1980s. Within their first year, HEAL leaders broadened their focus, using weekly meetings and print publications to introduce PWAs to homeopathy, Reiki, chiropractic, herbalism, acupuncture, attitudinal healing, and countless other unorthodox health systems.[13] Rather than emphasize any one healing paradigm, discussion coordinators tasked themselves with providing avenues and approaches whereby PWAs could directly engage their condition on their own terms, nurturing a hope that they could survive their diagnosis. Group facilitators made clear that they possessed no panaceas and promised only health-affirming strategies for individuals seeking to "stave off the specter of death" by focusing on strategies for healthful living.[14]

Given the fraught relations between mainstream biomedicine and unorthodox health movements through the twentieth century, readers may be surprised to learn that many mainstream AIDS activists viewed HEAL's early work as uncontroversial. Yet through the mid-to-late 1980s, orthodox biomedicine remained largely impotent against AIDS. In this setting, orthodox gatekeepers lacked sufficient social or political capital to decry alternative remedies as quackery. As one later HEAL leader would remark of the early 1980s, "No one had anything, so nobody objected."[15] Furthermore, HEAL literature went to great pains to make clear that unorthodox health interventions were best viewed as complementary to mainstream medical therapeutics. One early informational packet counseled its readers, "If you have any one of the 29 diseases which are included in the Acquired Immune Deficiency Syndrome, HEAL advises that you follow the best procedure to treat it, which may well include prescription drugs . . . Once your prescription medicine has done the job, HEAL can supply suggestions on how to rebuild your immune system."[16] In a 1986 *PWAC Newsline* article, HEAL leader Alan Burns reiterated this sentiment, stating that "the holistic therapies discussed at HEAL do not rule out medicine."[17] Rather than attempt to persuade individuals that unorthodox therapeutics were superior to an ineffectual or dangerous mainstream practice, HEAL leaders conceived of PWAs as autonomous agents capable of making their own decisions.

HEAL's early focus on PWA empowerment harmonized well with PWAC's initiatives, with both groups decrying universal fatality narratives and striving to cultivate amongst PWAs a belief in their capacity to persevere through their diagnosis. Through the 1980s, the leaders of both groups contributed opinion pieces to each other's publications. One 1986 *PWAC Newsline* article, for example, featured HEAL leader Tom Cunningham condemning the "conspiracy of hopelessness" pervading mainstream biomedical discourse.[18] In 1989, PWAC cofounder Michael Callen penned a piece in HEAL's *Quarterly Bulletin* wherein he identified several traits shared by long-term survivors of AIDS. HEAL leaders were pleased to point out that the first two items in Callen's list underscored the frequency with which long-term survivors sought recourse in alternative and holistic approaches to healing.[19]

The support HEAL enjoyed from its more mainstream colleagues extended beyond leaders' joint publication in group newsletters. In the late 1980s, as HEAL endeavored to secure funding for its burgeoning services—which by then included weekly meetings, dinners, and an informational hotline—it obtained letters of support from other prominent AIDS service groups. In one such letter penned in 1988, the executive director of the PWAC declared, "I find the basic philosophies of HEAL to be consistent and complementary to our own—namely, that all people need to [be] allowed to be responsible for their own lives and health. The right to retain control over how their bodies are treated and to choose alternative healing methods is fundamental to PWA Coalition's philosophy of self-empowerment."[20] Even the GMHC—viewed by many as a more orthodox AIDS service organizations—voiced its support, with one representative writing, "[HEAL] provides information on alternative therapies for AIDS-related illness, a necessary balance to the Western-medicine options touted by most other hotlines, and does so in a responsible manner."[21] The strongest word of endorsement came not from an AIDS service organization but from a New York City Department of Health agency, with the director of the city's official AIDS hotline declaring,

> On behalf of the counselors and supervisors here at the Department of Health's AIDS Hotline, I would like to commend you for HEAL's continued and invaluable contributions to all those living with HIV disease . . . Many of our clients request information regarding the non-traditional and holistic approaches that are not routinely studied by the medical community. HEAL's explorations of alternative therapies and other approaches to healing has met these clients' needs . . . You continue to remind us all of the importance of empowering those living with HIV to investigate different therapies wherever and whenever possible.[22]

For HEAL leaders, the most cherished testimonials for the group's work came from its members. These letters, anonymized versions of which appeared in the group's informational packets, tell of PWAs wracked with despair who found, in HEAL, the will necessary to continue fighting. In one letter, the author reflects, "[W]hen I walked into the doctor's office for a routine physical, I wasn't ready for the diagnosis of ARC[23] I received, or the doctor's encouraging words: 'There's nothing you can do . . . come back in three months.' Finding HEAL has made me feel as good as I did before I saw the doctor."[24] A second handwritten letter tells the story of a young man who, upon receiving an HIV positive test result, mailed his diplomas to his parents in preparation for death. He credited a chance encounter with a HEAL pamphlet with transforming his life. "I read it page by page, line by line. Making notations, writing down questions for the next meeting . . . I went from a basket case to a human being again."[25] Another individual would write to thank HEAL for freeing him from victimhood, referring to the group's unorthodox services as "balm to my troubled soul."[26]

HEAL would remain a largely uncontroversial voice within the larger AIDS service community through the late 1980s and early 1990s, even as mainstream biomedicine concretized its response to AIDS. The growing focus within professional circles on viral AIDS etiologies—propelled by Health and Human Service Secretary Margaret Heckler's 1984 announcement of the discovery of HTLV-III/LAV—strained a holistic paradigm that challenged reductive, unicausal etiological models. However, because it would be another three years before the viral model bore therapeutic fruit, holistic health advocates found sufficient space to promote their philosophies without contradicting mainstream practice. Moreover, as discussed in chapter 4, not every member of New York City's gay community agreed with the viral etiological AIDS models. In addition to the *PWAC Newsline*, through the mid-to-late 1980s, the *New York Native*—the same outlet that had published Larry Kramer's call to arms at the start of the epidemic—promulgated an array of unorthodox etiological AIDS theories.[27]

HEAL's holistic health activism assumed a more outwardly confrontational stance in 1987 when the FDA granted expedited approval of AZT, the first antiretroviral developed to treat AIDS. While group leaders had previously endorsed the use of mainstream therapies for opportunistic infections, many could not bring themselves to support AZT. One HEAL leader, for example, noted that group members who took the drug suffered for little apparent gain: "[P]eople would come to our meetings with black fingernails, vomiting, and diarrhea. [AZT] had no effect on T-cells increasing whatsoever."[28] In the PWAC's *Surviving and Thriving with AIDS*, one recently diagnosed PWA recalled attending a HEAL meeting only to feel overwhelmed and "freaked out" by the group's anti-AZT platform.[29] Furthermore, HEAL members occasionally engaged in public acts of resistance referred to as "zaps"—term popularized in the 1970s-era gay liberation movement. On one occasion, HEAL members zapped a conference of physicians assembled by AZT manufacturer Burroughs Wellcome to challenge what they deemed pharma's stranglehold over the medical profession.[30]

While HEAL's early critiques of AZT were, at times, strident, they were not enough to brand the group as dangerous. Indeed, the representatives of the PWAC, GMHC, and New York City's Department of Health all penned their letters of support for HEAL years after AZT's approval. In these early years, the drug was simply too controversial to marginalize those who questioned its cost-benefit ratio and toxicity profile.[31] Furthermore, although individuals disagreed when it came to the drug's benefits, most agreed that it was no panacea. Indeed, even those who would come to question HEAL's later activism conceded the positive contributions the group made in challenging mainstream etiological and therapeutic parochialism. In a 1996 *Out Magazine* article, for example, AIDS activist Bob Lederer harshly critiqued the group's mid-1990s-era work while acknowledging that, in its earlier years, HEAL had provided "an important antidote to the widely accepted simple-minded one-bug/one-drug line."[32]

Yet points of disagreement, at times, forced rifts between HEAL and other AIDS service organizations. As groups such as GMHC professionalized, they dedicated increasing attention to the promotion of research into biomedical cures for AIDS. For some of their leaders, HEAL's pursuit of alternative therapies and critiques of biomedical orthodoxies was a distraction. When Fedorko suggested to GMHC that macrobiotics were preferable to AZT regimens, he encountered rigidity from Executive Director Richard Dunne. "I could tell immediately that he was hostile to the idea of macrobiotics . . . we didn't click," Fedorko recalled.[33] Both Fedorko and Fouratt, furthermore, reported similar resistance from ACT UP's Treatment and Data Committee, particularly when HEAL challenged ACT UP's efforts to secure greater access to AZT and, later, the second antiretroviral approved by the FDA, ddI.[34]

Some of the disagreements between HEAL and GMHC stemmed from class-based differences in the two groups' membership bases. HEAL, in Fedorko's opinion, had been comprised of artists and free spirits—a creative group of nonconformists who were "clever in putting together a regimen and a belief system to at least get them through the near future in a healthy way." This population differed from that of GMHC, which he argued had been created by and for "the bourgeois white boys,"[35] or ACT UP, which he believed contained its own highly vocal "white pro forma contingent."[36] In his estimation, these more mainstream groups represented a shirt-and-tie "homocracy"—a society of professional homosexuals that viewed itself as superior to HEAL's free spirited homosexual proletariat.[37] Fedorko's bifurcation of the AIDS service landscape based upon class is fascinating, particularly because he associated HEAL's alternative health activism with a nonprofessional social class, thereby challenging a scholarly bias that locates alternative health movements within the bourgeoisie.[38]

While differences between membership bases would, at times, bubble over, through the 1980s and early 1990s, HEAL remained a respected member of New York's larger AIDS service community. By the mid-1980s, the city's AIDS service organizations had been forced to develop strategies for collaborating through differences of opinion. As the epidemic raged on through the late 1980s and 1990s, and it became clear that Fedorko's Dark Ages would not yield to a Renaissance of curative therapeutics, many PWAs could make a legitimate claim to the benefits of a multifocal, multifaceted activist response.

Yet at some point in the early-to-mid 1990s, mainstream groups' tolerance for HEAL's unorthodox activism reached its breaking point, with the holistic health group eventually becoming radicalized and ostracized by its peers. The same group that had once robed its support for holistic health paradigms in the language of therapeutic complementarity would vehemently denounce the biomedical mainstream. One 1996 HEAL informational packet, for example, decries the mainstream viral etiological model and antiretroviral drugs it yielded, arguing, "as far as 'AIDS' goes, we have been subject to the most heinous and genocidal fraud in medical history."[39] A second column went further still, arguing that biomedical professionals had intentionally misled the public in their response to AIDS. Its author argued that HEAL members had, by the late 1980s, become "aware that the public was being intentionally misled about the causes, size and very nature of AIDS . . . We could not in good conscience ignore the emerging connection between all those nice AIDS doctors and all those dead AIDS patients."[40] In perhaps the clearest sign of the group's departure from its earlier embrace of therapeutic complementarity, in the mid-1990s it began stamping its literature with a new slogan pithily conveying its radical condemnation of biomedicine: "Fire your doctor."[41]

To date, no scholarly work has chronicled HEAL's transformation from a consonant-if-contrarian health activist group to a radicalized dissident organization. The AIDS historiography includes virtually no works analyzing the group's early history as a broadly complementary health support group. The rare analyses that mention HEAL often reduce the group to its mid-1990s–era dissidence. Some scholars go a step further, dismissing HEAL's dissidence as a byproduct of the firebrand activism of University of California retrovirologist Peter Duesberg.[42] The author of one recent scholarly work on AIDS dissidence, for example, briefly mentions HEAL within a section titled "AIDS Activism Meets Denialism." Demonstrating an incomplete understanding of the group's history, it suggests that HEAL existed as a bounded activist organization that, at some point, veered into the orbit of Duesbergian denialism, only to become irrevocably trapped within its gravitational pull.[43]

There is irony in such reductions, for they treat Duesberg—a man who argued that HIV was insufficient to cause AIDS—as a necessary and sufficient cause of the larger dissidence movement. Yet HEAL did not exist as a consonant and complementary therapeutic movement only to become infected by Duesberg's dissidence in the late 1980s. In fact, the transformations witnessed in HEAL's activism by the early-to-mid 1990s were, themselves, a consequence of a radicalization of the same holistic health principles the group endorsed through the 1980s. Thus, HEAL was not infected by the Berkeley retrovirologist, but rather embraced its own expression of AIDS dissidence as a result of the radicalization of its operating principles. In time, that perspective became informed and influenced by Duesberg in key ways. AIDS activism, in short, did not "meet" AIDS denialism; it helped give birth to it.

I maintain that this radicalization of health holism resulted from HEAL's embrace of increasingly unorthodox interpretations of two core holistic health principles. The first of these principles, which I term the "multifactoriality" of health and disease, is similar to the theory of multifactoriality discussed in chapter 4. Many PWAs viewed the principle as empowering, as it posited an ever-increasing number of avenues whereby they could strive to bolster their health. However, by the mid-1990s, a small faction within HEAL expanded the group's holistic multifactorial discourse to explicitly include questions of AIDS etiology, at which point it collided with a mainstream biomedical community that had rallied behind a viral etiological model. This move ultimately exposed HEAL to many of the same criticisms Joseph Sonnabend and Michael Callen endured in their endorsement of multifactorial etiological models.

HEAL leaders and members would also come to radicalize a second holistic health principle that emphasized the intrinsic interdependency of the physical, psychological, social, environmental, and spiritual domains of life. As in the case of holistic multifactoriality, the principle of interdependency proved broadly empowering to PWAs when applied to questions of therapeutics. However, some within HEAL would expand it to consider questions of disease etiology. This radicalization led these leaders to pursue controversial positions, contributing toward HEAL's conspiratorial rejection of mainstream biomedical practice.

The Radicalization of Health Holism: A Divisive Multifactoriality

To understand HEAL's turn toward a radicalized health holism, it is essential that we first review the holistic health movement out of which its early outreach grew. As discussed in chapter 4, this is no easy task. Over the course of the past several decades, myriad professionals and lay individuals alike have adopted the term "health holism" to connote a wide variety of beliefs and practices, and as a result, no single definition of the movement exists. In his 2016 volume *To Fix or to Heal: Patient Care, Public Health, and the Limits of Biomedicine*, sociologist Joseph E. Davis argues that, at its core, health holism embraces "a systematic concern with the whole organism, a focus on the interconnected effects of the larger physical or social environment, and attention to population-level variation."[44] As Davis notes, virtually all premodern health systems qualify as holistic based upon this definition.[45] Indeed, advocates of health holism frequently frame their beliefs as a return to an idealized and bucolic past.[46] However, it is erroneous to suggest that the holistic health movement as we know it today is premodern in origin, for it was promulgated as an antipode and antidote to modern biomedicine. Where biomedicine has come to rely upon increasingly advanced diagnostic and therapeutic technologies, holism invokes a simpler past; where biomedicine seeks to reduce disease to its constituent causes, holism speaks of the irreducible links between the mind, body, and environment; and where biomedicine—in some estimations—dehumanizes patients, holism claims to humanize them.

As discussed in chapter 2, by the mid-twentieth century, the groundswell of therapeutic successes biomedicine logged in the earlier part of the century had begun to dry up, with intractable chronic conditions replacing infectious diseases as major sources of morbidity and mortality in the developed world. The same magic bullets that had successfully treated pneumonia and tuberculosis proved largely ineffectual against cancer, heart attack, and stroke. As lay and professional commentators had long intuited, these diseases stemmed not from infection with single agents but from a nebulous web of interconnected biological, behavioral, social, and environmental variables.[47] The holistic health movement flourished in these years, developing complex, multifactorial models for responding to chronic disease while, in the case of conditions such as cancer, resisting heroic biomedical interventions.[48]

It has become almost cliché to discuss AIDS as the century's great anachronism—a terrifying epidemic that lurched society from the limbo of chronicity back into the hell of plague. Yet our tendency in the developed world to divide AIDS history into an era of infectious disease (1982–1996) and an era of chronic disease (1996 to present) blinds us to a wide array of activist traditions organized in the earliest days of the epidemic.[49] As described in chapters 2 and 3, for those diagnosed with AIDS through the early 1990s, life did not map neatly onto an infectious disease narrative. Indeed, in some cases, AIDS was directly related to chronic disease discourse, from the early term "gay cancer,"[50] to Kaposi sarcoma, to the virus U.S. researchers initially implicated in the disease.[51]

Deeper connections reveal themselves when one considers the ambiguity that attends most uses of the term "chronic disease." The websites for many state departments of health avoid defining the term entirely, speaking instead of chronic conditions by way of example. The Department of Health for Illinois is one exception to this rule, although even it vaguely defines a chronic disease as one that "persists over a long period of time."[52] The U.S. National Center for Health Statistics is somewhat more precise, defining as chronic those diseases lasting three months or longer,[53] while another recent work suggests a duration "measured in months and years, not days and weeks." The definition and bounds of chronicity, in short, differ based upon the disease under consideration.[54] This ambiguity is relevant to early AIDS history, for the PWA empowerment movement arose out of a desire to challenge universal fatality narratives and argue that PWAs could survive long term with their condition. To say that AIDS was an infectious disease pre-1996 is, thus, to prioritize epidemiological history over social history, thereby obscuring the lived experience of countless PWAs who fought tirelessly to reframe their condition through a chronic disease lens.[55] It was among these PWAs—and not the epidemiologists—that health holism, a movement more commonly associated with chronic conditions such as cancer, established a following.

As Davis and others have argued, a key component of the mid-twentieth century's holistic health movement was its shift away from modern biomedicine's penchant for reducing disease to unicausal origins. Instead, holistic health practitioners argued that conditions such as cancer resulted from the multiplicative effects of numerous variables. HEAL would embrace a similar conceptualization of therapeutic multifactoriality, arguing that AIDS resulted from the combined effects of myriad forms of antigenic assault spanning all domains of life. It is important to note that this early embrace of multifactoriality was not, in fact, born out of a dissident contrarianism. Instead, group leaders believed that multifactorial AIDS models yielded a wider array of therapeutic interventions PWAs could embrace in their efforts to gain control over their bodies and their disease. In describing this approach to health, HEAL Executive Board member Andrew Cort exalted, "This is good news! If there are many factors involved in illness, then there are many things which can be done to regain and/or maintain health. We do not have to wait for a 'magic bullet,' we do not have to count on just one treatment. Instead, we can deepen our own personal responsibility toward all aspects of our health and well-being."[56] Consistent with this belief, HEAL literature abounded with explorations of alternative health modalities including macrobiotics, herbalism, chiropractic medicine, hypnotherapy, Reiki, and attitudinal healing.[57]

While many would see in HEAL's early embrace of multifactorial disease paradigms a vehicle for PWA empowerment, by the mid-1990s, the situation had changed considerably. A review of the archive reveals that at approximately this time, a small faction of HEAL members under the leadership of Michael Ellner shifted the group's discourse. Early in the group's history, HEAL members invoked multifactoriality as a means to an end: the promulgation of an ever-increasing number of avenues for therapeutic intervention. Ellner instead viewed it as an end in itself, presenting multifactoriality as an etiological philosophy in conflict with biomedicine. This turn toward a rigid etiological multifactoriality was, in part, a response to the consolidation of mainstream biomedicine's support behind a "killer virus" theory. Indeed, throughout the 1980s, AIDS researcher Robert Gallo betrayed little patience for activists who challenged the notion that HIV was both necessary and sufficient to cause AIDS, which in turn inspired Ellner and his colleagues to challenge mainstream unicausal models even more strongly.[58]

Relying upon lay, informal analyses of HEAL members, Ellner argued that AIDS resulted from the additive effects of severe antigenic stresses amongst gay men, specifically identifying as the main culprits repeated infections with sexually transmitted agents, persistent recreational drug use, and long-term use of antibiotics. By the late 1980s and early 1990s, the sexual practices of gay men garnered attention in HEAL informational packets, with one naming "repeated traumatic sex acts and multiplicity of sexual partners engaging in anal sex" as a major factor underlying AIDS.[59] Ellner was the most vocal HEAL leader to implicate gay male "promiscuity" in AIDS, arguing that nearly all PWAs he met in HEAL meetings had engaged in such behavior through the 1970s and 1980s. "They were looking to live wild and high and die young and beautiful," he argued, "having sex in numbers that I don't think were ever possible historically because you didn't have so many people in the same place."[60] HEAL advisor Frank Buianouckas echoed many of Ellner's positions, invoking PWAC cofounder Michael Callen's medical history to argue that as a result of repeated infections with STIs, the immune systems of many gay men had come to resemble that of an individual living in a pre-industrial society.[61]

While Ellner presented his multifactorial arguments as more intrinsically empowering than unicausal viral models, many gay men regarded his views as not only disempowering but bigoted. Such accusations pained the HEAL member, a self-described "child of the '60s" who, while identifying as straight, prided himself on his fervent support for gay rights and sexual liberation.[62] In Ellner's view, his embrace of multifactoriality protected the hard-won victories of sexual liberation by challenging the notion that a single unlucky act of sexual intercourse shared between two people could transmit a virus and cause AIDS.[63] Yet, in rejecting a primary causal role for HIV, he bore the burden of enumerating sexual practices sufficient to transmit immunodeficiency. Thus, to protect sexual freedom, he painted PWAs as having engaged in extreme acts of sexual excess, making statements that enraged many gay men. Consider, for example, a response Ellner gave in a 1994 episode of *Tony Brown's Journal* when asked which gay male sexual practices caused immune collapse: "I would think it would have a violent atmosphere around it; be very, very brutalizing to the person—the receptive partner, in this case. And I think another component would be volume, the number of partners; that anal sex, in and of itself, is not what's the danger. It's if you have a number of exposures, and continuous exposures, and a lot of antigenic assaults on your health, that really is the danger."[64]

Some HEAL contributors also focused attention on recreational drug use by gay men. Ellner was particularly supportive of *New York Native* journalist John Lauritsen's claims that AIDS was caused, in part, by gay men's use of amyl nitrite inhalants ("poppers").[65] The two activists collaborated frequently: Lauritsen penned columns in HEAL publications,[66] he and Ellner appeared together on *Tony Brown's Journal*,[67] and at one point, Ellner described Lauritsen as capable of "walk[ing] on water."[68] Other HEAL contributors echoed the claim that recreational drug use among gay communities underlie AIDS. One 1995 HEAL white paper, published by controversial physician Robert Willner, claimed that 96 percent of gay men surveyed had used nitrile inhalants, 90 percent used marijuana, 60 percent amphetamines, 55 percent cocaine, 50 percent Quaaludes, and 50 percent lysergic acid.[69]

By the 1990s, HEAL expanded its discussion of the immune burden of drugs to include more explicit attacks on mainstream pharmaceutical agents. Willner, for example, argued that the use of "street drugs" and medicines such as AZT together "correlate virtually 100% with the development of AIDS in Europe and the United States."[70] A *HEAL Info Page* circulated among members pointed to the use of prescription medicines, over-the-counter remedies, and adulterated street drugs to argue that PWAs had turned their bodies into a "human toxic dump site."[71] Some linked the risks of sexual intercourse with pharmacological stressors by arguing that gay men in the 1970s exposed themselves to numerous STIs and treated them with copious amounts of antibiotics, resulting in a cycle of immune degradation.[72] The group's occasional forays into discussions of AIDS among injection drug–using populations were no less controversial. In one particularly incendiary HEAL article, Frank Buianouckas invoked images of "drug addicts shooting up in dank abandoned buildings, living off Captain Crunch, if they have any money left after they have bought their dope, cigarettes and booze—otherwise they exist on sugar packets stolen from wherever possible."[73]

As HEAL discourse became increasingly dominated by multifactorial antigenic assault brought upon by recreational drug use, medicinal drug use, and sex, the notion that PWA empowerment was predicated upon individuals reclaiming responsibility for their lives took on more moralistic undertones. By the 1990s, some members began to suggest that those who sought magic bullet solutions to AIDS were looking for quick fixes to avoid engaging in a holistic examination of their lives.[74] In one early 1990s article in a HEAL informational packet, Lese Dunton argues, "Some people will never allow themselves to stop and look, and they will die . . . The concept that you're responsible for everything that happens to you—some people resist that greatly."[75] Similarly, in the aforementioned episode of *Tony Brown's Journal*, Ellner's attempt to explain the controversy surrounding lifestyle modification campaigns suggests a level of judgment. "I think [PWAs] don't want to hear that message," he explained. "They want a pharmaceutical solution. They're not looking to change their lives. What they're looking for is, 'Give me a medicine, so I can go back and do these behaviors.'"[76]

By the early 1990s, Ellner and others within HEAL sharpened their critiques of pharmaceutical solutions, arguing even more forcefully that the biomedical system itself was directly contributing to AIDS. Two medical advances catalyzed this radicalization of the multifactorial model. The first was the FDA's acknowledgment that the initial dosage regimen for AZT had been too high, prompting it to decrease the recommended dose from 1,200 milligrams to 600.[77] While many in the AIDS community saw this as a triumph, Ellner and others took it as evidence that AZT was indeed toxic and had contributed to the immune degradation among PWAs. It also led the group to claim that Burroughs Wellcome had known of AZT's toxicity but ignored it to insulate their earnings.[78]

The second issue that contributed to HEAL's radicalization precipitated the dissolution of HEAL's greater membership and drove a wedge between the group and the PWAC. Through the 1980s, Callen waged a battle to convince biomedical leaders that asymptomatic PWAs could prevent the contraction of AIDS-related conditions through the prophylactic use of medications. Attributing his long-term survival to Sonnabend's decision to treat him prophylactically with agents such as Bactrim, Callen fought tirelessly to convince the FDA that his approach could save lives, finally achieving success in the early 1990s. For Ellner, who viewed mainstream biomedical treatments as intrinsically dangerous and one of many factors contributing to AIDS, the prophylactic use of medicines amongst asymptomatic PWAs was anathema.[79] Through the 1990s, he engaged in a bitter critique of prophylaxis and, in some cases, directly criticized Callen, who died of AIDS-related conditions in December of 1993. In one video aired on Manhattan's cable news network, Ellner commented that as a result of Callen's prophylactic drug use, "He didn't even look human for the last six or seven months" of his life.[80] Another author would, in 1997, describe Callen as, "the AIDS 'survivor' 12 years after diagnosis, defying the pronouncements of the authorities that salvation lies in AZT but preaching the false gospel of 'prophylactic' use of antibiotics, holding up his sandwich bag of pills, 56 of which he took every day."[81]

While HEAL's multifactorial health activism had endured criticism, Ellner's attempts to invoke it to condemn prophylactic treatments was the last straw for the group's longstanding members, many of whom resigned in protest by 1992.[82] Among the defectors was Eugene Fedorko, who helped organize the group and once served as president. In a 1995 interview with AIDS activist Bob Lederer, Fedorko explained, "HEAL's message that all Western medicine is bad—and particularly not to take antibiotics—is horribly oversimplified. Sure, there are toxicities to consider and counteract. But the big killer infections like *Pneumocystis carinii* pneumonia (PCP) can't be treated with less than antibiotics or the person will die."[83] As Fedorko's comments suggest, when the group pursued an increasingly radicalized rejection of mainstream medicine, it ostracized itself from other unorthodox health activists. HEAL member Tom DiFerdinando underscored this point in a 1997 article wherein he lambasted the unorthodox AIDS community for acquiescing to a mainstream unicausal etiological model. In his opinion, the larger alternative health community had come to use HIV as "an unspoken and socially sanctioned closet door behind which one can hide . . . absolv[ing] themselves of responsibility as a participant in their environment or situations."[84]

Thus, as activists embraced radical multifactoriality as an alternative to a mainstream, unicausal viral paradigm, they came to ostracize not only practitioners of biomedicine but alternative health activists as well. Yet this radical turn does not fully explain HEAL's marginalization as an AIDS service organization. For its leaders would also adapt a second holistic health principle—the notion that all variables underlying health and disease are interdependent—to arrive at newer, more radical theories of AIDS etiology. It is to this second health principle that I now turn.

The Radicalization of Health Holism: From Holistic Interdependency to an Isolating Dissidence

As health scholar Michael H. Cohen has observed, health holism "attempts to account for patients as whole persons, exercising autonomous choices and seeking health in terms of a larger pursuit toward an irreducible, unified, physical, emotional, mental and spiritual wholeness."[85] This emphasis on the interdependence of physical, emotional, environmental, and spiritual spheres generally confers upon the holistic health movement an aura of harmonious, New-Age free-spiritedness. Popular representations of health holism reinforce such associations, conjuring images of idealistic hippies and high-flying health gurus who spent their time, in Frank Zappa's immortal words, "jiving with that cosmik debris."[86]

Yet the holistic health movement jived with far more than cosmik debris; it also jived with mainstream theories of social development. This was, after all, the dawn of globalization wherein technology, commerce, and information transfer were poised to collapse the boundaries that had divided societies.[87] A globalized world was one defined by interconnection. Correspondingly, for some commentators, the early-to-mid twentieth century's fixation with specialization, segmentation, atomization, and rigidly mechanistic etiological models began to appear anachronistic. In his bestselling 1982 text *The Turning Point*, for example, Fritjof Capra argued: "[W]e are trying to apply the concepts of an outdated world view—the mechanistic world view of Cartesian-Newtonian science—to a reality that can no longer be understood in terms of these concepts. We live today in a globally interconnected world, in which biological, psychological, social, and environmental phenomena are all interdependent. To describe this world appropriately we need an ecological perspective which the Cartesian world view does not offer."[88]

If holistic interdependence was a dialect, it was one many people by the 1980s had come to understand, which helps explain HEAL's early success in appealing to PWAs. As in the case of the multifactorial health model, the group's early endorsement of holistic interdependency was linked directly to its wide-ranging therapeutic initiatives. By the early 1990s, HEAL had come to argue that physical, somatic illnesses such as AIDS could be treated through interventions aimed at modulating individuals' psychological or emotional states. Ellner, whose own alternative health practice was in the field of hypnotherapy, believed that the mind played a crucial role in AIDS prognosis. Through the 1980s, he held many workshops advocating the use of "hypnoimmunotherapy" to treat PWAs.[89] HEAL also organized communal Reiki and attitudinal healing seminars, introducing members to traditions such as the AIDS Mastery and Louise Hay's therapeutic approach.[90] Ellner's approach also directly invoked spirituality: he identified as an interfaith minister and used the title Reverend.

Had HEAL maintained its emphasis on holistic therapeutics, we likely would remember it today as a benign, idealistic exponent of the early integrative medicine movement. The strongest accusation scholars would level against it would be allegations of fringe quackery like the ones that greeted Louise Hay's psychotherapeutic response to AIDS.[91] However, by the 1990s, Ellner and his colleagues had shifted the group's holistic health discourse away from questions of therapeutics to ones dealing more directly with etiology. More specifically, he endorsed an increasingly radical view holding that AIDS resulted from the aggregate effects of emotional and psychological trauma. In this view, the mind served as a conduit that translated socially mediated, structural, and symbolic forms of violence onto the body. AIDS thus became the fault of the systems of power within society, which imprinted themselves on the body through the intercession of the mind.

Students of public health may recognize overlaps between Ellner's embrace of holistic interdependency and the fields of social epidemiology and social medicine. Both, for example, challenge reductive conceptualizations of disease, viewing illness instead as the results of complex webs of causation.[92] While Ellner's embrace of holistic interdependency differs from social epidemiology in key regards—including, for example, his disregard for Cartesian dualism—the two models provide languages which allow individuals affected by disease to impugn larger structural forces that often escape biomedical inquiry.

Ellner was far from the first to position the mind as a nexus linking bodily disease with structural violence. In 1956, for example, Margaret Meade penned a *New York Times* column wherein she discussed the popular notion that social change begat anxiety among members of the public which, in turn, begat disease. "This is what we have arrived at with all our vaunted progress, our great technological advances, our great wealth," Meade wrote. "[E]veryone goes about with a burden of anxiety so enormous that, in the end, our stomachs and our arteries and our skins express the tension under which we live."[93] Lay and professional audiences alike have long afforded anxiety a special role in registering the stresses of society onto the body, be it amongst nineteenth-century individuals diagnosed with neurasthenia or mid-twentieth century individuals diagnosed with heart disease.[94]

For those who viewed anxiety as a translator of social stresses onto the body, it had a great deal to translate through the mid-to-late twentieth century. This was, after all, an era poet W. H. Auden famously called the "Age of Anxiety" in his Pulitzer Prize–winning eclogue of the same title. Written some three decades before the dawn of the AIDS pandemic, it is remarkable for the ways in which Auden—himself a closeted gay man—portends the anxieties of the AIDS epidemic: "They swallowed and sank, ceased thereafter / To appear in public; exposed to snap / Verdicts of sharks, to vague inquiries / Of amoeboid monsters, mobbed by slight / Unfriendly fry, refused persistence. / They are nothing now but names assigned to / Anguish in others, areas of grief," he wrote. "Many have perished; more will."[95]

Ellner's early interest in the mind's role in AIDS led him to a radical theory first proposed by Casper G. Schmidt in a 1984 *Journal of Psychohistory* article titled "The Group-Fantasy Origins of AIDS." This piece, largely ignored in AIDS scholarship, exists as one of the earliest dissident etiological AIDS treatises.[96] Described by Ellner as a Renaissance man, Schmidt relocated to New York from his native South Africa to open a psychoanalytic practice and is credited with articulating a holistic critique of HIV before the virus was named.[97] In his 1984 article, he wrote, "Against the grain of monoetiological thinking and an unconsciously held Cartesian dualism, I posit that AIDS is a bio-psycho-social disorder. I argue that a sequence of group psychological events in the U.S. has shamed—and mercilessly so—the homosexuals and the drug addicts, giving rise to an epidemic of shame-induced depression."[98] In Schmidt's biopsychosocial model, AIDS was an example not of an infectious disease spread by germs, but rather a "contagious form of psychological disturbance . . . spread by suggestion."[99]

His unorthodox perspective maintained that AIDS represented a crystallization of the entrenched symbolic violence promulgated by the Moral Majority against gay men through the 1970s and early 1980s. As Schmidt saw it, gay men had become the scapegoats of a shamed and penitent society, the "whipping boys" of a "sadistic" New Right who self-righteously condemned its members to death as a means of reinforcing its own sense of virtue and sanctity.[100]

Schmidt's theory is provocative, flying in the face of not only mainstream biomedical theory but also the theories we today associate with AIDS dissidence. "The Group-Fantasy Origins of AIDS" is, furthermore, noticeably thin on the types of support modern audiences have come to expect from etiological models, with most of Schmidt's evidence appropriated from non-AIDS related epidemiological studies and anthropological research of pre-industrial societies.[101] In place of mechanistic discussions of disease pathways, for example, Schmidt cites the shaming taboos of New Guinean tribal societies, practices which he argues carried the capacity to cause death. He acknowledged this shortcoming in his model, promising to publish a companion article dedicated to matters of pathology and biology. However, he would die of AIDS-related complications in 1994, never having completed the piece.[102]

Setting aside the shortcomings of Schmidt's model, his 1984 article is interesting as an expression of applied social theory. For the biopsychosocial paradigm presents us with a world wherein deep, structurally mediated inequities directly yield fatal infectious disease through their work on the human psyche. In this frightening worldview, power is made flesh, as individuals plagued by trenchant sources of symbolic violence experience emotional trauma which, in turn, causes a breakdown in their somatic organ systems. Schmidt's world is one wherein the gaze of the empowered, the hate of the oppressors, and the inequities of the majority act directly on individuals, yielding immunodeficiency. We know very little of Schmidt's history or background. However, it is interesting to note that the psychoanalyst penned his works during roughly the same time that Michel Foucault and Pierre Bourdieu first articulated their microphysics of power and symbolic power theories.[103]

While it is incorrect to argue that AIDS activists endorsed Schmidt's model in its most literal form, many endorsed perspectives that intersected aspects of his work. *New York Native* journalist John Lauritsen, for example, granted that psychological effects could influence AIDS, arguing that gay men regularly "experienced terror, owing to the war waged against gay men by the Moral Majority."[104] Moreover, the HEAL archive is rife with articles claiming that the stress and anxiety placed upon gay men by a discriminatory society played a direct role in AIDS, with many authors listing chronic stress among the variables impugned in multifactorial AIDS etiological models.[105] However, no single individual was influenced more by Schmidt's theories than Ellner. In a 2009 interview, he focused on the fatalistic hysteria pulsing through society through the

1980s: "[I]t occurred to me because I was trained in hypnosis, that the power of suggestion and the level of hysteria was enough to make someone ill, possibly kill them, if they really got caught up in it."[106]

Through the 1980s and 1990s, Ellner adapted Schmidt's paradigm, incorporating it into a broad, multifactorial etiological AIDS model that impugned multiple factors. While he continued to recognize Schmidt's emphasis on homophobia, Ellner echoed Callen and Navarre's critiques in arguing that it was the anxiety wrought through AIDS universal fatality narratives that caused the most harm to PWAs. In one article published in the 1980s, he extolled, "We have been led to believe that HIV is synonymous with AIDS, and that AIDS equals death. The hopelessness these beliefs engender is as damaging to the immune system as any virus."[107] For Ellner, anxiety over universal fatality narratives and hysteria over anti-gay stigma together yielded a "trance state" wherein PWAs uncritically accepted mainstream theories and practices.[108] By the mid-1990s, he referred to this state as the "AIDS Zone," which he described as "a virtual community center where everyone either goes to die or is encouraged to die; an ideological framework within which expression of the crisis mentality is not only sanctioned but also actively encouraged."[109] He believed that the only way to escape the AIDS Zone was to break free of the cultural hypnosis wrought through the "hidden, spontaneous, accidental and unrecognized forms of power of suggestion" which held that "HIV=AIDS=DEATH."[110]

As mainstream biomedical professionals coalesced around the HIV etiological model and developed antiretrovirals such as AZT and ddI, Ellner intensified his critique of the AIDS Zone. In his opinion, physicians and PWAs alike had become entranced by the HIV=AIDS=DEATH paradigm, and by perpetuating the notion that the only viable response to AIDS was treatment with antiretrovirals, had themselves contributed to the spread of immune deficiency. One 1990 HEAL article titled "Psychological Genocide: The Push for AIDS Testing" decried mainstream calls for individuals to consent to HIV blood tests by invoking language reminiscent of Schmidt's. "The framing of AIDS as universally fatal, and HIV=AIDS," Ellner argued, "is like a shaman bone pointing and causing death."[111] Through the 1990s, Ellner and his supporters continued to condemn biomedicine's HIV/AIDS model and the antiretrovirals it wrought, arguing that the PWA community was "being terrorized by the HIV dogma."[112] In his view, all of society had become entranced into accepting the notion that PWAs were helpless victims in need of pharmacological intervention. Consider, for example, an article he penned in 2000 expanding the borders of the AIDS Zone:

> If you're HIV+ your part is to get sick and die; if you are a doctor your role is to test for an antibody, make healthy people sick and sick people die, and then blame a virus; if you're a gay AIDS activist your role is to insure that unproven treatments get into everyone's body and that everyone wear a condom as if everyone's

> at risk; if you're an AIDS organization your role is to deliver HIV+'s to the pharmaceutical ovens and silence anyone who questions the insanity; and if you're not in any of these groups your role is to wear a red ribbon, a latex condom and act like you care. AIDS works because everyone has something to do. It all serves to keep us all from looking at what's truly going on in the world. The rampant death and subsequent social cleansing artificially absolves everyone of the repressed tension generated by the preexisting social conditions.[113]

Thus, in the radically incendiary expansion of the holistic health model, biomedicine itself represents a form of tyranny blinding individuals to the deep, structural origins of disease. For Ellner, by giving everyone a scripted role, the biomedical response to AIDS forestalled their engagement with the world while creating the impression that they were making progress against the disease. Medicine's magic bullets thus served as an equivalent to Marx's "opium of the people," palliating their pain while robbing them of the incentive to organize for broad structural change.

This stance, complete with allegations of genocide on the part of physicians, incontrovertibly alienated HEAL from the larger PWA community—and it is not hard to see why. The same group that began in the 1980s by welcoming diverse therapeutic responses to AIDS had, by the mid-1990s, rejected mainstream therapeutic efforts. In time, group leaders would not only challenge biomedical interventions, but harshly judge PWAs who pursued them. Such was the case in an early-1990s volume penned by HEAL Executive Board Member Andrew Cort arguing that, by failing to acknowledge the holistic underpinnings of AIDS and instead buying into pharma's treatments, PWAs had squandered their opportunity for life-changing empowerment.[114] Thus, in HEAL's radicalization of the holistic health paradigm, we find the group's ultimate rejection of the borderland health model, with group leaders critiquing PWAs for adopting mainstream therapeutic modalities.

This underscores the ultimate irony of HEAL's mid-1990s era embrace of holistic interdependency. While individuals such as Ellner sought to underscore broad, structural sources of violence, they ultimately expressed their activism in reductive, individualistic terms. Within HEAL columns, it is the PWA who incurs a personal moral obligation to challenge larger systems of structural violence by rejecting mainstream biomedical nostrums. What began as a model focused upon fundamental inequities, structural violence, and symbolic violence devolved into a moralistic assessment of PWAs' willingness to stand up to these entrenched systems of inequity and violence. This phenomenon bears striking resemblance to the operationalization of Ivan Illich's theories, which, as discussed in chapter 3, critics alleged began from a position of radical humanism before inverting into "petty conservatism."[115] So too does it remind us of the history of social epidemiology and social medicine. For these movements were defined by efforts to identify the fundamental social correlates of health and disease and yet, by the late twentieth century, had become reduced to initiatives focused upon modulating individual risk behaviors. These overlaps further suggest that the orthodox and the unorthodox are not nearly as dissimilar as the fringe-mainstream metaphor would have us believe.

By the mid-to-late 1990s, with the group's core gay male membership base abandoning HEAL, Ellner and his colleagues fully committed themselves to dissident activism.[116] Although the period would mark the decline of the New York group's membership, it also saw the consolidation of HEAL's influence in the nascent AIDS dissidence movement. By the mid-1990s, as the Internet facilitated grassroots organization, small, independent grassroots HEAL chapters had taken root in Arizona, California, Florida, Michigan, Minnesota, New Hampshire, Oregon, Vermont, and Washington, as well as in Argentina, Australia, Canada, England, and Mexico.[117] In a 2009 interview, Ellner claimed that, at one point, twenty-three autonomous HEAL chapters were in operation throughout the world, making HEAL an early hub of the dissident movement—though all of these chapters were small, independent, grassroots initiatives using the group's name. The most successful splinter group was HEAL Los Angeles, formed in 1995 by Christine Maggiore, who would go on to play a significant role in the U.S. AIDS dissident movement. HEAL's New York activism also persisted, even as the group shrank to include little more than Ellner and a handful of supporters. Through the late 1990s, HEAL aired its views on an international stage, with Ellner penning articles in the United Kingdom's dissident *Continuum Magazine*,[118] and for a time it hosted its own public access cable television show in Manhattan.[119] It also used these fora to comment on international affairs, as when South African President Thabo Mbeki endorsed HIV dissident perspectives during his 1999–2008 tenure in office.

By the early 2000s, HEAL's activism had largely ceased. Christine Maggiore died of AIDS-related conditions in 2008, and though Ellner would continue to espouse contrarian perspectives beyond 2010, the group atrophied. By this point, the dissident movement had become firmly associated with Duesberg, who published articles and volumes throughout the 1990s and early 2000s, several of which HEAL members cited in the group's literature.

Interestingly, while Ellner would, through the 1990s, invoke Duesberg's contributions to dissident discourse, by the late 1990s and early 2000s, the HEAL leader began to express concern with the degree to which dissidence had transformed into a battle waged within the borders of biomedicine. For, unlike HEAL, Duesberg did not seek to supplant all of biomedicine with a radically holistic health paradigm. Rather, he intended to underscore what he perceived to be AIDS researchers' failures to satisfy biomedicine's own standards.[120] This divergence troubled the longtime HEAL president, who in 2009 decried, "I think that a lot of the people involved in the dissident movement now have a certain level of integrity issues. I think they're invested in maintaining biotechnology, maintaining molecular biology and just making HIV, AIDS an isolated situation. It's not isolated. There [are] problems with that whole branch of science and that ties into cancer research as well. They're all interconnected."[121] Thus, Ellner longed for an AIDS dissidence defined not by the language and tools of biomedicine, but by a radically contrarian holistic health model that challenged Western biomedicine writ large. Yet by 2010, that dissidence had become a thing of the past, its support eroded not only by advances in mainstream biomedicine that made AIDS treatable within the developed world, but also by the redefinition of dissidence itself as an expression of Duesbergian denialism.

AIDS DISSIDENCE: COLLABORATION IN THE BORDERLANDS

As HEAL's activism became increasingly dissident, opportunities for movement within the therapeutic borderland faded. Ultimately, activists painted orthodox medicine as inherently incompatible with unorthodox healing approaches. The borderlands, once dynamic spaces of interexchange, transformed into no man's lands. Walls were erected, borders policed, and forays into the wilderness branded as fringe.

Yet, even as the walls rose, we find expressions of dynamic interexchange—albeit of a different form. The very dissidence that forestalled opportunities for dynamic interrelations with orthodox biomedicine provided opportunities for communication between different groups. One important and understudied expression of such collaboration was the relationship formed between New York City's AIDS activist organizations, African American leaders, the gay press, and the African American press over a shared embrace of unorthodox AIDS perspectives.

Through the mid-1980s, by some estimates, over half of all U.S. pediatric AIDS cases occurred among Black communities while upwards of 40 percent of all cases occurred in Black and Latinx populations.[122] When clinicians and public health professionals advocated increased discussion of AIDS risk factors among Black populations, the stigma associated with both homosexuality and AIDS posed significant hurdles.[123] Yet the dissident movement demonstrated an ability to move beyond these obstacles, forging collaborations between the city's gay and Black institutions—although the result of these collaborations were not always in line with public health goals.[124]

For example, through the late 1980s and early 1990s, HEAL—still largely associated with the gay community—hosted outreach events in Harlem. These included sessions similar in structure to their downtown meetings in addition to targeted food kitchens and holistic living workshops. In the early 1990s, the group was even recognized by the US Department of Health and Human

Services for this work.[125] Many of these outreach initiatives were spearheaded by Cliff Goodman, a HEAL member who described himself as, "a 32-year-old, Gay man of African descent, born in the southwest Bronx . . . and raised in North Central Harlem. I am a veteran (peacetime, 1976–1979 U.S. Army—Korea/Germany), a college dropout (Lehman College, Bronx) a Buddhist, a Hypnotist, a member of NA/AA. I'm also poor, HIV+, but sexy and happy!"[126]

In addition to the Harlem outreach, Goodman hosted workshops for prisoners in the city's carceral system, many of whom were members of minority communities. In 1992, he organized one such session in the women's ward at Riker's Island, noting, "The women present were eager to hear alternative information other than the usual propaganda about AZT. Many decided to stop taking their AZT on the spot. [They] are determined to do their best even while incarcerated, to eat healthy meals, exercise and develop spiritually."[127] While Goodman's work demonstrates the presence of intersectional activism within the unorthodox AIDS movement, it should not be taken to mean that his efforts were openly accepted by all HEAL members. In an article published in a circa-1991 HEAL packet, he observed, "There was some concern from an associate that I should 'tone down' the language of this editorial! He felt that it was 'too emotional' for you to understand and he had the nerve to ask me will I 'move it to the back' (people of color section) of the HEAL newsletter."[128]

Despite these points of tension, in time, HEAL's outreach initiatives resulted in dialogue with leaders in the city's African American community. In 1998, the Reverend Al Sharpton's National Action Network invited HEAL to participate in an AIDS conference in Harlem. In it, African American leaders joined with the representatives of several groups to discuss alternative AIDS theories. Ellner and Maggiore presented dissident perspectives impugning the viral etiological model alongside others who believed that HIV was designed by the U.S. government to decimate minority populations.[129] Standing before a room of over 150 audience members, Ellner argued that the "AIDS fantasy" had been concocted to decimate gay populations and that powerful forces were using the same tactics against African Americans.[130] Meanwhile, Maggiore drew applause from the crowd when she announced that she refused to take antiretrovirals.[131] *New York Times* journalist David France reported on the event, expressing exasperation at its content: "At times, the thrust of the six-hour gathering seemed to be an emotional plea to anyone with HIV to stop taking their medication. Lynn Gannett, who identified herself as a data processor on an early research trial of the AIDS drug AZT, spoke in a quavering voice as she beseeched the audience. 'Please,' she said, 'if you are on these pills or if your baby is taking them, stop, I beg you. The drugs can kill you.'"[132]

AIDS dissidence also facilitated collaboration between communities as expressed by coverage in the city's gay and African American media outlets. For example, in 1985, the city's best known gay newspaper, *The New York Native*, argued, "We feel that the current AIDS epidemic shares more than a few factors with the Tuskegee syphilis experiment."[133] Two years later, one of the newspaper's columns declared, "Bad blood, AIDS, syphilis, gays, blacks, the Division of Venereal Disease Control, the Centers for Disease Control. A remarkably similar cast of characters."[134]

These direct comparisons between communities' experiences also appear in works of creative art published during the 1980s. In 1987, *Christopher Street,* a literary-themed sister publication to the *Native,* printed a poem composed by Sean Lawrence. In it, he describes having watched a news program wherein people living in Africa, where the AIDS-related death toll was extremely high, were seen praying. The image prompted Lawrence to reflect on how he would respond to a diagnosis of AIDS. "I'm not gonna let the clap doctors / of Greenwich Village play / immunology with my disco body," he wrote. Instead, he decided that he would go to Africa to join the deathwatch of the tribes of Nairobi or die with a caravan of nurses in Rwanda. His closing lines poignantly capture the legacies of biomedical distrust shared by both queer communities and communities of color: "I remember someone at / the Centers for Disease Control / telling me that AIDS / was their way of / getting rid of the blacks. / If I get it / I'm gonna go to Africa / and get rid of me with them."[135]

Sometimes, newspapers facilitated direct collaborations between communities. In 1987, for example, New York's *Amsterdam News* republished a letter the *Native's* publisher had drafted to the mayor of New York.[136] With it, the newspaper's editors included a comment endorsing the gay publication for articulating views impugning the integrity of biomedicine: "Given the history of the US Public Health Service, when it comes to Blacks, the 40 year syphilis experiment conducted at Tuskegee makes it very easy to believe that AIDS is man-made, and could possibly be another 'test.' *New York Native,* the foremost Gay newspaper in the country, raises this most important issue in a front page letter to Edward I. Koch that is reproduced on this page. The prospect of this is frightening, as well as entirely possible."[137]

By the 1990s, the *Native* and *Christopher Street* had come under attack from mainstream activist groups such as ACT UP, who challenged the radical theories its editors endorsed.[138] In a sign of continued collaborations between Black and gay media outlets, several prominent African American journalists defended the gay press. Tony Brown, a leading African American journalist and the host of the longest-running national public affairs PBS television show, offered a defense of the *Native's* publisher in one of the nation's oldest and largest Black newspapers, the *Los Angeles Sentinel.* In it, he began, "This column is a tribute to a White man who is a homosexual." He went on to argue, "If ever there was a time when the gay community and the Black community need one another, it is now . . . On this particular issue of survival, we must put down our petty biases and identify the real enemy."[139]

The distrust in biomedicine voiced in the pages of *Amsterdam News* and dissident texts influenced countless individuals at risk of contracting HIV. One indication of such influence is registered in the writings of David Gilbert, a White ally of the Black Liberation Army who was sentenced to life imprisonment in a 1981 robbery wherein two police officers and a guard were killed. Beginning in 1986, Gilbert worked to educate prisoners about AIDS and decry the state of disinformation within prisons. In a piece published in the mid-1990s, he called conspiracy myths "the main internal obstacle . . . to concentrating on thorough and detailed work on risk reduction."[140] As Gilbert explained, "What's the use, believers ask, of making all the hard choices to avoid spreading or contracting the disease if the government is going to find a way to infect people anyway? . . . [S]uch theories provide an apparently simple and satisfying alternative to the complex challenge of dealing with the myriad of social, behavioral, and medical factors that propel the epidemic."[141]

Gilbert sought to dispel these claims, arguing that the conspiracy theories upon which they were premised were rooted in ultra-right ideologies. At the same time, he urged readers to focus their attention on the structural racism and neglect that consigned Black and Brown communities to death. In a column section titled, "Fight the Power/Fight the Plague," he argued, "We don't need to be led on a wild goose chase searching for the little men in white coats in a secret lab—which we will never find—which only leads us away from confronting the colossal crimes of malign neglect that are right in front of our faces, that can be documented, that are completely rooted in racism, homophobia, and profiteering."

The unorthodox views Gilbert strove to combat differed from those that filled the pages of HEAL literature. Yet, despite their points of contradiction, they were able to coexist under a common roof, as when Ellner and Maggiore presented their anti-HIV perspectives alongside speakers who believed HIV was manufactured by the government as a form of social control. For unorthodox AIDS activism was defined not by a bounded, internally consistent etiological or therapeutic model but by a diverse network of complex and contradictory perspectives and philosophies. Furthermore, the legacies of distrust and anti-authoritarianism it channeled created opportunities for collaboration between communities, harmonizing in fascinating and poorly understood ways.

CONCLUSION: REMEMBERING HEAL

As this analysis underscores, HEAL was a complex and controversial group whose organizing goals and principles changed over the course of a changing epidemic. Respected and lauded as a member of the larger AIDS service community through the 1980s, by the mid-1990s, HEAL became isolated and radicalized, replacing a complementary therapeutic focus with a divisive and contrarian etiological philosophy. This turn was not a result of the group's "infection" with

Duesberg's theories. Instead, HEAL's dissidence stemmed from a radicalization of the principles of multifactoriality and interdependency underlying the holistic health model. Historians of health and medicine would do well to heed HEAL's history, for it demonstrates the complex ways in which alternative health movements—and, more specifically, holistic health movements—may become radicalized.

Nothing about HEAL's history is straightforward, and readers cannot be faulted for experiencing a certain exasperation with the principles its members endorsed through the 1990s and early 2000s. For those accustomed to neat and ordered etiological models, HEAL's activism is frustrating. The same individuals who impugned sexual practices as a primary cause of AIDS also blamed the medical community's prescription of AZT, while simultaneously indicting the anxiety bubbling within the gay community as a result of homophobia and AIDS fatalism. Furthermore, HEAL leaders spoke at community events alongside others whose unorthodox views differed markedly from their own. Yet, where some find internal inconsistency, others will find a complex activist tradition that underwent profound transformations as its members pursued an increasingly radicalized and oppositional stance toward mainstream biomedicine. By remembering forgotten grassroots activist groups such as HEAL, we stand to learn a great deal about not only unorthodox health movements, but orthodox health movements as well. For, as this analysis suggests, these grassroots groups often reflect principles and philosophies that reverberate through the mainstream.

CONCLUSION

Listening to and Learning from the Sounds of Furious Living

By APPENDING TO the historical register the unorthodox AIDS activism embraced by members of the PWAC and HEAL, we arrive at a more complete representation of AIDS activism. The picture that emerges also challenges broad assumptions regarding patient responsibility and empowerment in the domain of health and disease. As such, this volume offers lessons both for the scholars tasked with studying the history of healing and the healers we entrust with keeping us well.

THE SOUNDS OF FURIOUS LIVING: LESSONS FOR THE PRACTICE OF HISTORY

In their 1979 volume *Health Care in America: Essays in Social History*, David Rosner and Susan Reverby write of the need to move historical practice away from celebratory chronicles of ennobled physicians. In their new social history of public health, they transformed the patient, who had long served as the object of medicine, into the subject of historical analysis.[1] Several years later, Roy Porter made his own contribution to this historiographic discourse, advocating a "history from below" prioritizing the perspectives of patients over that of biomedical experts.[2]

At roughly the same time, a second group of scholars tasked themselves with writing histories of health movements previous historians had marginalized.[3] Thus, beginning in the mid-twentieth century, we find the proliferation of historical research looking anew at healing systems such as homeopathy, hydropathy, chiropractic medicine, and Thomsonian medicine. Inspired by a desire to move beyond dismissive critiques of such healing systems, these scholars endeavored to replace hagiographies of biomedical leaders with nuanced analyses of the disempowered and marginalized. Yet by focusing on bounded therapeutic philosophies and schools of practice, these histories often remained beholden to professional taxonomies. The result is a scholarly tradition that, while seeking to capture the experience of the forgotten, often substitutes one group of professionals for another.

In this volume, I have argued that the appropriation of a borderland construct can aid historians in our endeavor to craft social histories of health and disease. In this model, historians conceive of patients as individuals capable of locating themselves within and between multiple lay and professional systems of healing, existing in the nebulous borderlands formed between medical sects. When faced with disease—be it acute, chronic, infectious, noninfectious, or of unknown duration or origin—individuals within these borderlands selectively adopt etiological models and therapeutic modalities from different systems, generating syncretic practices that defy classification. This conceptual model is, in fact, consistent with evidence compiled by David Eisenberg, Patricia Barnes, and the Institute of Medicine, suggesting that individuals frequently borrow from both orthodox and unorthodox healing systems, creating their own healing amalgams.[4] Thus, by examining individuals' engagement with different healing modalities and philosophes, historians of medicine move one step closer to accomplishing a social history of health attuned to the complex ways in which power aggregates and manifests in society—what Michel Foucault termed the "microphysics of power."[5]

What, then, are the lessons historians may glean from this reconceptualization of patient empowerment? First, by interpreting individuals' movements within and between healthcare borderlands as expressions of agency, we reject the claim that those who embrace alternative medicine have, in every instance, been hoodwinked into doing so. Students of the history of medicine are well acquainted with the colorful charlatans who lurk in the fringes of society, capitalizing on desperation to peddle their wares. Yet histories of unorthodox health movements focused only upon quacks are no more histories from below than accounts of orthodox medicine focused upon the part played by the physician.

This volume also challenges the notion that a social history of unorthodox health activism reads as an interminable struggle between marginalized irregular sects and a hegemonic biomedical profession. For patients, in fact, weave together orthodox and unorthodox healing systems. Although PWA activists such as Michael Callen argued that biomedicine's methods of knowledge production had become dogmatic and dangerous, we identify in such activism a belief in a reimagined and reconstituted biomedicine. A similar phenomenon presents itself for some members of HEAL who fiercely condemned biomedicine while simultaneously invoking the tools and language of biomedicine to make their case. Furthermore, in both groups, PWAs combined mainstream and alternative healing systems in their effort to find meaning and order amidst uncertainty.

We might say that even the most impassioned advocates of unorthodox healing waged two battles—one against the hegemony of orthodox systems of knowledge production and the other against the hegemony of the unknown itself. The need to stanch the suffering visited upon their communities led patients to creatively engage that which they condemned, all in an effort to glean knowledge amidst uncertainty.[6] The historical account that emerges from this analysis is far less neat and ordered than enumerations of professional battles waged in the pages of competing medical journals. But then again, life is seldom as carefully curated as in professional journals.

This exploration of everyday forms of resistance furthermore demonstrates that individuals' hybridizations of healing systems have been motivated by more than those systems' etiological models or therapeutic nostrums. Many PWAs explored alternative healing systems due to frustration with how biomedicine framed and discussed AIDS. Some, for example, inveighed against universal fatality narratives, arguing that they were innately disempowering. This belief, in turn, motivated unorthodox healing approaches, with advocates of Louise Hay and the AIDS Mastery maintaining that psychoemotional stressors could, themselves, contribute to AIDS. Even seemingly innocuous issues such as healers' designation of AIDS as an infectious or chronic disease became contested facets of narrative construction. For these terms communicated messages of desperation or hope, thus influencing individuals' migrations within the healthcare borderlands.

The histories of the PWAC and HEAL also counsel scholars to look anew at patients' conceptualizations of personal responsibility for health and disease, demonstrating that PWAs engaged in a complex reinterpretation of responsibility facilitated by the term's multiple meanings. When conservative factions argued that gay men with AIDS incurred moral responsibility for their disease, some PWAs translated this moral responsibility discourse into causal responsibility discourse. Some among them further translated notions of etiological responsibility into paradigms of therapeutic responsibility, claiming a responsibility for effecting their own treatment through engagement with alternative healing systems. Thus, in moving between and hybridizing different healing systems, some PWAs may have been partaking in more than therapeutic experimentation; they may have been engaging in secular acts of atonement facilitated by the multiple meanings of responsibility.[7]

Even as we identify acts of empowerment effected by individuals facing disease, so too must we recognize limits to that power. For patients do not act as absolute free agents charting courses through the healthcare borderland. The paths they take are influenced by numerous constraining variables. Socioeconomic status, for example, likely plays a role in facilitating individuals' abilities to experiment with healing strategies.[8] Future research is needed in this arena, particularly for groups whose memberships differ from the PWAC and HEAL.

I have argued that the everyday forms of resistance effected by queer communities through the mid-twentieth century helped facilitate unorthodox expressions of health resistance in the setting of AIDS. Future research should investigate whether other groups, such as African American communities, have adapted and translated resistance strategies in this way. What is clear is that members of the African American community affected by AIDS did indeed engage in everyday forms of resistance expressed through their migration in the healthcare borderlands. Even the archives of the relatively homogenous PWAC and HEAL reveal such migrations.

Other sources offer additional advice of these migrations. In the 1991 volume *Brother to Brother: New Writings by Black Gay Men*, for example, African American PWA and poet Craig G. Harris memorializes a recently departed PWA, explaining, "he swore no virus would beat him / armed with rose quartz and amethyst / homeopathic remedies / Louise Hay tapes / and the best doctors / at San Francisco General." The man, we are told, fought AIDS valiantly, "like a copperhead going / against a mongoose." When he died, Harris tells us that his friends prepared his death bed with crystal shields and thoughts of Icarus, the mythical hero who famously flew too close to the sun.

As scholars explore these rich engagements with unorthodox AIDS activism, we should heed the lessons revealed by the borderland model. For although, when viewed from one perspective, the young man in Harris's haunting poem was disempowered and desperate, from another he was a copperhead going against a mongoose. His fearless, furious life is the stuff of more than legend: it is the stuff of history.[9]

THE SOUNDS OF FURIOUS LIVING—LESSONS FOR THE PRACTICE OF PUBLIC HEALTH AND MEDICINE

Historians are lens makers, honing prisms through which society can come to better understand its past and present. Historians of medicine and health, moreover, offer a particular type of lens that may inform medical and public health policies. What lessons, then, can we glean from this analysis of unorthodox health activism?[10]

For one, it suggests that health professionals would do well to recognize that individuals do not always respect the borders delineating bounded systems of knowledge production. Just because we recognize the existence of formal schools of healing does not mean that patients responding to disease ally themselves with those systems. Inquiring into individuals' creative amalgamations of healing systems may encourage physicians to move beyond notions of noncompliance by focusing less on the distance patients stray from biomedical practice and more on the complex landscape of intersecting theories and practices they choose to explore.

Over the past forty years, progress has been made in this arena, particularly in mainstream medicine's embrace of complementary medicine. By calling health modalities complementary, these physicians sought to link them to mainstream practices, thereby suggesting a synergy between different healing systems. While an important sign of professional and institutional flexibility, we must be careful not to construe the existence of complementary health discourse as proof that mainstream medicine understands the expressions of power articulated by individuals in their migrations within the healthcare borderland. Cynics, for example, would maintain that the complementary health movement resembles historical efforts by regular physicians to subsume osteopathic practice into mainstream medicine. In this model, orthodox professionals welcome irregular health systems into their fold by subjecting them to the legitimizing tools of mainstream biomedicine (e.g., double blind clinical trials and epidemiological review.)[11] This process of accepting the unorthodox by way of the orthodox is not the chosen avenue through which all people, particularly those who distrust biomedicine's systems of knowledge production, amalgamate healing systems.

In addition, this volume may help physicians understand how their actions and inactions influence patient behavior. Consider, for example, the power imbued by the narratives clinicians utilize when discussing disease. Far too often, language becomes a tool wielded by biomedical professionals in the struggle to effect positive health outcomes. Such was the case, for example, when biomedical leaders portrayed AIDS as universally fatal to increase public concern and pressure for research funding. Painting AIDS as ineluctably fatal suggested that society was sacrificing those living with the disease; people who have lost faith in a health system's commitment to their healing have little reason to yoke themselves to it.

This analysis also suggests that health officials' proliferation of moral responsibility narratives may, through the translation of these narratives into causal responsibility discourse, motivate individuals' migration within the healthcare borderlands. If future research demonstrates that this translation of moral culpability narratives also applies in the context of other diseases, it demands consideration by those who design public health campaigns. For it would mean that health policies seeking to improve engagement with the healthcare system by shaming individuals may, in fact, engender opposite responses.

More broadly, *The Sounds of Furious Living* raises difficult questions regarding the proper aims of clinical and public health interventions and the relationship between health and patient empowerment. In many cases, PWA self-empowerment led individuals to eschew biomedically verified treatment regimens in favor of interventions later found to be ineffective. How, then, should health professionals reconcile expressions of empowerment born out of individuals' engagement with their healthcare with the disempowerment that results from their development of preventable disease?

On the surface, the relationship between health and power seems straightforward. Few, for example, would disagree that a society is empowered by virtue of the enactment of policies positively impacting the health of its members. Correspondingly, we grant that a society riddled with preventable disease is disempowered. Yet in this analysis of everyday forms of resistance, we find the expression of a different type of power. Here, power is manifest through individuals' direct engagement with their care—a power born out of praxis that brings them into contestation with orthodox norms. Whereas the first formulation assesses power as a function of a measurable outcome—the health status of individuals or communities—the second is more nebulous.

Imagine, for example, a society that decrees health by fiat, endorsing policies that coerce, stigmatize, and shame individuals with the goal of improving their health. Even if such a society achieved maximal health outcomes, few would conceive of it as one that truly empowers its members. Conversely, consider the community whose leaders warn of a coming epidemic, counseling its members to take precautionary measures to safeguard their health. If the community chooses to ignore these warnings and is decimated by a preventable disease, we may understandably ask whether its members were empowered in any meaningful sense of the word.

We need not limit our analysis to hypotheticals. Public health campaigns, for example, often utilize shame, stigma, and blame to motivate individuals into making healthy life choices—with such initiatives aimed at reducing tobacco use, obesity, and alcohol consumption, among other behaviors.[12] While such campaigns are a far cry from the society that decrees health by fiat, they raise analogous questions. If we value open and free engagement with health, then to what extent can tactics that emotionally coerce individuals to improve their health truly empower them?

Further, what of the community whose expressions of empowerment lead its members to ignore or resist state efforts to protect them from epidemics? Virtually this same issue arises among communities of "anti-vaxxers" who argue that the harms wrought through vaccines outweigh their benefits. If this pursuit of a direct engagement with healthcare leads people to make decisions that systematically endanger themselves through exposure to preventable disease, should we consider them empowered? The example of anti-vaxxers raises additional questions regarding society's obligation to defend the rights of others, for one person's decision to refuse vaccination impacts the greater community. These are more than academic questions, as evidence suggests that the anti-vaccination movement has grown in recent years, with vaccination rates correspondingly declining.[13]

While unorthodox AIDS activism did not influence as many people as the contemporary anti-vaccination movement, it very likely contributed to preventable deaths. As this analysis reveals, it changed the minds of people, be it PWAs who wrote into the PWAC and HEAL to say their publications encouraged them to refuse antiretroviral treatments or world leaders who invoked dissident perspectives to resist biomedical practice. Max Essex, for example, has impugned Peter Duesberg's brand of dissidence, calling him "the biggest disaster imposed on us."[14]

This underscores an important point: While I have endeavored to argue that unorthodox health activism is a legitimate topic of historical inquiry, this should not be taken to mean that such activism is always compatible with social norms. If anything, this analysis suggests that, by studying unorthodox health activism through an historical lens, we find ourselves faced with uncomfortable questions regarding those very norms and how precisely biomedicine ought to advance them. Is the aim of public health and medicine to improve people's health or to improve their engagement with their health? Furthermore, what exactly are the metrics by which we assess patient empowerment?

Research conducted in the second decade of the AIDS pandemic underscores the need for a more nuanced power analysis in public health and clinical practice. In 1997, Meredith Smith and colleagues examined reasons underlying PWAs' failure to adhere to treatment regimens utilizing AZT (also known as zidovudine, or ZDV). Their analysis of the literature paints a startling image: "Among individuals offered ZDV, those accepting it have been shown to view: the drug as being highly beneficial to their health, be highly susceptible to other people's opinions, and possess great confidence in the ability of 'powerful others' to affect health outcomes. In contrast, those declining ZDV have been shown to be: highly internally motivated; concerned with possible disruption of their current lifestyle; fearful of potential ZDV-related side effects or toxicity; resentful of ZDV distribution and pricing policies; and likely to deny having any need for treatment."[15] How should health professionals interpret the power differential between the "highly susceptible" individuals who accepted ZDV and the "highly internally motivated" ones who refused it? How should they reconcile this data with the verified benefits of ZDV, particularly following dosage reductions in the early 1990s? What does it mean, in short, to empower people to take ownership over their health?

In 1986, PWA Bob Carver Jr. penned a poem that appeared in a collection of works copublished by Northern Lights Alternatives, the creators of the unorthodox AIDS Mastery Workshop. In it, he speaks of PWAs fighting to survive, with each breath marking a victory, even if the end of their battles brought death. For

Carver, these PWAs were forgotten heroes: "No laurel makes their temple bright / None honor them on bended knee / They lived and die in infamy / Alone and solaced of the night."[16] By shining a light on these individuals, we illuminate a complex world defined by lives lived furiously and lost prematurely. Furthermore, in studying their activism, we do not endorse its every expression as compatible with societal norms. Rather, it is by studying it that we better understand, interrogate, and clarify those norms. Indeed, unorthodox health activism may teach us a great deal about what our society aspires to be. It shall fall to those who claim a part in the study of the history of health and disease, and those tasked with safeguarding the health of populations, to heed its lessons.

UNORTHODOX HEALTH ACTIVISM AND TWENTY-FIRST-CENTURY PANDEMICS: COVID-19

It is difficult to examine unorthodox activism arising in response to one of the twentieth century's last major pandemics without calling to mind public responses to one of the twenty-first-century's first pandemics. SARS-CoV-2 and HIV are very different viruses, the former transmitted through casual contact whereas the latter is not. Yet just as COVID-19 has restructured virtually all aspects of society, so too has it posed important questions regarding the limits of individual empowerment in the setting of infectious disease.

We find expressions of unorthodox COVID-19 activism in virtually every part of the world. Such engagement is often characterized in the scientific literature as examples of complementary medicine.[17] While this framing captures the syncretic nature of healthcare decision making, it simplifies the complex—and at times fraught—relationship between mainstream medicine and unorthodox health systems. Consider, for example, the case of a purported COVID-19 tonic developed in Madagascar and touted by several world leaders. Biomedical professionals warned that widespread use of the drug, which was derived from the same sweet wormwood plant used to develop an antimalarial agent, could contribute to the proliferation of drug-resistant malaria. Yet the alternative therapy developed a following among communities distrustful of Western biomedicine. As a 2020 *Science* article noted, "The embrace of an 'African' therapy for COVID-19 comes amid a climate of deep distrust of Western medical science in parts of African societies. Press stories frequently warn about experimental treatments being tested on hapless Africans; in March, a media storm erupted after French scientists suggested a coronavirus vaccine could be trialed on the continent."[18]

Furthermore, unorthodox COVID-19 activism is not limited to patient use of alternative treatments. It also influences people's conceptualization of the etiology of COVID-19 and the risk SARS-CoV-2 poses. Some Americans, for example, deny the pandemic's existence entirely while others believe that biomedical leaders "oversold" the science.[19] As Michael Gerson writes in a 2022 *Washington Post* article, "[M]ost Americans still float down covid river, living in denial of the rocks ahead: new variants, long covid, continuing deaths. Who would have predicted that so many people's response to an existential crisis should be folk cures and complacency?"[20]

Some scholars have warned that society's response to COVID-19 is symptomatic of a deeper anti-intellectual movement that critiques the authority of elite institutions of knowledge production. Such anti-intellectualism intersects many of the same historical currents that have attended the proliferation of unorthodox health activism throughout U.S. history—particularly anti-authoritarian currents. These sentiments found an advocate in U.S. President Donald Trump who, at various times, denied public health officials' analyses of COVID-19, dismissed its severity, offered divergent interpretations of epidemiological data, contradicted scientific recommendations regarding public safety measures, and suggested the benefits of unproven treatment modalities.[21] In some cases, Trump articulated these views while standing just feet away from public health leaders such as Anthony Fauci, who began his career helping to manage the U.S. response to AIDS. As the pandemic raged on, tensions between the President and his scientific advisors intensified.[22] In 2020, the Union of Concerned Scientists issued a stark warning regarding attacks on scientific expertise: "The Trump Administration's unprecedented attacks on science highlight an urgent need for the next president to restore integrity in science-based decision making. This administration has sidelined scientific guidance from experts inside and outside of agencies, directly censored scientists, suppressed federal scientific reports, and created a chilling environment that has demoralized federal scientists and led to self-censorship of their work."[23]

In addition to these anti-authoritarian and anti-elite narratives, in COVID-19 we find the proliferation of antimodern discourse. These narratives glorify humankind's dynamic relationship with nature and suggest that the solution to COVID-19 is to be found not in public health restrictions or clinical remedies but in an embrace of "natural" processes. Popularized by opponents of vaccination policies and in direct opposition to mainstream biomedical knowledge, they argue that herd immunity will vanquish the pandemic, obviating the need for vaccines.[24] Others argue that COVID-19 lockdowns endanger our health by robbing us of "natural" exposure to immune system-enhancing pathogens.[25] Here, mainstream policies are framed as health-denying, iatrogenic exercises that produce harm by forestalling natural processes.

On occasion, critics also have questioned etiological models linking SARS-CoV-2 infection with COVID-19. In October 2020, for example, a protestor challenged the Deputy Prime Minister of New Zealand to prove that SARS-CoV-2 satisfies Koch's postulates. The Minister responded with exasperation, saying that such expressions of denialism were to be expected from Americans and not

New Zealanders.[26] More common are charges that SARS-CoV-2 was manufactured by researchers and introduced to populations either accidentally or intentionally, highlighting longstanding popular distrust in biomedical institutions.[27]

How do these historical musings inform our understanding of unorthodox COVID-19 activism? For one, they contextualize the complex etiology of U.S. resistance to biomedical authority. For as long as we have had "regular medicine," we have had resistance to it. That resistance has been propagated across time, buoyed by currents of antiheroism, antidogmatism, anti-authoritarianism, and antimodernism. The raw stuff of resistance is, therefore, woven through our history and culture, ingrained in our ideals, and propagated through the clouded perspective of collective, communal, and familial memory. Among communities wherein the specter of past abuse is felt most strongly, resistance to biomedicine likely flows most readily. For others, additional factors amplify the currents. In the case of both AIDS and COVID-19, U.S. Presidents have served as unorthodox amplifiers: Reagan through his absence of compassionate leadership and Trump through his ever-present promulgation of anti-elitist and unorthodox interpretations of the pandemic.[28]

Unorthodox COVID-19 activism also poses important questions regarding the limits of empowerment in the setting of public health emergencies—particularly those involving easily transmissible infectious diseases. If public health professionals hope to implement policies that will minimize the harm wrought through the embrace of unorthodox perspectives, we must develop a far more nuanced understanding of the behavior itself. Indeed, perhaps the greatest endorsement of unorthodox health activism would be to ignore it.

Finally, throughout this volume, I have argued that in examining individuals' embrace of unorthodox health systems, historians ought to shift our attention away from larger-than-life hucksters and quacks to instead focus on individuals making decisions in times of great uncertainty. Correspondingly, we ought to recognize that the decisions individuals make under the duress of disease are oftentimes expressions of agency. However, we may grant this point while also acknowledging that hucksters and quacks do indeed influence people's actions, and circumstances may exist wherein their influence undermines an individual's free choice. Consider, for example, a hypothetical scenario wherein a huckster is hegemonic, feeding an individual propaganda that fuels his own arguments while depriving her of alternative perspectives. In such a scenario, we may question the notion that the individual is freely choosing to adopt the huckster's views.

Some might argue that as we approach the close of the first quarter of the twenty-first century, the huckster has very nearly become hegemonic. They might hold that we are no longer the society reading the pages of the *PWAC Newsline* and amalgamating our own etiological and therapeutic models for disease. They might argue that we have become increasingly siloed, our perceptions of the world crafted by algorithms designed to reinforce our ideas and amplify our distrust of those with whom we disagree. They might maintain that each day, we interact with devices that purport to present a free marketplace of ideas but instead mine our psyche to prey upon our wants and fears.[29] These concerns ought to give historians and health professionals alike pause. For as virtual life and reality collapse into one another, virtual hegemonies become real ones. Those who believe that COVID-19 is a hoax, that it was manmade as a form of social control, or that it is best treated with unproven experimental therapies have those views reinforced in ways that not even the most charismatic nineteenth-century huckster could dream of concocting.

Not everyone agrees with such assessments of the echo chamber effect of modern-day social media. But evidence has emerged to support the theory, including one recent study investigating perspectives regarding COVID-19 among over 230,000 Twitter users. It found that, on the platform, "communication is not just falsely manipulated, but also hindered, by communication bubbles segregated by partisanship." Furthermore, information rarely travels in or out of echo chambers, particularly those defined by right-leaning beliefs.[30]

This debate suggests that any conceptualization of empowerment must recognize the importance of the free availability of ideas. For, in the setting of informational hegemonies, not every migration within the healthcare borderlands is a true expression of empowerment. We therefore require a power metric that is nuanced enough to differentiate free from manipulated movement but that is not itself rejected as an expression of orthodox power systems.

THE PROMISE AND PERIL OF FURIOUSLY LIVED LIVES: BEYOND HEALING

This chapter has focused on questions of lay empowerment in the context of healthcare decision-making, counseling scholars and health professionals to develop a more nuanced approach to examining expressions of empowerment deriving from individuals' engagement with their health. However, my analysis merely scratches the surface of a much larger issue, the reach of which extends beyond matters of health. For just as individuals command and express empowerment through their engagement with unorthodox healing systems, so too do they express shifting allegiances to unorthodox perspectives in disciplines as wide ranging as science, politics, history, and journalism. People, in short, engage with their world in a multiplicity of ways, and that engagement, at times, generates consternation on the part of those entrusted by society with ensuring its health, safety, and well-being.

We might consider, for example, the case of the individual who vehemently disagrees with claims—meticulously articulated and supported by scientists—that human activity has played a role in the warming of the planet. The easy response is to argue that such an individual is not truly informed. We may argue, for example, that she has been manipulated into rejecting mainstream scientists' pronouncements by political and industrial forces intent on maintaining the status quo. There is, indeed, evidence to support this claim, as the previous section's discussion of social media echo chambers underscores.[31] However, let us, for a moment, set aside the echo chamber and consider the person who fervently disputes our claim that she has been manipulated, who chronicles and indexes support for her ideas, demonstrating what Richard Hofstadter might characterize as an "almost touching concern with factuality."[32] This individual forces us to answer an uncomfortable question: To what extent may individuals legitimately derive power through the rejection of the codified systems of knowledge production society relies upon for the generation of truth—and for the implementation of policies premised upon that truth?

This issue cuts to the core of very real dilemmas, particularly as public distrust in the scientific process is at an all-time high. One recent Pew Research Poll found marked discord between lay and professional perspectives on a wide variety of scientific matters. Whereas 87 percent of scientists contend that humans contribute to global climate changes, only 50 percent of the lay public concur. Similarly, although 88 percent of scientists argue that genetically modified foods are safe for human consumption, a mere 37 percent of the public agrees. Even in the case of a topic many view as settled—the theory that humans descended from apes—we find a significant delta between scientific support for the principle (98%) and lay support (65%).[33] Assume, for a moment, that at least some of the individuals who disagree with these scientific principles freely engaged diverse perspectives before reaching their conclusions. Assume further that important policies turn upon the acceptance of these positions (a circumstance plainly true in the case of global warming). We thus are left with the same dilemma we encountered in our analysis of everyday expressions of health activism. Namely, to what extent would we say that the dissenters are empowered?

For some authors, these data point to a larger and deeper problem—a sign that society has entered a period defined by a glorification of obliviousness. A 2015 article in the *Washington Post*, for example, argued, "America risks drifting into a new Age of Ignorance. Even as science makes unparalleled advances in genomics to oceanography, science deniers are on the march—and they're winning hearts and minds more successfully than the academic experts whose work they deride and undermine."[34] How do we reconcile the individual who actively engages his world through the dissemination of contrarian ideas challenging orthodox systems of knowledge production? How do we compare him to the individual who absents himself entirely from any dialogue surrounding world events, but who acquiesces to the interpretations of events consistent with orthodox systems of knowledge production? To return to a familiar question, what is the metric of empowerment?

Work remains to be done before we can answer these questions. Historians must commit to further examining the avenues through which lay individuals have sought and attained empowerment in the case of healthcare decision-making and in other domains as well. The same level of analysis rendered in this volume is necessary for other expressions of contrarian resistance. In our analyses, we must seek to elucidate the variables that conspire to influence individuals' migration between orthodox and unorthodox positions, paying particular attention to the roles played by historically mediated resistance to orthodoxies. So, too, must we explore the structural constraints that limit individuals' migration between systems of knowledge production, including limitations in educational opportunity. It is only by employing the tools of social historical analysis in this way that we may understand how power operates among communities embracing contrarian and unorthodox perspectives. Furthermore, it is only with this understanding that we may hope to develop a morality of empowerment itself powerful enough to guide us through the turbulent waters we face.

ACKNOWLEDGMENTS

This book is derived from research I conducted while pursuing my PhD in Sociomedical Sciences from Columbia University. I would like to thank the members of my orals and dissertation committees, including Ronald Bayer, Merlin Chowkwanyun, James Colgrove, Amy Fairchild, Steven Mintz, and David Rosner in addition to Matthew Connelly and Mary Marshall Clark. Their mentorship and support were invaluable through all stages of my training and research. I also am grateful to Andrea Constancio, NiTanya Nedd, and Yasmin Davis for their help through my studies.

None of this research would have been possible were it not for the wisdom and kindness of the many archivists and librarians who aided me in my efforts, including Rich Wandel at the Lesbian, Gay, Bisexual, and Transgender Community Center Archives; Tal Nadan at the Brooke Russell Astor Reading Room for Rare Books and Manuscripts of the New York Public Library; and Hillary Dorsch Wong at Cornell University's Rare Books and Manuscripts Collection. So too must I thank the editors at Rutgers University Press, particularly Peter Mickulas, and the anonymous reviewers who provided feedback on my text. Last but certainly not least, I owe a note of most sincere thanks to my family, friends, colleagues, and peers who provided support and inspiration during the time I spent researching and drafting this book.

NOTES

INTRODUCTION

1. Jacqueline Thomason, "AIDS Organizations, U.S.," in *Encyclopedia of Lesbian and Gay Histories and Cultures, Volume II*, ed. George E. Haggerty (New York: Garland Publishing, Taylor & Francis Group, 2000), 50.
2. Observations made based on Internet search of "AIDS Activism 1990" using Google image archive, accessed February 8, 2015.
3. See, for example, Michael P. Brown, *RePlacing Citizenship: AIDS Activism and Radical Democracy* (New York: The Guilford Press, 1997) and Deborah B. Gould, *Moving Politics: Emotion and ACT UP's Fight Against AIDS* (Chicago: University of Chicago Press, 2009).
4. See, for example, Peter F. Cohen, "'All They Needed': AIDS, Consumption, and the Politics of Class," *Journal of the History of Sexuality* 8, no. 1 (July 1997).
5. James C. Scott, "Everyday Forms of Resistance," *Copenhagen Papers* 4, no. 1 (May 1989): 33.
6. A complete discussion of ACT UP's protest methodology is beyond the scope of this analysis. Interested readers may consult Brown, *RePlacing Citizenship*; Cohen, "'All They Needed'"; and Gould, *Moving Politics*.
7. I have chosen the descriptor "unorthodox" because it conveys variation from a norm while remaining relatively free from association with sectarian practices through history. The terms "alternative" and "irregular," for example, have their own complicated historiographical uses. However, the term is not without controversy. Some critics allege that it is pejorative, with at least one claiming that it is wielded as an insult to biomedicine by AIDS dissidents. See Jeanne Bergman, "The Cult of HIV Denialism," *Achieve: A Quarterly Journal on HIV Prevention, Treatment and Politics* (Spring 2010): 16.
8. We see this tension between unorthodox and mainstream AIDS activists within the structure of ACT UP itself. Many members of the group advocated a focus on "drugs into bodies" campaigns while others attempted, largely unsuccessfully, to direct the group's energies to the exploration of alternative and experimental therapies, such as Compound Q. See, for example, Gould, *Moving Politics*, 337.
9. See, for example, Dennis Altman, *AIDS in the Mind of America* (Garden City: Anchor, 1986); Ronald Bayer, *Private Acts, Social Consequences: AIDS and the Politics of Public Health* (New York: Free Press, 1989); Ronald Bayer and Gerald Oppenheimer, *AIDS Doctors: Voices from the Epidemic; An Oral History* (New York: Oxford University Press, 2002); Jennifer Brier, *Infectious Ideas: U.S. Political Responses to the AIDS Crisis* (Chapel Hill: University of North Carolina Press, 2009); Brown, *RePlacing Citizenship*; Susan M. Chambré, *Fighting for Our Lives: New York's AIDS Community and the Politics of Disease* (New Brunswick: Rutgers University Press, 2006); Cohen, "'All They Needed'"; Douglass Crimp, ed., *AIDS: Cultural Analysis, Cultural Activism* (Cambridge: MIT Press, 1988); Gould, *Moving Politics*; Elizabeth Fee and Daniel M. Fox, eds., *AIDS: The Burdens of History* (Berkeley: University of California Press, 1988); Elizabeth Fee and Daniel M. Fox, eds., *AIDS: The Making of a Chronic Disease* (Berkeley: University of California Press, 1991); Mirko D. Grmek, *History of AIDS: Emergence and Origin of a Modern Pandemic* (Princeton: Princeton University Press, 1993); David L. Kirp, *Learning by Heart: AIDS and Schoolchildren in America's Communities* (New Brunswick: Rutgers University Press, 1990); Marita Sturken, *Tangled Memories: The Vietnam War, the AIDS Epidemic, and the Politics of Remembering* (Berkeley: University of California Press,

1997); and Paula Treichler, *How to Have Theory in an Epidemic: Cultural Chronicles of AIDS* (Durham: Duke University Press, 1999).

10. Epstein explains that his volume is dedicated to analyzing "tendencies toward professionalization within social movements that engage with expert knowledge." Though he notes the existence of alternative health movements, they are not his primary focus. Steven Epstein, *Impure Science: AIDS, Activism, and the Politics of Knowledge* (Berkeley: University of California Press, 1996), 234. Emphasis removed. See also 41; in a 2017 article, Justin Abraham Linds articulates the need for further analysis of alternative avenues of AIDS activism. Using records from ACT UP's Alternative and Holistic Treatment committee, he analyzes efforts by PWAs to pursue the curative potential of microbes in the form of fermented foods. Justin Abraham Linds, "Ferments and the AIDS Virus: Interspecies Counter-Conduct in the History of AIDS," *Medical Humanities* 45, no. 4 (August 2019): 435–442.

11. This quote is from Mark Harrington, Cofounder of the Treatment Action Group (TAG). See Mark Harrington, "AIDS Activists and People with AIDS," in *Tactical Biopolitics: Art, Activism and Technoscience,* eds. Beatriz da Costa and Kavita Philip (Cambridge: MIT Press, 2008).

12. HCM Strategists, "Back to Basics: HIV/AIDS Advocacy as a Model for Catalyzing Change," 27, accessed November 17, 2016, http://hcmstrategists.com/wp-content/themes/hcmstrategists/docs/Back2Basics_HIV_AIDSAdvocacy.pdf.

13. As I note throughout this volume, this elision is not absolute, because some scholars, including Steven Epstein, Susan Chambré, and Martin Duberman, have contributed to our understanding of individuals and groups who played a part in unorthodox AIDS activism. However, to date, no research has examined the broader unorthodox AIDS activism movement or explored its historical roots.

14. Scott describes a similar phenomenon when he posits that a seemingly individual act of resistance—peasant desertion—has consequences for states attempting to conscript armies. Scott, "Everyday Forms of Resistance."

15. Naomi Abrahams, "Towards Reconceptualizing Political Action," *Sociological Inquiry* 62, no. 3 (July 1992): 327–347.

16. Deborah G. Martin, Susan Hanson, and Danielle Fontaine, "What Counts as Activism?: The Role of Individuals in Creating Change," *Women's Studies Quarterly* 35, no. 3/4 (Fall–Winter 2007): 78–94.

17. See, for example, Rhys H. Williams, "The Cultural Contexts of Collective Action: Constraints, Opportunities and the Symbolic Life of Social Movements," in *The Blackwell Companion to Social Movements,* eds. David A. Snow, Sarah A. Soule, and Hanspeter Kriesi (Malden, MA: Blackwell Publishing, 2004), 101.

18. David Rosner and Susan Reverby, eds., "Beyond the Great Doctors," in *Health Care in America* (Philadelphia: Temple University Press, 1979); Roy Porter, "The Patient's View: Doing Medical History from Below," *Theory and Society* 14, no. 2 (1985); Other authors who contributed to social historical analysis of health and health care include Nancy Tomes and Karen Buhler-Wilkerson.

19. As sociologist Cynthia Fuchs Epstein notes, "[R]eal people are quite capable of vastly contradictory behaviors and transformations that stem from different elements of themselves." Epstein advocates moving away from rigid interpretations of identity and instead toward models that recognize the "seeming paradoxes of 'odd combinations' of identity elements and subselves, even those 'mutually irreconcilable.'" Cynthia Fuchs Epstein, "The Multiple Realities of Sameness and Difference: Ideology and Practice," *Journal of Social Issues* 53, no. 2 (Summer 1997): 273.

20. As Richard Hofstadter writes, "One of the impressive things about paranoid literature is the contrast between its fantasied conclusions and the almost touching concern with factual-

ity it invariably shows." Richard Hofstadter, "The Paranoid Style in American Politics," *Harper's Magazine*, November 1964).

21. Michel Foucault, *Discipline and Punish: The Birth of the Prison* (New York: Pantheon Books, 1977); For a discussion of the micro-physics of power, see Robert S. Leib, "Spaces of the Self: Foucault and Goffman on the Micro-Physics of Discipline," *Philosophy Today* 61, no. 1 (Winter 2017): 189–210.

22. Some authors presume that dissidence began with or was defined by the pronouncements of rogue scientists, most notably University of California Berkeley retrovirologist Peter Duesberg. Seth C. Kalichman, for example, argues that, "In every respect, HIV denialism starts and ends with Peter Duesberg." See Seth C. Kalichman, *Denying AIDS: Conspiracy Theories, Pseudoscience, and Human Tragedy* (New York: Copernicus Press, 2009), 175. See also Bergman, "The Cult of HIV Denialism."

23. Harish Naraindas, Johannes Quack, and William S. Sax, "Introduction: Entangled Epistemes," in *Asymmetrical Conversations: Contestations, Circumventions, and the Blurring of Therapeutic Boundaries* (New York: Berghahn Books, 2014), 6.

24. For a discussion of subaltern history, see Dipesh Chakrabarty, "Minority Histories, Subaltern Pasts," *Postcolonial Studies* 1, no. 1 (February to March 1998).

25. Lindsay Abrams, "BBC Staff Ordered to Stop Giving Equal Airtime to Climate Deniers," *Salon*, July 16, 2014, https://www.salon.com/2014/07/06/bbc_staff_ordered_to_stop_giving_equal_air_time_to_climate_deniers/.

26. Numerous authors have defined and analyzed paternalism, with perhaps the most famous analysis provided by John Stuart Mill. A more straightforward definition, published at the height of the early AIDS pandemic, comes from Paul Turner Hershey, who argues, "An action, initiated by a human individual or group with regard to another human individual or group, is paternalistic if, and only if, (1) the action is primarily intended by the initiator to benefit the recipient, and (2) the recipient's consent or dissent is not a relevant consideration for the initiator." Paul Turner Hershey, "A Definition for Paternalism," *J Med Philos* 10, no. 2 (1985): 171–182.

27. Susan Chambré, *Fighting for Our Lives*; Martin Duberman, *Hold Tight Gently: Michael Callen, Essex Hemphill, and the Battlefield of AIDS* (New York: The New Press, 2016), 120.

28. HEAL's archives remain largely unexplored, having been stored by group members in various garages and closets for decades. Several archives house editions of the *PWAC Newsline*, a volume consulted in chapter 4. Sources cited throughout this volume are from the New York Public Library Manuscripts and Archives Division (NYPL-MAD), the Lesbian, Gay, Bisexual and Transgender Community Center National History Archive (LGBT-NHA), the New York Public Library, Science Industry and Business Branch (NYPL-SIB), and the Cornell University Library Rare and Manuscript (CUL-RMC).

PART I THE SOILS OF UNORTHODOXY

1. H. E. MacDermot, "Notes on the Early Editions of Osler's Textbook of Medicine," *Annals of Medical History* 6, no. 4 (May 1934): 224.

2. Harvey Cushing, *The Life of Sir William Osler* (Oxford: Clarendon Press, 1926), 349.

3. Robert L. Martensen, "Infections and Inequalities: The Modern Plagues," *The New England Journal of Medicine* 342 (May 2000): 1374. I do not mean to suggest that my use of the seed and soil metaphor is identical to Osler's, but rather that his use of it to describe an infectious disease informs this volume's analysis of a social movement that arose in response to an infectious disease.

CHAPTER 1 SITUATING UNORTHODOX AIDS ACTIVISM WITHIN THE HISTORY OF MEDICINE IN THE UNITED STATES

1. Allan M. Brandt, "AIDS in Historical Perspective: Four Lessons from the History of Sexually Transmitted Diseases," *American Journal of Public Health* 78, no. 4 (April 1988).
2. This discussion intersects debates regarding culture as an empowering and constraining force. See, for example, Ann Swidler, "Culture in Action: Symbols and Strategies," *American Sociological Review* 51, no. 2 (April 1986).
3. See, for example, Harish Naraindas, Johannes Quack, and William S. Sax, eds., *Asymmetrical Conversations: Contestations, Circumventions, and the Blurring of Therapeutic Boundaries* (New York: Berghahn, 2014). Here, in discussing hegemony, I borrow a formulation articulated by Sara Mills: "[H]egemony is a state within society whereby those who are dominated by others take on board the values and ideologies of those in power and accept them as their own; this leads to them accepting their position within the hierarchy as natural or for their own good." Sara Mills, *Michel Foucault* (New York: Routledge, 2003), 75.
4. Jayanta Mahapatra, *Relationship* (New York: The Greenfield Review Press, 1980), 10.
5. Mahapatra, 19.
6. This quote of Woolf's is a favorite of many historians. Virginia Woolf, *A Room of One's Own* (Oxford: Oxford University Press, 1998), 58.
7. Norman Gevitz, ed., "Three Perspectives on Unorthodox Medicine," in *Other Healers: Unorthodox Medicine in America* (Baltimore: Johns Hopkins University Press, 1988).
8. In a 1913 article in the *Journal of the American Medical Association*, physician John Benjamin Nichols wrote of his concern: "When . . . we contemplate the zeal, enthusiasm, and faith of the devotees of the pseudomedical sects; when we consider the large numbers of their adherents; when we appreciate that their following comes from the most reputable, most substantial and most intelligent sections of the community—from the better rather than the lower classes of society—then we should begin to realize that these popular beliefs are not the product of perversity or wickedness or ignorance, but result from powerful cause deeply rooted in human nature . . . we should look on medical sectarianism as a psychologic phenomenon presenting a definite scientific problem, and study its causes, nature and manifestations in precisely the same dispassionate way as we would investigate any other pathology condition." John Benjamin Nichols, "Medical Sectarianism," *Journal of the American Medical Association* IX, no. 5. (February 1913): 331.
9. For a discussion of this historiographic turn, see Geoff Eley, "Dilemmas and Challenges of Social History since the 1960s: What Comes after the Cultural Turn?" *South African Historical Journal* 60, no. 3 (2008); An early work in the history of alternative medicine whose approach was roughly consistent with this turn was Walter I. Wardwell, "The Reduction of Strain in a Marginal Social Role," *American Journal of Sociology* 61, no. 1 (July 1955).
10. Martin Kaufman notes that regular medicine's battles with homeopathy led to a shift away from heroic medical techniques such as bleeding and mercury. Martin Kaufman, *Homeopathy in America: The Rise and Fall of a Medical Heresy* (Baltimore: Johns Hopkins University Press, 1971); Susan Cayleff highlights the contributions hydropathy made in establishing a place for women in the practice of American medicine. Susan E. Cayleff, *Wash and Be Healed: The Water-Cure Movement and Women's Health* (Philadelphia: Temple University Press, 1991).
11. Robert C. Fuller, *Mesmerism and the American Cure of Souls* (Philadelphia: University of Pennsylvania Press, 1982); John S. Haller, Jr., *The History of American Homeopathy: From Rational Medicine to Holistic Health Care* (New Brunswick: Rutgers University Press, 2013); John S. Haller, Jr., *Kindly Medicine: History of Physio-Medicalism in America, 1836–1911*

(Kent, OH: Kent State University Press, 1997); John S. Haller, Jr., *Medical Protestants: The Eclectics in American Medicine, 1825–1939* (Carbondale: Southern Illinois University, 1994); John S. Haller Jr., *The People's Doctors: Samuel Thomson and the American Botanical Movement: 1790–1860* (Carbondale: Southern Illinois University Press, 2001); Kaufman, *Homeopathy in America*; Anne Taylor Kirschmann, *A Vital Force: Women in American Homeopathy* (New Brunswick: Rutgers University Press, 2004); Naomi Rogers, *An Alternative Path: The Making and Remaking of Hahnemann Medical College and Hospital of Philadelphia* (New Brunswick: Rutgers University Press, 1998); and James C. Whorton, *Nature Cures: The History of Alternative Medicine in America* (Oxford: Oxford University Press, 2002).

12. David Rosner and Susan M. Reverby, eds., "Beyond the Great Doctors," in *Health Care in America* (Philadelphia: Temple University Press, 1979); Roy Porter, "The Patient's View: Doing Medical History from Below," *Theory and Society* 14, no. 2 (March 1985).

13. See, for example, Nancy Tomes, *The Gospel of Germs: Men, Women and the Microbe in American Life* (Boston: Harvard University Press, 1999); Wendy Kline, *Bodies of Knowledge: Sexuality, Reproduction, and Women's Health in the Second Wave* (Chicago: University of Chicago Press, 2010).

14. Gloria Anzaldúa, *Borderlands: La Frontera, The New Mestiza* (San Francisco: Aunt Lute Books, 1987); Kelly Lytle Hernández, "Borderlands and the Future History of the American West," *Western Historical Quarterly* 42, no. 3 (Fall 2011).

15. The Oxford Learner's Dictionary defines fringe medicine as "any type of treatment which is not accepted by many people as being part of Western medicine, for example one using plants instead of artificial drugs." Thurstan B. Brewin writes, "[F]ringe is a crisp one syllable title, covering alternative, unconventional, complementary, natural and holistic . . ." Thurstan B. Brewin, "Logic and Magic in Mainstream and Fringe Medicine," *Journal of the Royal Society of Medicine* 86, no. 12 (December 1993), 721. In a separate piece, Brewin warns against "fraternizing with the fringe." Thurstan B. Brewin, "Fraternizing with Fringe Medicine," *British Journal of General Practice* 44, no. 383 (June 1994). See also Gina Kolata, "On Fringes of Health Care, Untested Therapies Thrive," *New York Times*, June 17, 1996.

16. Therapies studied included herbal medicine, massage, megavitamins, self-help groups, folk remedies, energy healing, and homeopathy. David Eisenberg et al., "Trends in Alternative Medicine Use in the United States, 1990–1997: Results of a Follow-up National Survey," *Journal of the American Medical Association* 280, no. 18 (1998): 1569–1575.

17. This statistic includes individuals who used prayer to treat disease; excluding this practice, over a third of all adults had still employed complementary or alternative healing methods, with the most common being natural products, breathing exercises, meditation, chiropractic care, yoga, massage, and diet-based therapies. See Patricia Barnes et al., "Complementary and Alternative Medicine Use among Adults: United States," *Advance Data from Vital and Health Statistics*. U.S. Department of Health and Human Services (May 2004): 1–19.

18. Institute of Medicine, Committee on the Use of Complementary and Alternative Medicine by the American Public, *Complementary and Alternative Medicine in the United States* (Washington, DC: National Academies Press, 2005), 34.

19. The history of the term "heroic medicine" is murky, with at least one scholar tracing it to the carnage of Civil War–era military hospitals. However, as the cited examples illustrate, the term predates the Civil War by at least a generation and generally carried a pejorative connotation. Nortin M. Hadler, *Worried Sick: A Prescription for Health in an Overtreated America* (Chapel Hill: University of North Carolina Press, 2008), 198.

20. William Fullerton Cumming, *Notes of a Wanderer in Search of Health: Through Italy, Egypt, Greece, Turkey, up the Danube, and Down the Rhine, Volume I* (London: Saunders and Otley, 1839); See also "Literary Register," *Tait's Edinburgh Magazine* VI (1839), 342.

21. The alternate spelling of R.A.C. pills here was likely a typographic error. The letters communicate the pills' ingredients: rhubarb, aloe, and calomel.
22. The physician author of the quoted section clarified that in attacking calomel, he meant no disrespect to the creator of R.A.C. pills, Professor John Esten Cooke: "I respect the Professor; at the same time I am convinced of his delusion." E. F. Bouchelle, "Practical Remarks on Congestive Fever," *Southern Medical and Surgical Journal* (June 1847), 358.
23. Ralph B. "Monty" Leonard, "The Calomel Rebellion," *Southern Medical Journal* 80, no. 5 (1987): 638.
24. James Whorton, *Nature Cures*, 32.
25. B.F.W. Stribling, "Fogyism," in *Poems for the Old and Young* (Beardstown, IL: L.U. Reavis, 1857), 68; While hydropathy and Thomsonian medicine did not employ high doses of toxic drugs such as calomel, their treatments were not always gentle. Thomson relied heavily upon lobelia, an herb affectionately referred to as "pukeweed" while hydropaths regularly submerged themselves in freezing water.
26. Mark Twain, *Tom Sawyer's Conspiracy*, 1897. See Mark Twain, *Huck Finn and Tom Sawyer among the Indians* (Berkeley: University of California Press, 2011), 157.
27. William Rothstein, *American Physicians in the Nineteenth Century: From Sects to Science* (Baltimore: Johns Hopkins University Press, 1972), 180–181.
28. C. W. Kellogg, "Calomel, Its Uses and Abuses," Read at Meeting of the San Joaquin Valley Medical Society (March 11, 1902). *Occidental Medical Times* XVI, no. 4 (1902).
29. See, for example, William Murray, *Rough Notes on Remedies*, 4th ed. (London: HK Lewis, 1901).
30. See David J. Hess, "CAM Cancer Therapies in Twentieth Century North America," in *The Politics of Healing: Histories of Alternative Medicine in Twentieth Century North America*, ed. Robert D. Johnston (New York: Routledge, 2004).
31. I highlight the perseverance of heroic discourse in the context of cancer because of the intersections between popular understanding of AIDS in the early-to-mid 1980s and cancer. The case of childhood autism is also interesting, because unorthodox activists have maintained, despite scientific evidence to the contrary, that mercury in vaccine preservatives plays a role in autism. See Dan Olmsted and Mark Blaxill, *The Age of Autism: Mercury, Medicine, and a Man-Made Epidemic* (New York: St. Martin's Griffin, 2011).
32. Gary Null and Robert Houston, "The Great Cancer Fraud," *Penthouse* (September 1979).
33. In commenting on dominant medical responses to cancer, one author noted, "[W]e [doctors] radiated, we lashed, burned, and poisoned." She went on to argue, "I think we'll look back on this era and think we were totally crazy that we did these barbaric things." Amy Sue Bix, "Engendering Alternatives," in *The Politics of Healing: Histories of Alternative Medicine in Twentieth-Century North America*, ed. Robert D. Johnston (New York: Routledge, 2004), 161; Susan Sontag's essays furthermore underscore the frequency with which metaphors present mainstream treatments as dangerous. In summarizing lay framings of cancer, for example, she noted that "patients are 'bombarded' with toxic rays" and "chemotherapy is chemical warfare, using poisons." Susan Sontag, *Illness as Metaphor and AIDS and Its Metaphors* (New York: Picador, 2001), 65. Sontag's earlier essay was published as *Illness as Metaphor* (New York: Farrar, Straus and Giroux, 1978).
34. Some authors were direct in linking critiques of biomedical responses to AIDS with historic instances of heroic medicine. Consider, for example, the reflections of South African AIDS denialist Anthony Brink: "It took four centuries before medicine finally recognised that calomel (mercurous chloride) couldn't cure, only kill, and dumped it from its pharmacopoeia. Until then, notwithstanding its manifest poisonousness, doctors had advocated it, some with poetic fervour, as a panacea for gout, headache, menstrual pain, syphilis, and no

end of other ailments. No modern doctor . . . would dream of ladling mercury salts down their patients' throats nowadays. When is the penny going to drop with AZT?" Anthony Brink, "AZT and Heavenly Remedies" (1999), accessed March 20, 2015, http://www.virusmyth.com/aids/hiv/abazt2.htm.

35. Richard H. Shryock, "Empiricism Versus Rationalism in American Medicine," *Proceedings of the American Antiquarian Society* 79, no. 1 (1969).

36. Shyrock, "Empiricism," 105.

37. "Proceedings of the Meeting," *Report of the Third Meeting of the British Association for the Advancement of Science* (London: John Murray, 1834), xxii.

38. One 1883 medical journal noted, "[L]et us note that the word empiricism is a much abused word among physicians who deny that they are empiricists. The word means experiment, or a conclusion derived from trial. Empiricism is, therefore, a word which covers in its meaning the expressive basis of the foundation of all sciences—even medical science." The author goes on to decry that empiricism had become besmirched in its association with "quackery." Romaine J. Curtiss, "Medical Empiricism, Homeopathy and Codes," *Western Lancet* XII, no. 8 (1883): 352.

39. Richard Shryock argues, "Galen, in comparing the two schools, invoked a plague on both their houses since in the end both commonly used the same remedies." He added: "since empiricism is attacked by some dogmatists as . . . unscientific, while again the empiricists attack rationalism as being plausible but not true, the result is . . . [an] argument . . . elaborated at great length as they refute and defend each other in great detail." Shryock, "Empiricism," 101.

40. Owen Whooley, *Knowledge in the Time of Cholera: The Struggle over American Medicine in the Nineteenth Century* (Chicago: University of Chicago Press, 2013), 79.

41. Roberta Bivins notes that Hahnemann added one caveat: "unless he is feigning illness." Roberta Bivins, *Alternative Medicine?: A History* (Oxford: Oxford University Press, 2007), 93.

42. T. A. Ashby, "Editorial," *Maryland Medical Journal* (December 12, 1885): 129.

43. Though they professed an openness to different clinical approaches, there remained one school of medicine for which many Eclectics could not hide their contempt: the regular school. The cited quote is from *The American Journal*, an Eclectic medical journal. "Editorial," *The American Medical Journal* XXV, no. 12 (1897): 569.

44. J. M. Taylor, "Antiseptic Surgery in Country Practice," *The Medical and Surgical Reporter* LIX, no. 23 (1888): 704.

45. Taylor, "Antiseptic Surgery," 705.

46. Taylor, "Antiseptic Surgery."

47. Taylor, "Antiseptic Surgery," 706.

48. Taylor would also critique the use of bichloride of mercury to kill germs, calling it "a most virulent poison." Taylor, "Antiseptic Surgery," 705.

49. Marcus Boon and Kate Hunter, "Dr Joseph A Sonnabend Takes a Look: An Interview," *PWA Coalition Newsline* 72 (December 1991): 28.

50. In the early 1980s, a debate waged between American and French researchers regarding the identity of the virus that causes AIDS. American researchers headed by Robert Gallo advocated a role for the HTLV-III, while French researchers headed by Luc Montagnier advocated a role for the lymphadenopathy associated virus (LAV). In 1986, the International Committee on the Taxonomy of Viruses settled the dispute, naming the causative agent the human immunodeficiency virus.

51. Michael Callen, "Why I Don't Believe that HIV is the Cause of AIDS and Why I Think It Matters at All," *PWA Coalition Newsline* 29 (December 1987), 35.

52. Callen is quoted in a letter written by a Mr. Schick. Mr. Schick, "Letter to the Editor," *PWA Coalition Newsline* 37 (October 1988), 13. The letter is almost certainly written by Rob

Schick, who would later become a regular columnist for the *Newsline*. Similarly, in 1988, Max Navarre, an editor of the *Newsline*, wrote, "The medical love affair with AZT is particularly alarming to those of us who remain unconvinced that HIV is 'the cause' of AIDS. Every time I hear HIV referred to as the 'AIDS virus,' my teeth start to grind." Max Navarre, "AIDS in '88—An Editorial," *PWA Coalition Newsline* 30 (January 1988), 16.

53. Michael A. Flannery, "The Early Botanical Medical Movement as a Reflection of Life, Liberty, and Literacy in Jacksonian America," *Journal of the Medical Library Association* 90, no. 4 (October 2002): 449.

54. Flannery, "The Early Botanical," 445.

55. Nadav Davidovitch, "Negotiating Dissent," in *The Politics of Healing: Histories of Alternative Medicine in Twentieth Century North America*, ed. Robert D. Johnston (New York: Routledge, 2004).

56. Mark Twain, "Remarks on Osteopathy," in *Mark Twain Speaking*, ed. Paul Fatout (Iowa City: University of Iowa Press, 1978), 384–388, 386.

57. See Anne Taylor Kirschmann, "Making Friends for 'Pure' Homeopathy," in *The Politics of Healing: Histories of Alternative Medicine in Twentieth Century North America*, ed. Robert D. Johnston (New York: Routledge, 2004).

58. The rise of bioethics was informed and influenced by several intersecting factors, including concerns with an increasingly technologized biomedical practice, harms posed by pharmaceutical agents, violations committed on the part of researchers and clinicians, and debates surrounding brain death. For a discussion of these topics, see David J. Rothman, *Strangers at the Bedside: A History of How Law and Bioethics Transformed Medical Decision Making* (New York: Basic Books, 1992) and Robert Baker, "Explaining the Birth of Bioethics, 1947–1999," in *Before Bioethics: A History of American Medical Ethics from the Colonial Period to the Bioethics Revolution* (Oxford: Oxford University, 2013), 274–318.

59. Lerner also cites as evidence of this tension a statement made by Franz Ingelfinger, editor of the *New England Journal of Medicine* and creator of the so-called "Ingelfinger rule" which stipulated that the journal would not publish findings that had been published in other journals or by other media outlets. In 1980, Ingelfinger declared, "a certain amount of authoritarianism, paternalism, and domination are the essence of the physician's effectiveness." Although Ingelfinger died shortly after the publication of this comment, the Ingelfinger rule influenced debates regarding AIDS activists' demands for access to scientific findings prior to publication. In 1991, the journal's editor wrote that the press' premature publication of unverified scientific claims regarding the use of cyclosporine and ribavirin to treat AIDS had violated the Ingelfinger rule, resulting in confusion and harm. Ingelfinger quoted in Barron H. Lerner, "From Careless Consumptives to Recalcitrant Patients: The Historical Construction of Noncompliance," *Social Science and Medicine* 45, no. 9 (1997): 1428.

60. This trend has, for the most part, continued with minor variations. Between the years 2010 and 2014, approximately 1700 articles including the term "autonomy" were published per year, compared with 4589 including "noncompliance." Figures calculated using PubMed's "Results by Year" feature, accessed March 21, 2015. PubMed.gov. U.S. National Library of Medicine, National Institutes of Health.

61. For a discussion of the creation of lay expertise in response to AIDS, see Steven Epstein, *Impure Science: AIDS, Activism, and the Politics of Knowledge* (Berkeley: University of California Press, 1996).

62. Michel Foucault, "La Fonction Politique de l'intellectuel," in *Dits et Écrits*, Vol. II: 1976–1988, eds. Daniel Defert and Francois Ewald (Paris: Gallimard, 2001): 112; Colin Gordon, "The Political Function of the Intellectual," *Radical Philosophy*, 17 (Summer 1977): 13; Daniele Lorenzini, "What is a 'Regime of Truth'?" *Le Foucaldien* 1, no. 1 (Feb 2015): 1–5.

63. I locate the roots of antimodernity earlier than Lears's period of focus (1880–1994). T. J. Jackson Lears, *No Place of Grace: Antimodernism and the Transformation of American Culture, 1880–1920* (Chicago: University of Chicago Press, 1994).
64. Readers interested in a recounting of the rational foundations of Graham's system of health may consult Stephen Nissenbaum, *Sex, Diet and Debility in Jacksonian America: Sylvester Graham and Health Reform* (Chicago: The Dorsey Press, 1980).
65. While the vagaries of Graham's health system are largely forgotten, his name is still attached to a popular bread product: the Graham cracker. Nissenbaum, *Sex, Diet and Debility*, 7.
66. One can identify parallels between Graham's attack on the impersonal dimensions of modernity and Max Weber's theories. This relationship, however, is complex, for while Weber criticized the forces of capitalism, he also attacked asceticism commanded by Puritan teachings, which "descended like a frost" on civilization. See Robert Bocock, *Consumption* (New York: Routledge, 1993), 8; Nissenbaum, *Sex, Diet and Debility,* 135; Michael S. Goldstein, *Alternative Health Care: Medicine, Miracle, or Mirage?* (Philadelphia: Temple University Press, 1999), 139–141.
67. This formulation of disease was consistent with the "seed versus soil" arguments of the day. These metaphors were used to explain the preferential action of particles or germs (the seed) upon a body made susceptible by lifestyle or environmental conditions (the soil). Graham expanded upon such metaphors considerably. See Nissenbaum, *Sex, Diet and Debility,* 96.
68. Lears, *No Place of Grace,* 142.
69. White formed her own health institute headed by James Harvey Kellogg, whose beliefs shared much in common with Graham's.
70. Kirschmann, *A Vital Force,* 129.
71. Twain's testimony was published in multiple sources. One, the *World Review*, began with, "Mark Twain believes in liberty and wants every fellow given a free hand in his trial in the world." "Liberty in Healing," *The World Review* I (March 9–August 31, 1901).
72. The Emmanuel Movement was closely associated with the nascent field of psychotherapy. See Eric Caplan, *Mind Games: American Culture and the Birth of Psychotherapy* (Berkeley: University of California Press, 1998); see also Whorton, *Nature Cures,* 123.
73. Roy Porter, "Thomas Gisborne: Physicians, Christians and Gentlemen," in *Doctors and Ethics: The Earlier Historical Setting of Professional Ethics,* eds. Andrew Wear, Johanna Geyer-Kordesch, and Roger French (Atlanta: Rodopi, 1993), 267; See also Jonathan B. Imber, *Trusting Doctors: The Decline of Moral Authority in American Medicine* (Princeton: Princeton University Press, 2008), 219.
74. For a discussion of Mather's integration of religious and medical systems of thought, see Margaret Humphreys Warner, "Vindicating the Minister's Medical Role: Cotton Mather's Concept of the Nishmath-Chajim and the Spiritualization of Medicine," *Journal of the History of Medicine* 36, no. 3 (July 1981).
75. One interesting exception is Oliver Wendell Holmes. Discussing Mather's involvement in inoculation debates, Holmes wrote, "In 1721, [smallpox], after a respite of nineteen years, again appeared as an epidemic. In that year it was that Cotton Mather, browsing, as was his wont, on all the printed fodder that came within reach of his ever-grinding mandibles, came upon an account of inoculation as practised in Turkey, contained in the 'Philosophical Transactions.' He spoke of it to several physicians, who paid little heed to his story; for they knew his medical whims, and had probably been bored, as we say now-a-days, many of them, with listening to his 'Angel of Bethesda,' and satiated with his speculations on the Nishmath Chajim." See Oliver Wendell Holmes, *Medical Essays: 1842–1882* (Boston: Houghton, Mifflin and Company, 1883), 346.

76. See Whorton, *Nature Cures*, 58.
77. Hahnemann's description won homeopathy the endorsement of several influential individuals, including leading Transcendentalists. See Robert C. Fuller, *Alternative Medicine and American Religious Life* (Oxford: Oxford University Press, 1989), 25–26.
78. Robert Fuller has explicitly located several such awakenings in U.S. history, including during the period wherein Thomsonian, Grahamian, and homeopathic healing systems prospered. Fuller, *Alternative Medicine*, 19.
79. Imber, *Trusting Doctors*.
80. See, for example, Thomas Lawrence Long, *AIDS and American Apocalypticism: The Cultural Semiotics of an Epidemic* (Albany: State University of New York Press, 2005).
81. In documents produced in PWAC and HEAL literature, Callen noted that most long-term survivors of AIDS he had interviewed embraced alternative medicine alongside religious practices. Michael Callen's "7 Very Important Qualities" was printed in both HEALING AIDS (June 1988) and the HEAL Quarterly 1, no. 1 (Fall 1989).
82. The leader in question was Michael Ellner of Health Education AIDS Liaison (HEAL).
83. Anonymous, "The Family with AIDS," in *Surviving and Thriving with AIDS: Collected Wisdom, Volume II*, ed. Michael Callen (New York: People with AIDS Coalition, 1988): 180, emphasis in original.

CHAPTER 2 A BROKEN MODEL

1. This is not to say that scholars have failed to examine how societies conceive of disease over time. Charles Rosenberg, for example, has described four stages of the "pestilential drama." See Charles E. Rosenberg, *Explaining Epidemics: And Other Studies in the History of Medicine* (Cambridge: Cambridge University Press, 1992); see also Philip Strong, "The Pestilential Apocalypse: Modern, Postmodern and Early Modern Observations," in *Meddling with Mythology: AIDS and the Social Construction of Knowledge*, eds. Rosaline S. Barbour and Guro Huby (New York: Routledge, 1998).
2. In the early 2000s, researchers discovered that *Pneumocystis carinii* caused disease in rats while a separate strain of the fungus caused disease in humans. As a result, the scientific community began referring to the human pathogen as *Pneumocystis jirovecii*. This is the term in use today.
3. The article won the American National Association of Science Writers' Science-in-Society Award for 1985 and was reissued in a volume published by Picador and Pan Books in 1986. It begins with a chapter titled "Magna Mortalitas," a reference to the term written in fourteenth-century monastic chronicles to denote interruptions in transcriptions during the years of the bubonic plague. David Black, *The Plague Years: A Chronicle of AIDS, the Epidemic of Our Times* (New York: Simon and Schuster, 1986).
4. See, for example, the following *New York Times* articles: Vincent Canby, "Manhattan's Privileged and the Plague of AIDS," May 11, 1990, C16; Steven Erlanger, "A Plague Awaits," July 14, 1991, SM24; Jill Johnston, "Gay Politics Goes Mainstream," November 1, 1992, SM14; Clifford J. Levy, "Grief over AIDS Spurs Gifts to Neediest," January 14, 1993, B3. For other uses of the term, see Rodger Streitmatter, *From "Perverts" to "Fab Five": The Media's Changing Depiction of Gay Men and Lesbians* (New York: Routledge, 2009), 64; see also Antony A. Vass, *AIDS: A Plague in Us; A Social Perspective* (Cambridge: Venus Academica, 1986).
5. Sue Cross, "Jerry Falwell Calls AIDS a 'Gay Plague,'" *Washington Post*, July 6, 1983, B3; Norman Podhoretz, "AIDS Education Should be Truthful: The Disease is a 'Gay Plague,'" *Minneapolis Star Tribune*, November 2, 1987, 12A; *Charlotte Observer*, May 20, 1983; "'Gay plague' is epidemic in US," *Irish Times*, July 16, 1982, 7; Christine Doyle, "The Gay Plague," *Times of*

India, May 15, 1983; "Across Canada Gay Plague Confirmed," *Globe and Mail*, July 21, 1982, 9; "Alert over 'Gay Plague,'" *Daily Mirror*, May 2, 1983; "'Gay Plague' May Lead to Blood Ban on Homosexuals," *Daily Telegraph*, May 2, 1983; William Scobie, "'Gay Plague' Sets Off Panic," *The Observer*, June 26, 1983, 10.

6. Steven F. Kruger, "Medieval/Postmodern: HIV/AIDS and the Temporality of Crisis," in *Queering the Middle Ages*, eds. Glenn Burger and Steven F. Kruger (Minneapolis: University of Minnesota Press, 2001), 260. The term "plague" maintains a narrow, historically rooted connotation unlike words such as "epidemic." As Charles Rosenberg has argued, the latter once denoted discrete episodes of disease, but through the twentieth century, came to take on diffuse meanings. Consider, for example, discussions of the epidemics of substance use disorder and automobile accidents. Charles Rosenberg, *Explaining Epidemics and Other Studies in the History of Medicine*, 278–279.

7. The Los Angeles cartoon was published in the *Los Angeles Times* in 1986. See *AIDS: Plague or Panic?*, ed. Oliver Trager (New York: Facts on File, 1988); The London cartoon was created by Kevin Kallaugher and published in the *Sunday Telegram* circa 1992. For a presentation of this and other cartoons cited here, see *Cartooning AIDS around the World*, eds. Maury Forman and David Horsey (Dubuque, IA: Kendall Hunt, 1992).

8. Forman and Horsey, *Cartooning AIDS*.

9. Forman and Horsey, *Cartooning AIDS*.

10. Ed Rowe, *Homosexual Politics: Road to Ruin for America* (Washington, DC: Church League of America, 1984).

11. See Hans Johnston and William Eskridge, "The Legacy of Falwell's Bully Pulpit," *Washington Post*, May 19, 2007.

12. Fogel's description of a Fourth Great Awakening is not accepted by all scholars. See Robert William Fogel, *The Fourth Great Awakening and the Future of Egalitarianism* (Chicago: University of Chicago Press, 2002).

13. Compare Falwell's condemnations to those delivered by Reverend Edward Anderson, who in 1832 maintained that cholera was a "national scourge" sent by God in response to tyranny, licentiousness, discontent, infidelity, and pride. Edward Anderson, "The Plague Stayed," in the *Christian Guardian* (London: L.B. Seeley and Sons London, 1832), 259. Reprinted from sermon given March 21, 1832.

14. Randall Balmer, "C. Everett Koop and the Religious Right," *Christian Century*, March 6, 2013, https://www.christiancentury.org/blogs/archive/2013-03/c-everett-koop-and-religious-right.

15. In the article, Koop responds to the effects of stigma and prejudice on children with AIDS. "Ray Boys' Treatment Criticized," *Ocala Star Banner*, September 13, 1987; Larry Kramer also compared the public response to AIDS to medieval abuses: "And, once in [hospitals], patients are now more and more being treated like lepers as hospital staffs become increasingly worried that AIDS is infectious." See Larry Kramer, "1,112 and Counting," *New York Native*, March 14–27, 1983.

16. Allan M. Brandt, "AIDS in Historical Perspective: Four Lessons from the History of Sexually Transmitted Disease," *American Journal of Public Health* 78, no. 4 (April 1988): 367–371.

17. Guenter B. Risse, "Epidemics and History: Ecological Perspectives and Social Responses," in *AIDS: the Burdens of History*, eds. Elizabeth Fee and Daniel Fox (Berkeley: University of California Press, 1988), 55.

18. Fee and Fox also note that in locating AIDS within infectious disease narratives, they ignored structural issues of great significance to the lived experience of people with AIDS: "Because the history of visitations of plagues was the only history that appeared relevant to the new epidemic, most people ignored the alternative historical models that were available.

For example, most of those who used historical analogies avoided the most pertinent aspects of the histories of venereal disease and tuberculosis, emphasizing issues of surveillance and personal control policy and ignoring the problems of housing, long-term care, public education, and the financing of palliative care for people suffering from chronic infections." Elizabeth Fee and Daniel Fox, eds., "Introduction: The Contemporary Historiography of AIDS," in *AIDS: The Making of a Chronic Disease* (Berkeley: University of California Press, 1991), 3–4.

19. This reasoning calls to mind Foucault's argument that, "Knowledge linked to power, not only assumes the authority of 'the truth' but has the power to make itself true." Michel Foucault, *Discipline and Punish: The Birth of the Prison* (London: Tavistock, 1977), 27.

20. Heckler's announcement was widely reported. See, for example, Gerald N. Callahan, *Infection: The Uninvited Universe* (New York: St. Martin's Press, 2006), 222.

21. As one journalist wrote in 1992, "Because of Salk's reputation, people with HIV clamored for his vaccine when it was just a rumor. Once it became available, they scrambled to be included in the nine clinical trials offered nation-wide . . ." Mary Flannery, "From the Man Who Beat Polio: Jonas Salk's Aids Vaccine is being Tested Here," *Philadelphia Daily News*, July 8, 1992.

22. Ronald Bayer, "Public Health Policy and the AIDS Epidemic: An End to HIV Exceptionalism?," *New England Journal of Medicine* 324 (May 1991): 1502; Ron Bayer, "HIV Exceptionalism Revisited," *AIDS & Public Policy Journal* 9, no. 1 (1994): 16.

23. As Caroline Hannaway writes, "We also have to consider the general wisdom of how much the study of past epidemics helps in considering AIDS. Has society changed in ways that are going to make such a discussion irrelevant? We historians do not want to think that this is the case, but we should consider the questions." Caroline Hannaway, "Commentary on Workshop 1: Before AIDS: An Overview of Previous U.S. Epidemics to Clarify the Administrative, Scientific, and Social Responses to Mass Disease," in *AIDS and the Historian: Proceedings of a Conference at the National Institutes of Health 20–21 March 1989*, eds. Victoria A. Harden and Guenter B. Risse. NIH Publication no. 91–1584 (March 1991), 30.

24. From *The Prelude*, a piece Wordsworth began in 1798. It was published shortly after his death in 1850.

25. See, for example, Julia H. Smith and Alan Whiteside, "The History of AIDS Exceptionalism," *The Journal of the International AIDS Society* 13, no. 47 (December 2010).

26. Smith and Whiteside, "The History of AIDS Exceptionalism." See also Dennis Altman, "Legitimation through Disaster: AIDS and the Gay Movement," in *AIDS, The Burdens of History*, eds. Elizabeth Fee and Daniel Fox (Berkeley: University of California Press, 1988) and Rolf Rosenbrock et al., "The Normalization of AIDS in Western European Countries," *Social Science & Medicine* 50, no. 11 (June 2000): 1607–1629.

27. Throughout U.S. history, some anticontagionist measures have been protested on the grounds that they interfered with freedom, though in earlier iterations, the freedom invoked was often economic. Sylvia Noble Tesh, for example, has argued that anticontagionists "called quarantines ineffective and charged that closing ports was mere mindless bureaucracy. In sum, they argued against contagionism on the grounds that it was inconsistent with the ideals of progress, individualism, and freedom that guided the Industrial Revolution." Tesh refers to Ackerknecht's well-known research on the topic. Sylvia Noble Tesh, *Hidden Arguments: Political Ideology and Disease Prevention Policy* (New Brunswick: Rutgers, 1996), 16.

28. This quote comes from the *Annual Report of the New York City Department of Health* (1961), quoted in James Colgrove, *State of Immunity: The Politics of Vaccination in Twentieth Century America* (Berkeley: University of California Press, 2006), 155.

29. Jeff Goldsmith, "The Paradigm Shift: Transforming from an Acute to Chronic Care Model," *Decisions in Imaging Economics* (1990). Other authors used similar language. See, for example, Robert E. McKeown, "The Epidemiologic Transition: Changing Patterns of Mortality and Population Dynamics," *American Journal of Lifestyle Magazine* 3, no. 1 Suppl. (July 2009): 19S–26S; see also Peter Piot and Shah Ebrahim, "Prevention and Control of Chronic Diseases," *British Medical Journal* 341 (November 2010): c4865.

30. Nancy Tomes, "Epidemic Entertainments: Disease and Popular Culture in Early-Twentieth-Century America," *American Literary History* 14, no. 4 (Winter 2002): 631; Not even the memory of the great influenza pandemic of 1918–1920 seemed capable of altering this transition, a point historian Alfred Crosby underscores in deeming the outbreak "America's forgotten pandemic." See Alfred Crosby, *America's Forgotten Pandemic: The Influenza of 1918*, 2nd ed. (Cambridge: Cambridge University Press, 2003). Tomes disagrees with Crosby's larger argument but concedes that anxieties persisted in "muted and indirect form(s)." See Tomes, "Epidemic Entertainments," 649–650.

31. See Nancy Tomes, *The Gospel of Germs: Men, Women, and the Microbe in American Life* (Cambridge: Harvard University Press, 1999), 252–255.

32. Rebecca Culyba, "Classification and the Social Construction of Disease in Medical Systems: A Historical Comparison of Syphilis and HIV/AIDS in the United States," PhD diss., (Northwestern University, 2008), 65.

33. Culyba, "Classification." 65–66.

34. "Conquering the Chronic Disease," *Science News* 116, no. 17 (October 1979), 277–278.

35. The issues include environmental pollution, smoking, drug use, poverty, race relations, the Vietnam War, campus unrest, and inflation. G. Ray Funkhouser, "The Issues of the Sixties: An Exploratory Study in the Dynamics of Public Opinion," *The Public Opinion Quarterly* 37, no. 1 (1973): 66.

36. One might argue that this transformation in discourse, in part, led society to almost universally overlook infectious epidemics of the 1970s, such as the burden presented by hepatitis. To my knowledge, we still lack a thorough understanding of the history of hepatitis in the United States.

37. Goldsmith argues, "Society has been perversely rewarded for its defeat of the past's most threatening diseases. We added almost 30 years to life expectancy. That's the good news. The bad news is that we now die of even more horrible illnesses later in our lives. The eradication of infectious disease made it possible for us to die from heart disease, cancer and Alzheimer's." Goldsmith, "The Paradigm Shift," 13.

38. Rachel Carson, *Silent Spring* (Boston: Houghton Mifflin Company, 1962).

39. Michael Harrington, *The Other America: Poverty in the United States* (New York: Macmillan Publishers, 1962).

40. Boston Women's Health Collective, *Women and Their Bodies: A Course* (Boston: Boston Women's Health Collective, 1970; for discussions of the Love Canal tragedy, see "Time Bomb in Love Canal," *New York Times*, August 5, 1978, 18; Michael H. Brown, "Love Canal, USA," *New York Times*, January 21, 1979, SM 6.

41. For a discussion of Dubos's legacy, see Heather L. Van Epps, "René Dubos: Unearthing Antibiotics," *Journal of Experimental Medicine* 203, no. 2 (February 2006): 259 and Carol L. Moberg, "Friend of the Good Earth: René Dubos (1901–1982)," in *Launching the Antibiotic Era*, eds. Carol L. Moberg and Zanvil A. Cohn (New York: Rockefeller University Press, 1990).

42. René Dubos, *So Human an Animal: How We Are Shaped by Surroundings and Events* (New York: Scribner, 1968).

43. Dubos railed against the constant exposure of children to "pollutants, noise, ugliness and garbage in the streets," arguing, "This constant exposure conditions children to accept public squalor as the normal state of affairs and thereby handicaps them mentally at the beginning of their lives." Paul L. Montgomery, "René Dubos, Scientist and Writer, Dead," *New York Times*, February 21, 1982; in his 1973 essay, "On the Limitations of Modern Medicine," John Powles echoes many of Dubos's ideas. Further, he combines them with evolutionary arguments, maintaining that degenerative diseases such as heart disease and hypertension were diseases of maladaptation, arising "because our earlier evolution has left us genetically unsuited for life in an industrialized society." See John Powles, "On the Limitations of Modern Medicine," *Science, Medicine and Man* 1, no. 1 (1973): 8.

44. For a discussion of this topic, see Elliot G. Mishler, "Viewpoint: Critical Perspectives on the Biomedical Model," in *Social Contexts of Health, Illness and Patient Care* (Cambridge: University of Cambridge, 1981).

45. Dubos, *So Human an Animal.*

46. Charles Rosenberg, "The Tyranny of Diagnosis: Specific Entities and Individual Experience," *The Milbank Quarterly* 80, no. 2 (June 2002): 243.

47. For a discussion of the successes of medicine during this period, see Paul Starr, *The Social Transformation of American Medicine* (New York: Basic Books, 1982).

48. Vijay Kumar Yadavendu, *Shifting Paradigms in Public Health: From Holism to Individualism* (New York: Springer, 2013), 64–65.

49. Iago Galdston, ed. *Beyond the Germ Theory: The Roles of Deprivation and Stress in Health and Disease* (New York: Health Education Council, 1954).

50. George L. Engel, "The Need for a New Medical Model: A Challenge for Biomedicine," *Science* 196, no. 4286 (April 1977): 129–136; George L. Engel, "A Unified Concept of Health and Disease," *Perspectives in Biology and Medicine* 3, no. 4 (1960): 459–485.

51. Allan Brandt and Martha Gardner, "Antagonism and Accommodation: Interpreting the Relationship between Public Health and Medicine in the United States during the 20th Century," *American Journal of Public Health* 90, no. 5 (2000): 707–715.

52. John Ehrenreich, ed., "Introduction: The Cultural Crisis in Modern Medicine," in *The Cultural Crisis of Modern Medicine* (New York: Monthly Review Press, 1978), 13.

53. Simmering beneath the surface in Ehrenreich's analysis were postwar apprehensions regarding the unchecked powers of science in medicine—an apprehension that, as sociologist M. L. Tina Stevens has argued, helped motivate the birth of American bioethics. See M. L. Tina Stevens, *Bioethics in America: Origins and Cultural Politics* (Baltimore: Johns Hopkins University Press, 2000), 9.

54. Ehrenreich, "Introduction: The Cultural Crisis," 13.

55. Ehrenreich invokes McKeown's thesis, arguing that it had been explicated earlier by René Dubos. Others have noted that Dubos maintained positions like McKeown's, albeit without the wealth of demographic data McKeown would cite. See, for example. Peter Conrad, ed., "The Social Production of Disease and Illness," in *The Sociology of Health and Illness, Critical Perspectives* (Waltham, MA: Worth Publishers, 2009), 6. Later, scholars critiqued McKeown's reasoning. See, for example, James Colgrove, "The McKeown Thesis: A Historical Controversy and Its Enduring Influence," *American Journal of Public Health* 92, no. 5 (2002): 725–729.

56. Science historian Laura Otis has explored this relationship in detail, concluding, "bacteriology served imperialist ideology." Laura Otis, *Membranes: Metaphors of Invasion in Nineteenth-Century Literature, Science, and Politics* (Baltimore: Johns Hopkins University Press, 1999).

57. In a 1997 volume, Charles Rosenberg argued, "[I]f the presumed value-free rationality of science could help justify the West's moral superiority, then opposition to the Cold War implied a willingness to question the authority and social impact of science and the scientific community." Charles Rosenberg, *No Other Gods: On Science and American Social Thought*

(Baltimore: Johns Hopkins University Press, 1997), xii. Rosenberg also cites David A. Hollinger, "Science as a Weapon in *Kulturkampfe* in the United States during and after World War II," *Isis* 86, no. 3 (1995): 440–54.

58. See, for example, John H. Knowles, "The Responsibility of the Individual," *Daedalus* 106, no. 1 (1977): 58; Some authors resisted efforts to make structural inequities the responsibility of the individual. In 1981, Sylvia Noble Tesh argued, "[W]hat does it mean to hold the individual responsible for smoking when the government subsidizes tobacco farming, permits tax deductions for cigarette advertising and fails to use its taxing power as a disincentive to smoking? What does it mean to castigate the individual for poor eating habits when the public is inundated by advertisements for 'empty-calorie' fast foods and is reinforced in present patterns of consumption by federal farm policy?" Sylvia Noble Tesh, "Disease Causality and Politics," *Journal of Health Politics, Policy and Law* 6, no. 3 (1981): 379–380.

59. Knowles wrote, "The cost of sloth, gluttony, alcoholic intemperance, reckless driving, sexual frenzy, and smoking is now a national, and not an individual, responsibility. This is justified as individual freedom—but one man's freedom is another man's shackle in taxes and insurance premiums. I believe the idea of a 'right' to health should be replaced by the idea of an individual moral obligation to preserve one's own health—a public duty if you will." Knowles, "The Responsibility of the Individual," 59.

60. Knowles, "The Responsibility of the Individual," 58.

61. Foucault argues that prior to the mid-twentieth century, the state's involvement in protecting health flowed from a desire to maintain strength, the work force, the capacity to produce, and so on. As such, the goals of medicine were nationalistic. He argues that, after World War II and the adoption of the Beveridge Plan, "health was transformed into an object of State concern, not for the benefit of the State, but for the benefit of individuals." Michel Foucault, "The Crisis of Medicine or the Crisis of Antimedicine?," trans. Edgar C. Knowlton, Jr., William J. King, and Clare O'Farrell, (the first of three lectures on social medicine, Rio de Janeiro State University, Rio de Janeiro, Brazil, October 1974).

62. Robert Crawford, "Individual Responsibility and Health Politics in the 1970s," in *Health Care in America: Essays in Social History*, eds. Susan M. Reverby and David Rosner (Philadelphia: Temple University Press, 1979), 247–268. See also Robert Crawford, "You are Dangerous to Your Health: The Ideology and Politics of Victim Blaming," *International Journal of Health Services* 7, no. 4 (1977): 663–680.

63. See Anthony Weston, "On the Body in Medical Self-Care and Holistic Medicine," in *The Body in Medical Thought and Practice*, ed. Drew Leder (Dordrecht, Netherlands: Kluwer Academic Publishers, 1992), 69–84.

64. See, for example, the work of Engel, who developed the biopsychosocial model. Engel, "A Unified Concept," 459–485. See also Elliot G. Mishler, "Viewpoint: Critical Perspectives." Tesh additionally discusses the web-like nature of disease causality, reminding audiences that multicausal models were quite old, appearing in the works of John Stuart Mill." See Tesh, *Hidden Arguments*, citing John Stuart Mill, *A System of Logic, Ratiocinative and Inductive* (New York: Cambridge University Press, 1843).

65. Ehrenreich wrote, "Modern medicine has been largely based on: (a) the doctrine of specific etiology: each disease is caused by a specific cause; if the cause (e.g. a germ) is present, the person will get the disease, if it is not, he or she will not; and (b) the machine model of the body: the body is conceived of as a machine made up of a group of interacting physical (and chemical) parts; the functioning of these parts is independent of the mind of the organism. These doctrines have provided the underpinnings for much of the advance of scientific medicine. However, their limitations, even in dealing with infectious disease, have become more and more evident. Dubos, Selye, and others have stressed a multiple–cause model of disease,

in which body, mind, and environment (including, but not limited to, exogenous microorganisms) *interact* to produce disease or to cure it; they have called for the re-exploration of more holistic approaches to health and disease." Ehrenreich, "Introduction: The Cultural Crisis." See also Ehrenreich, "Introduction: The Cultural Crisis," 27; see also Ehrenreich, "Introduction: The Cultural Crisis," 14.

66. René Dubos, *Man, Medicine, and Environment* (New York: The New American Library, 1968), 85.

67. Marilynn Preston, "Mind-body Link and 'Heal Thyself' are New Medicine 'Miracle Drugs.'" *Chicago Tribune*, September 23, 1976, A3.

68. For a discussion of the complex and controversial use of "noble savage" imagery in alternative medicine movements, see Jane Marcellus, "Nervous Women and Noble Savages: The Romanticized 'Other' in Nineteenth-Century US Patent Medicine Advertising," *Journal of Popular Culture* 41, no. 5 (September 2008): 784–808.

69. See Weston, "On the Body."

70. The mid-to-late twentieth-century popularity of the holistic movement coincided with revitalized interest in biological homeostasis. Through the 1960s–1980s, many authors expressed interest in the work of Claude Bernard who, in the nineteenth century, had originated the theory of milieu interieur, which informed later views of homeostasis. Iago Galdston, for example, invoked Bernard to support his environmental stress-based model of disease. In 1980, Elsevier published a 600-page centenary tribute to Bernard. H. Parvez and S. Parvez, eds., *Advances in Experimental Medicine: A Centenary Tribute to Claude Bernard* (New York: Elsevier/North-Holland Biomedical Press, 1989); In 1984, the volume *Stress, Immunity and Aging* reinforced similar concepts. Its cover depicted a brain held in a vice grip bearing the labels "nutrition," "emotional stress," "environmental stress," and "aging." Lightning bolts extend from the brain, giving rise to immune system cells and antibodies. Edwin L. Cooper, ed., *Stress, Immunity and Aging* (New York: Marcel Dekker, 1984).

71. In particular, the movement resonated with the women's rights movement. See Amy Sue Bix, "Engendering Alternatives," in *The Politics of Healing: Histories of Alternative Medicine in Twentieth Century North America*, ed. Robert D. Johnston (New York: Routledge, 2004); Historian Mark Jackson has further argued that holistic etiological models resonated in the Cold War era as the world sought to find balance between major world powers. See Mark Jackson, *The Age of Stress: Science and the Search for Stability* (Oxford: Oxford University Press, 2013), 13.

72. James S. Gordon, "Holistic Medicine: Advances and Shortcomings," *Journal of Western Medicine* 136, no. 6 (June 1982): 546.

73. See, for example, Kurt Butler, *Consumer's Guide to Alternative Medicine* (New York: Prometheus Books, 1992). Butler specifically refers to chiropractors in this manner, but his work is marketed as a broad discussion of fringe practitioners, "health pornographers," and the "quackery mafia."

74. Preston, "Mind-body Link," A3.

75. Lewis Thomas, "On Magic in Medicine," *New England Journal of Medicine* 299, no. 9 (August 1978): 461–463.

76. Thomas, "On Magic in Medicine," 462.

77. Joel Gurin, "The Changing Medical Model," *University of California San Francisco Magazine* 1, no. 2 (1978): 11; Additionally, in his 1982 piece, James S. Gordon argues that holistic medical practitioners had begun to focus too much on the responsibility of the individual to act to maintain their health. Gordon, "Holistic Medicine," 548, 551; A similar sentiment appeared in U.K. and Irish papers. In a 1981 *Irish Times* article, for example, one author argued, "The paramedical and the medical are getting more united in this concept of responsibility, which is stressed by many unorthodox practitioners too." Ronit Lentin, "Choosing Not to be Sick," *Irish Times*, July 6, 1981, 10.

78. These overlaps are further registered in the 1970s and 1980s–era scholarship of Robert Crawford. As mentioned earlier, Crawford critiqued Knowlesian moralization narratives as ignoring structural sources of illness. So, too, was he critical of the health holism movement, arguing that it similarly located solutions to structural problems in individual behavior: "Nonetheless, holistic health appears to be burdened by the ideology of healthism [defined as the preoccupation with personal health as the primary focus for the definition and achievement of well-being]. Even though whole persons and their experience regain a new attention and multiple causation replaces the medical theory of specific etiology, and even though the mind-body dualism is renounced . . . the healthism formulation still situates the problem at the level of the individual mind and body." Robert Crawford, "Healthism and the Medicalization of Everyday Life," *International Journal of Health Services* 10, no. 3 (1980): 365–388, 374.

CHAPTER 3 A BROKEN TRUST

Epigraph: A modified version of this quote appears in Irving Kenneth Zola, "Medicine as an Institution of Social Control," *The Sociological Review* 20, no. 4 (April 1972): 500. Here, I use the original passage from C. S. Lewis, *The Abolition of Man* (Oxford: Oxford University Press, 1943).

1. John H. Knowles, "The Responsibility of the Individual," *Daedalus* 106, no. 1 (Winter 1977): 57–80, 58.

2. In a footnote to a 2007 volume, Charles Rosenberg writes, "Although it is conventional to see the bioethics movement as having its late-twentieth-century origins in Nuremberg, it is equally conventional to see it crystallizing as a self-conscious movement in the 1960s as in part a response to those social currents that produced a more general sensitivity to individual rights—of women, of prisoners of sexual and racial minorities—and of an antiauthoritarian skepticism toward credentialed expertise." Charles E. Rosenberg, *Our Present Complaint: American Medicine, Then and Now* (Baltimore: Johns Hopkins, 2007), 184, n10. Authors such as M. L. Tina Stevens, furthermore, link bioethics to the anti-authoritarian climate of the 1960s. M. L. Tina Stevens, *Bioethics in America: Origins and Cultural Politics* (Baltimore: Johns Hopkins University Press, 2000); For discussions of the factors that contributed to bioethics' rise, including concerns with technological development, the dangers of pharmaceutical agents, and discourse surrounding the definition of brain death, see Albert Jonsen, "A History of Bioethics as Discipline and Discourse," in *Bioethics: An Introduction to the History, Methods, and Practice*, 3rd ed., eds. Nancy S. Jecker et al. (Toronto: Jones and Bartlett Learning, 2012); David Rothman, *Strangers at the Bedside: A History of How Law and Bioethics Transformed Medical Decision Making* (New York: Basic Books, 1992); Robert Baker, "Explaining the Birth of Bioethics, 1947–1999," in *Before Bioethics: A History of American Medical Ethics from the Colonial Period to the Bioethics Revolution* (Oxford: Oxford University, 2013).

3. Rothman, *Strangers at the Bedside.*

4. Rothman describes bioethicists as, "Ph.D.s, often trained in philosophy, many with a Catholic background, who typically followed conventional life-styles, [who] may not have been personally comfortable with still more left-leaning, agnostic, and aggressive advocates committed to alternative life-styles." Rothman, *Strangers at the Bedside*, 245.

5. Rothman, *Strangers at the Bedside.*

6. For discussions of bioethics' contributions, see Rothman, *Strangers at the Bedside*; Stevens, *Bioethics in America*; Albert R. Jonsen, *The Birth of Bioethics* (Oxford: Oxford University Press, 2003); John H. Evans, *The History and Future of Bioethics: A Sociological View* (Oxford:

Oxford University Press, 2014); Wesley J. Smith, *Culture of Death: The Assault on Medical Ethics in America* (San Francisco: Encounter Books, 2000).

7. Chase Madar, "The People's Priest," *American Conservative* 9, no 2. (February 2010): 24–26.

8. Anthony Weston, "Toward a Social Critique of Bioethics," *Journal of Social Philosophy* 22, no. 2 (Fall 1991): 109–118.

9. Daniel Callahan, "Bioethics and Policy—a History," in *From Birth to Death and Bench to Clinic: The Hastings Center Bioethics Briefing Book for Journalists, Policymakers, and Campaigns*, ed. Mary Crowley (Garrison, NY: The Hastings Center, 2008), ix–x.

10. Arthur L. Caplan, "'Who Lost China?' A Foreshadowing of Today's Ideological Disputes in Bioethics," *Hastings Center Report* 35, no. 3 (May–June 2005): 13.

11. Christine Overall, "Reflections of a Sceptical Bioethicist," in *Philosophical Perspectives on Bioethics*, eds. L. Wayne Sumner and Joseph Boyle (Toronto: University of Toronto Press, 1996), 166–167; In the introduction to the inaugural issue of the *International Journal of Feminist Approaches to Bioethics*, Mary C. Rawlinson writes that many bioethicists dismissed the rise of feminist bioethics, arguing that feminists tackled issues already considered by mainstream bioethics or that their efforts constituted a special interest discipline centered upon women's health issues. Similarly, philosopher Laura M. Purdy has noted that, "Analyses sensitive to gender and other markers of disadvantage often have been rejected as uninteresting, bad scholarship, biased, ideological, or 'political,' thus having no place in a serious intellectual endeavor like bioethics." See Mary C. Rawlinson, "Introduction," *The International Journal of Feminist Bioethics* 1, no. 1 (Spring 2008), 1; Laura M. Purdy, "Good Bioethics Must Be Feminist (and Allied Liberationist) Bioethics," in *Philosophical Perspectives on Bioethics*, eds. L. Wayne Sumner and Joseph Boyle (Toronto: University of Toronto Press, 1996): 144.

12. Arthur W. Frank and Therese Jones, "Bioethics and the Later Foucault," *Journal of Medical Humanities* 24, no. 3/4 (December 2003): 184.

13. Bruce Jennings, "Biopower and the Liberationist Romance," *Hastings Center Report* 40, no. 4 (July–August 2010); Stevens describes bioethics as a "midwife" to biomedicine, while Michael McKinnie refers to it as an "affirmative institution." See Stevens, *Bioethics in America*, xiii and Michael McKinnie, "A Sympathy for Art: The Sentimental Economies of New Labour's Arts Policy," in *Blairism and the War of Persuasion: Labour's Passive Revolution*, eds. R. Johnson and D. L. Steinberg (London: Lawrence and Wishart, 2004). See also Stuart J. Murray and Dave Holmes, "Introduction: Towards a Critical Bioethics," in *Critical Interventions in the Ethics of Healthcare*, eds. Stuart J. Murray and Dave Holmes (Farnham, England: Ashgate, 2009), 2.

14. Medical sociologist Renee Fox raises many of these points. David Rothman dismisses her structural critiques, arguing that bioethicists transcended such problems by recognizing individuality across class. See Rothman, *Strangers at the Bedside*, 245. Yet this response ignores the ways in which autonomy and rights are constructed and operationalized among disempowered groups.

15. Several publications articulating a feminist critique of bioethics appeared throughout the 1990s. See, for example, Susan Sherwin, *No Longer Patient: Feminist Ethics and Health Care* (Philadelphia: Temple University Press, 1992); Helen Bequaert Holmes and Laura M. Purdy, eds., *Feminist Perspectives in Medical Ethics* (Indiana University Press, 1992); Susan Wolf, *Feminism and Bioethics: Beyond Reproduction* (Oxford: Oxford University Press, 1996); Rosemarie Putnam Tong, *Feminist Approaches to Bioethics: Theoretical Reflections and Practical Applications* (Abingdon, England: Routledge, 1996).

16. Stevens cites a 1972 Hastings Center Board of Directors meeting wherein those assembled "reached an informal conclusion: the institute should make an effort to elect more members with a pro-technology bias." Stevens, *Bioethics in America*, 61; For further discussion of

Stevens's work and a criticism of her conclusions, see Ruth Macklin, "The New Conservatives in Bioethics: Who Are They and What Do They Seek?" *Hastings Center Reports* 36, no. 1 (January–February 2006); For other discussions of the motives of bioethical practice, see Caplan, "Who Lost China?"; John Sexton, "The Hollowness of Radical Bioethics," *The New Atlantis: A Journal of Technology and Society* 40 (Fall 2013): 89–103; Stuart J. Youngner and Robert Arnold, "Who Will Watch the Watchers?" *Hastings Center Report* 32, no. 3 (May–June 2002): 21–22; Albert W. Dzur, *Democratic Professionalism: Citizen Participation and the Reconstruction of Professional Ethics, Identity and Practice* (University Park, PA: Pennsylvania State University, 2008), 212.

17. Albert R. Jonsen, "Beating up Bioethics," *Hastings Center Report* 31, no. 5 (September–October 2001): 42.

18. M. L. Tina Stevens, "Letters," *Hastings Center Report* (January–February 2002): 5.

19. Jonsen, "Beating up Bioethics," 44.

20. I suspect that critics branded Illich's work as polemical for two reasons. First, rather than communicating in the language of academic detachment, he spoke in outrage. Second, his target audience was the general public. As H. Jack Geiger writes, "The ultimate target of his blame is not the professionals but the rest of us—all of us, at once eager consumers and the passive slaves of industrialism, and, therefore, the willing participants in our own dehumanization. [Illich] wants us—the world's biggest medical-care users and spenders—to think about our implicit beliefs in salvation through science and immortality through medical care." H. Jack Geiger, "Medical Nemesis: The 20th Century's Leading Luddite Turns to Medicine," *New York Times*, May 2, 1976; See also Madar, "The People's Priest."

21. See, for example, Allan Parachini, "Medical Iconoclast Attacks the 'Holistic' Path," *Los Angeles Times*, April 15, 1986.

22. Otto H. Kahn, "Capital and Labor: A Fair Deal," *Pere Marquette Magazine*, November 26, 1919. The magazine published excerpts from an address Kahn gave before the Carnegie Institute in Pittsburgh, PA.

23. Louis C. Lasagna, ed. "Introduction," in *Controversies in Therapeutics* (Philadelphia: W. B. Saunders, 1980), 3.

24. John P. Morgan, "The Politics of Medication," in *Controversies in Therapeutics*, ed. Louis C. Lasagna (Philadelphia: W. B. Saunders, 1980), 16.

25. Morgan, "The Politics of Medication," 16–17.

26. Philip R. Lee, "America is an Overmedicated Society," in *Controversies in Therapeutics*, ed. Louis C. Lasagna (Philadelphia: W.B. Saunders, 1980), 4.

27. Lasagna, "Introduction," 3.

28. John M. Firestone, *Trends in Prescription Drug Prices* (Washington, DC: American Enterprise Institute for Public Policy Research, 1970).

29. Edward M. Brecher and Consumer Reports Editors, *Licit and Illicit Drugs: The Consumers Union Report on Narcotics, Stimulants, Depressants, Inhalants, Hallucinogens, and Marijuana—Including Caffeine, Nicotine and Alcohol* (Boston: Little Brown, 1973). Illich cites this report and Firestone, *Trends in Prescription Drug Prices* in Ivan Illich, *Medical Nemesis: The Expropriation of Health* (New York: Pantheon, 1976), 69.

30. Morton Mintz, *By Prescription Only: A Report on the Roles of the United States Food and Drug Administration. . . .* (Boston: Beacon Press, 1967). *By Prescription Only* was a revised publication of an earlier Mintz work, titled *The Therapeutic Nightmare* (Boston: Houghton Mifflin Co., 1965).

31. Illich, *Medical Nemesis*, 67.

32. Mintz, *By Prescription Only*, 107.

33. Mintz, *By Prescription Only*, 160.

34. Rachel Carson, *New York Times Book Review*, December 2, 1962, quoted in Mintz, *By Prescription Only*, xii.
35. As a 1963 article in the *Journal of New Drugs* explained, "If the thalidomide experience is to make a lasting contribution to drug safety, it will be through the recognition of the importance of the Dr. Kelseys to the nation's health. These are the people we need more of: trained and responsible scientists in government, in industry and in the profession." *Journal of New Drugs* 3 (1963): 149.
36. Barbara Seaman, *The Doctor's Case Against the Pill* (Alameda: Hunter House, 1995); In 1996, following the twenty-fifth anniversary republication of the volume, a *JAMA* review reflected, "This is a strange view and not particularly recommended." Carl J. Levinson, "The Doctor's Case Against the Pill," *JAMA* 272, no. 2 (July 1996): 165–166.
37. Planned Parenthood would later bemoan that the AMA refused the package inserts on the grounds that they undermined a doctor's relationship with "his" patients. See Planned Parenthood, "The Birth Control Pill: A History," accessed July 10, 2022, https://www.plannedparenthood.org/files/1514/3518/7100/Pill_History_FactSheet.pdf.; See also Judy Norsigian, "Our Bodies Ourselves and the Women's Health Movement in the United States: Some Reflections," *American Journal of Public Health* 109, no. 6 (May 2019): 844–846.
38. For the Health-PAC Bulletin Digital Archives, see http://www.healthpacbulletin.org.
39. National Women's Health Network. *DES (Diethylstilbestrol)*, (Washington, DC: 1980).
40. For a discussion of the tensions that can arise from activist traditions that seek to pursue structural reform while also empowering body knowledge, see Susan M. Reverby, "Feminism & Health," *Health and History* 4, no. 1 (2002): 5–19.
41. Loretta J. Ross and Rickie Solinger, *Reproductive Justice: A History* (Oakland: University of California Press, 2017).
42. See Charles B. Inlander, Lowell S. Levin, and Ed Weiner, *Medicine on Trial: The Appalling Story of Ineptitude, Malfeasance, Neglect and Arrogance* (New York: Prentice Hall Press, 1988), 123.
43. Mintz, *By Prescription Only*, 37.
44. In February of 1986, the U.S. Department of Justice issued a report wherein it noted the substantial rise in malpractice cases through the 1980s. While many causes of this increase are considered, of particular interest here were early-to-mid 1960s changes wherein the "twin pillars" upon which tort law had been based—deterrence and compensation—were rejected in favor of "more enlightened theories based largely on concepts of societal inductance and risk spreading." The report cites the New Jersey Supreme Court decision Beshada v. Johns-Manville Products Corp., 90 NJ 191, 447 A.2d 539 (1982) holding that, "[E]ven if the danger at issue was scientifically unknowable at the relevant time, defendants nonetheless were still liable for having failed to warn of an unknowable risk. As justification for its holding the Court relied heavily on risk spreading." U.S. Department of Justice, *Report of the Tort Policy Working Group on the Causes, Extent and Policy Implications of the Current Crisis in Insurance Availability and Affordability*, February 1986, 35–36, n23.
45. Sidney M. Wolfe, Christopher M. Coley, and the Health Research Group, *Pills That Don't Work: A Consumers' and Doctors' Guide to over 600 Prescription Drugs That Lack Evidence of Effectiveness* (New York: Farrar Straus Giroux, 1981), 1.
46. Wolfe, Coley, and the Health Research Group, *Pills That Don't Work*, 3.
47. Andrea Pawlyna, "Readers Learning more about 'Pills that Don't Work,'" *Baltimore Sun*, December 27, 1981; As Sidney Wolfe observed, many individuals wrote to the publisher asking to purchase two copies of the book, one for themselves and the other to educate their physicians. One letter read, "[P]lease forward a copy to our pediatrician at the following address, since $6 is cheaper than an office visit for an ineffective prescription." Allan Parachini, "A Prescription Dilemma: 'Pills that Don't Work,'" *Los Angeles Times*, February 20, 1981.

48. Joel Kaufman, *Over the Counter Pills that Don't Work* (New York: Pantheon Books, 1983).
49. In his 1980 text, Temin endorsed the "sacred right to self medication." As it happens, Peter Temin was the brother of Howard Temin who, in 1975, shared the Nobel Prize with David Baltimore and Renato Dulbecco for the discovery of reverse transcriptase, the enzyme that facilitates HIV's replication. Peter Temin, *Taking Your Medicine: Drug Regulation in the United States* (Cambridge: Harvard University Press, 1980).
50. Jackson reviewed Temin's work alongside *Pills that Don't Work* and found the latter to be the superior text. Charles O. Jackson, "A Difficult Pill to Swallow," *Reviews in American History* 9, no. 4 (December 1981): 516–520.
51. For a detailed analysis of the rise of overmedication discourse pertaining to psychotropic drugs, see Susan Lynn Speaker, "Too Many Pills: Patients, Physicians, and the Myth of Overmedication in America, 1955–1980," PhD diss., (University of Pennsylvania, 1992). Throughout my research, I have benefited from the various sources Speaker cites in her analysis.
52. See Nicolas Rasmussen, "America's First Amphetamine Epidemic 1929–1971," *American Journal of Public Health* 98, no. 6 (June 2008): 974–985.
53. Gerald L. Klerman, "Policy Issues on Provision of Mental Health Services in Primary Care Settings: A Federal View," in *Mental Health Services in General Health Care, Volume I: Conference Report* (Washington, DC: National Academy of Sciences, 1979), 39; Dextropropoxyphene, deemed by some to be "the worst drug in history," was later pulled from the market. See Allison Gandey, "Physicians Say Good Riddance to 'Worst Drug in History,'" *Medscape Medical News*, February 2, 2011.
54. See Peter E. Bohm, "Drug Addiction," in *Adult Psychopathology*, ed. Francis J. Turner (New York: Free Press, 1984): 447; During a congressional investigation of diazepam, Senator Ted quipped, "Thousands of Americans are hooked and don't even know it." Richard Lyons, "Beneficial Valium Can Also Prove to Be Bad Medicine," *New York Times* (September 16, 1979).
55. Lyons, "Beneficial Valium."
56. Peter Tyrer, "The Benzodiazepines Bonanza," *The Lancet* 304, no. 7882 (September 1974): 710; A similar claim appeared approximately a year earlier in another *Lancet* article. A. L. Macnair, "Benzodiazepines: Use, Overuse, Misuse, Abuse?" *The Lancet* 301, no. 7812 (June 1973): 1101.
57. While these concerns recapitulated earlier fears regarding 1950s-era anxiolytic drugs, the tenor of conversation was far more sensational. For an example of 1950s-era anxiety concerning tranquilizing drugs, see "Anti-Worry Pills Posing Great Peril," *Philadelphia Tribune*, February 26, 1957, 8.
58. Arthur Gordon, "Happiness Doesn't Come in Pills," *Reader's Digest*, January 1957: 60–62.
59. Leslie Farber, "Ours is the Addicted Society," *New York Times Magazine*, December 11, 1966. Quoted in Speaker, *Too Many Pills*, 46.
60. Barbara Mikulski, "Challenge I," in *Census Bureau Conference on Issues in Federal Statistical Needs Relating to Women: Research Papers Based on the 1978 Conference with Agency Responses*, ed. Barbara B. Reagan (Washington, DC: U.S. Department of Commerce Bureau of the Census, 1979), 115–119.
61. Betty Friedan, *The Feminine Mystique* (New York: W. W. Norton and Co., 1963); See also D. L. Herzberg, '"The Pill You Love Can Turn on You': Feminism, Tranquilizers, and the Valium Panic of the 1970s," *American Quarterly* 58, no. 1 (March 2006): 79–103.
62. Keith Richard and Mick Jagger, "Mother's Little Helper," The Rolling Stones, recorded July 2, 1966, track 1 on *Aftermath*. The song peaked at number eight on the Billboards Singles Charts in 1966. At the end of the song, the mother dies of an overdose.
63. Elliot B. Tapper, "Doctors on Display: The Evolution of Television's Doctors," *Baylor University Medical Center Proceedings* 23, no. 4 (October 2010): 393–399.

64. This is a jaw-dropping claim, which Speaker makes in the context of discussions of perceptions of overmedication in the 1960s and 1970s. To my knowledge, she does not discuss her methodology for calculating the figure. Speaker, "Too Many Pills," 53. Other authors noted a turn in the popular perceptions of physicians. In a 1982 article in *Science*, John C. Burnham analyzes postwar distrust in medicine, which he observes was motivated, in part, by critiques of "not only priestly pretension but technical performance." John C. Burnham, "American Medicine's Golden Age: What Happened to It?" *Science* 215, no. 4539 (March 1982): 1474–1479.
65. Jeremy A. Greene and Scott H. Podolsky, "Reform, Regulation and Pharmaceuticals—The Kefauver-Harris Amendments at 50," *New England Journal of Medicine* 367, no. 16 (October 2012): 1481–1483.
66. Humphrey presided over Senate hearings investigating the FDA's failure to comply with the Kefauver-Harris Amendment. A trained pharmacist, he had worked as a young man in his family's farmer drugstore, which had generated some acclaim for selling patent medications promising to cure the ailments of people and pigs alike.
67. Edgar Berman, *The Solid Gold Stethoscope* (New York: Macmillan, 1976). In 1980, a *Harper's Bazaar* article told readers, "It's quite probably that your physician is part of your problem." See Elizabeth Whelan and Margaret Sheridan, "The Prescribed Addiction," *Harper's Bazaar* (January 1980): 100–101, quoted in Speaker, "Too Many Pills," 53.
68. Berman was a controversial figure who famously asserted that women were unable to hold leadership positions due to their "raging hormonal imbalance." A self-declared chauvinist, his apologists would argue that his vitriol was satirical. See, for example, Judy Klemesrud, "A Surgeon and Author Explains His Chauvinism," *New York Times*, August 22, 1982.
69. Berman, *Solid Gold Stethoscope*, 160.
70. This interpretation of physician behavior is reminiscent of Pierre Bourdieu's conceptualization of habitus, which he describes as, "society written into the body, into the biological individual." One's habitus structures her perception of the world in profound ways. According to Wendy Wiegmann, as a result of the fit between one's habitus and the fields in which they exist, "individuals develop a 'common sense' of what is doable and thinkable (or unthinkable) within society, and perceive these as being self-evident and natural. This common sense is defined as the orthodox or doxa of the field. Anything outside of a particular way of acting is unorthodox, a challenge to the status quo, and assumed to be forbidden, even when the status quo is oppressive or detrimental to the individual." Applying this concept to physicians, one might argue that they have come to accept as orthodox a system of legitimation—the requisite provisioning of pharmacological agents—that, in some cases, undermines their autonomy and authority. See Pierre Bourdieu, *In Other Words: Essays Toward a Reflexive Sociology* (Redwood City, CA: Stanford University Press, 1990), 63; Wendy Wiegmann, "Habitus, Symbolic Violence, and Reflexivity: Applying Bourdieu's Theories to Social Work," *Journal of Sociology and Social Welfare* 44, no. 4 (December 2017): 95–116, 97.
71. Edmund Pellegrino, "Prescribing and Drug Ingestion: Symbols and Substances," Paper presented at the American Association for the Advancement of Science Annual Meeting, Boston, MA, February 18–24, 1976, quoted in Lee, "America is an Overmedicated Society," 6. As a bioethicist, Pellegrino was committed to articulating the virtues that defined medicine and underpinned the doctor-patient relationship. However, he had little stomach for attacks on the healthcare system he viewed as radical or destructive, frowning upon Illich's *Medical Nemesis*. For a discussion, see Robert J. Barnet, "Ivan Illich and the Nemesis of Medicine," *Medicine, Health Care and Philosophy* 6 (October 2003): 273–286.
72. Here, Muller cites an unpublished manuscript by Stuart Albert. See Charlotte Muller, "The Overmedicated Society: Forces in the Marketplace for Medical Care," *Science* 176, no. 4034 (May 1972): 490.

73. "Doctors Need Tranquilizers," *Science Newsletter*, March 15, 1960, 148. See also "Prescribing Called Doctor Disease," *Science Newsletter*, February 6, 1960, 89, quoted in Speaker, "Too Many Pills," 37.

74. While Freidson argued that this bias pervades standard practice, it was provoked and exacerbated by the work of "moral entrepreneurs"—physicians who strove "to create in the public mind profound pity and horror at [their] own specially chosen human failing." In his analysis, Freidson interrogates theories formulated earlier by Timothy J. Sheff. Eliot L. Freidson, *Profession of Medicine: A Study of the Sociology of Applied Knowledge* (New York: Dodd, Mead and Company, 1975): 253–256.

75. Freidson, *Profession of Medicine*, 257. Freidson cites Harry Bakwin, "Pseudodoxia Pediatrica," *New England Journal of Medicine* 232 (June 1945): 691–697; Some sixty years after the publication of Bakwin's tonsillectomy research, John Ayanian and Donald Berwick replicated the study. Invoking Freidson's "bias toward action" model, they confirmed an activist intervention for pediatricians assessing children for two common clinical and diagnostic interventions interventions: tympanostomy tube placements and radiographies. John Z. Ayanian and Donald M. Berwick, "Do Physicians Have a Bias toward Action? A Classic Study Revisited," *Medical Decision Making* 11, no. 3 (July–September 1991): 154–158.

76. Louise Lander, *Defective Medicine: Risk, Anger, and the Malpractice Crisis* (New York: Farrar, Straus, and Giroux, 1978), 38, quoted in Inlander, *Medicine on Trial*, 201; John Ehrenreich would later argue, "The picture of the medical system that emerges from Freidson's description is that of some vast, expansionist, and itself uncontrolled regulatory apparatus . . . The ranks of the 'sick' swell, but there is no way that this army of 'deviants' can turn against the social order; each marches to a separate drummer, and submits to his or her own medical 'management.'" John Ehrenreich, ed., "Introduction: The Cultural Crisis in Modern Medicine," in The Cultural Crisis of Modern Medicine (New York: Monthly Review Press, 1978), 47.

77. John C. Burnham cites an incendiary comment made by popular author Evelyn Barkins in 1952: "Most patients are as completely under the supposedly scientific yoke of modern medicine as any primitive savage is under the superstitious serfdom of a tribal witch doctor." See Burnham, "American Medicine's Golden Age," 1475.

78. Jacob Needleman, *The Way of the Physician* (New York: Harper & Row, 1985).

79. For discussion of the rise of medical malpractice suits, see J. C. Mohr, "American Medical Malpractice Litigation in Historical Perspective," *Journal of the American Medical Association* 283, no. 13 (April 2000): 1731–1737.

80. J. Reese Daniels, "A Noble Profession: A Retort to Our Critics within the Bar," *American Bar Association Journal* 43 (February 1957): 119.

81. *American Magazine* 158 (1954): 47.

82. Rosemary Stevens, *American Medicine and the Public Interest* (New Haven, CT: Yale University Press, 1971), 421–422.

83. Herman Somers and Anne Somers, "The Paradox of Medical Progress," *New England Journal of Medicine* 266 (June 1962): 1253–1258.

84. Maurice Leven, *The Incomes of Physicians: An Economic and Statistical Analysis* (Chicago: University of Chicago Press, 1932): 50, quoted in William Weinfeld, "Income of Physicians, 1929–1949," *Survey of Current Business* (U.S. Department of Commerce, 1951), 14.

85. Stevens, *American Medicine*, 421–422; Speaker (1992) echoes this sentiment: "[W]ith seeming abandon, physicians used new drugs, new procedures and diagnostic testing, increasing the cost of even basic health care. But beneath the bottom line of dollar costs, Americans, according to public opinion polls, complained just as much about the social price, that is, the growing complexity and impersonal nature of modern medicine. The growth of medical knowledge, technology and specialization, while enabling better treatment, also encouraged 'the fragmentation of the patient into body parts, each with its own practitioners.'" Speaker, "Too Many Pills," 111.

86. Berman, *Solid Gold Stethoscope*, 12.

87. Seymour Bernard Sarason, *Caring and Compassion in Clinical Practice* (London: Jason Aronson, 1977), 50–51. He discusses an original survey he published in Seymour Bernard Sarason, *Work, Aging, and Social Change: Professionals and the One-Life-One-Career Imperative* (New York: The Free Press 1977).

88. Shaw's reflections on medicine were cited approvingly in Michael G. Michaelson, "The Coming Medical War," *New York Times Review of Books*, July 1, 1971, 32–38; See also Lester S. King, "Shaw and the Doctors," *Journal of the American Medical Association* 209, no. 10 (September 1969): 1531 and Roger Boxill, *Shaw and the Doctors* (New York: Basic Books, 1969).

89. Ingelfinger's comment includes a parenthetical imagining the depths to which physician advertisements would descend, writing, "Consult Dr. Paracelsus! Rapid Service, Accurate Diagnosis and Up-to-Date Treatment! No rectal or vaginal examinations or other unpleasant procedures. Attractive male and female assistants. See our latest Diagnostorama. All for only $25.00!" F. J. Ingelfinger, "Deprofessionalizing the Profession," *New England Journal of Medicine* 294, no. 6 (February 1976): 334–335.

90. N. D. Tomycz, "A Profession Selling Out: Lamenting the Paradigm Shift in Physician Advertising," *Journal of Medical Ethics* 32, no. 1 (January 2006): 26, 26–28.

91. Tomycz, "A Profession Selling Out," 27.

92. Waldemar Kaempffert, "The Case for Planned Research," *American Mercury* 57 (1943): 557, quoted in John C. Burnham, "American Medicine's Golden Age: What Happened to It?" *Science* 215, no. 4539 (March 1982): 1475.

93. Bernard DeVoto, "The Easy Chair: Letter to a Family Doctor," *Harper's Magazine* (January 1, 1951). DeVoto later gained fame as an authority on Mark Twain, whose colorful opinions on medicine were cited earlier in this volume.

94. DeVoto, "The Easy Chair," 57.

95. DeVoto, "The Easy Chair."

96. Richard Carter, *The Doctor Business* (Garden City, NY: Doubleday, 1958). The author who heralded Carter's work was a 1965 *Consumer Reports* columnist. For discussion, see Burnham, "American Medicine's Golden Age," 1475–1476.

97. Richard Harris, *A Sacred Trust* (New York: New American Library, 1966).

98. The books Michaelson reviews are Boxill, *Shaw and the Doctors*; Selig Greenberg, *The Quality of Mercy: A Report on the Critical Condition of Hospital and Medical Care in America* (New York: Anthenium, 1971); Ed Cray, *In Failing Health: The Medical Crisis and the AMA* (Indianapolis: Bobbs-Merrill Company, 1971); Harris, *A Sacred Trust*; Carol Lopate, *Women in Medicine* (Baltimore: Johns Hopkins University Press, 1968); Lee Cogan, ed., *Negroes for Medicine* (Baltimore: Johns Hopkins University Press, 1967); John C. Norman, ed., *Medicine in the Ghetto* (New York: Appleton-Century-Crofts, 1969); Robert S. Daniels, *Higher Education and the Nation's Health Policies for Medical and Dental Education: A Special Report and Recommendations by the Carnegie Commission on Higher Education* (New York: McGraw-Hill, 1970); Barbara and John Ehrenreich, *The American Health Empire: Power, Profits, and Politics* (New York: Random House, 1971).

99. John Knowles would become embroiled in the AMA's campaign against social medicine. Early in his presidency, Richard Nixon sought to appoint Knowles as assistant secretary of health, education, and welfare for health and scientific affairs, but the AMA blocked the move through Senator Everett Dirkson due to Knowles's support of "comprehensive, prepaid health insurance" provided by the federal government. For a discussion of the topic, see Dean

Kotlowsky, "The Knowles Affair: Nixon's Self-Inflicted Wound," *Presidential Studies Quarterly* 30, no. 3 (2000): 443–463.

100. See, for example, Zola, "Medicine as an Institution."

101. Thomas Szasz, *The Myth of Mental Illness* (New York: Harper & Row, 1961); See also a collection of Szasz's essays: Thomas Szasz, *The Medicalization of Everyday Life* (Syracuse, NY: Syracuse University Press, 2007) and a review of his work by Jeffrey Poland, *Metapsychology Online Review* 12, no. 35 (2008).

102. Thomas Szasz, "Thomas S. Szasz Cybercenter for Liberty and Responsibility," accessed June 12, 2016. http://www.szasz.com/manifesto.html.

103. The authors cite figures published by Carter, *The Doctor Business*; See Boston Women's Health Collective, *Women and Their Bodies: A Course* (Boston: Boston Women's Health Collective, 1970): 183. This was the initial name of *Our Bodies, Ourselves*.

104. They inquire of the reader, "How many remunerative testectomies do you think are done?" Boston Women's Health Collective, *Women and Their Bodies*, 183.

105. Here, they cite Dan Cordtz, "Change Begins in the Doctor's Office," *Fortune*, January 1970, 84; Michaelson argued that "pregnancy and childbirth are now treated by male doctors as routine diseases; the medical hierarchy is exclusively male-dominated; many hysterectomies and even mastectomies are performed without sound medical reasons; labor is too often induced, especially in the case of poor and black women, by oxytocin—an unsafe procedure when unnecessarily done—so that the woman will deliver at the doctor's convenience." Michaelson, "The Coming Medical War"; Ehrenreich (1978) discussed similar issues, citing allegations of structural racism directed at orthodox medicine through the late 1960s and 1970s. Ehrenreich, "Introduction: The Cultural Crisis."

106. This discussion of biomedicine challenges the common perception that physicians enjoyed tremendous respect through the mid-to-late twentieth century. Critics may highlight opinion surveys indicating that members of the public rated physicians high on prestige indices. However, as William A. Gamson and Howard Schuman have argued, prestige surveys likely mask more complicated assessments of professionals by the public. They argue, "It is the very people who rank the occupation of physician at the top of the prestige hierarchy who tend to show relatively more hostility toward doctors when the questioning shifts to concrete matters of occupational performance . . . [A]mbivalence may be the characteristic attitude of those who accord them the highest prestige." They furthermore point to a 1922 study conducted by Jacob Feldman wherein "doctors were described as rapacious, pompous, arrogant, inconsiderate, and so on . . . at a time when . . . the medical profession was supposedly accorded nothing but deification by a grateful populace." William A. Gamson and Howard Schuman, "Some Undercurrents in the Prestige of Physicians," *American Journal of Sociology* 68, no. 4 (January 1963): 463–470.

107. Others writing in a similar vein, as identified by E. Richard Brown, include Barbara and John Ehrenreich; Irving Kenneth Zola; Howard Waitzkin and Barbara Waterman; Thomas Szasz; and Talcott Parsons. See E. Richard Brown, *Rockefeller Medicine Men: Medicine and Capitalism in America* (Berkeley: University of California Press, 1979): 270, n103.

108. One of Illich's paroxysms held that, "Among murderous institutional torts, only modern malnutrition injures more people than iatrogenic disease in its various manifestations." Illich, *Medical Nemesis*, 26.

109. Madar, "The People's Priest."

110. Madar, "The People's Priest."

111. There is disagreement regarding Illich's move to Puerto Rico, as there is about many aspects of his life. See Henry Cox, "Appreciation: A Prophet, a Teacher, a Realistic Dreamer,"

National Catholic Reporter, December 20, 2002; Todd Hartch, *The Prophet of Cuernavaca: Ivan Illich and the Crisis of the West* (Oxford: Oxford University Press, 2015).

112. Todd Hartch recounts Illich's time in Cuernavaca. The title of his book inspired the title of this section. Hartch, *The Prophet of Cuernavaca*, 2015.

113. Cox, "Appreciation."

114. Illich, *Medical Nemesis*, 42.

115. Madar, "People's Priest."

116. Illich, *Medical Nemesis*, 40.

117. Illich, *Medical Nemesis*, 78.

118. Richard Smith has argued that while we may conceive of social iatrogenesis as harm wrought through the medicalization of life, cultural iatrogenesis arises through the medicalization of death. Quoting Illich, Smith notes, "[O]urs is a morbid society, where 'through the medicalisation of death, health care has become a monolithic world religion . . . Society, acting through the medical system, decides when and after what indignities and mutilations [the patient] shall die . . . Health, or the autonomous power to cope, has been expropriated down to the last breath.'" See Richard Smith, "Limits to medicine. Medical Nemesis: The Expropriation of Health," *The Journal of Epidemiology and Community Health* 57, no. 12 (2004): 928.

119. Illich would call the disempowering biomedical jargon "bureaucratic gobbledegook." Illich, *Medical Nemesis*, 41. As a result of this process, both suffering and healing outside the traditional biomedical patient role were deemed deviant.

120. Illich wrote, "The medical and paramedical monopoly over hygienic methodology and technology is a glaring example of the political misuse of scientific achievement to strengthen industrial rather than personal growth. Such medicine is but a device to convince those who are sick and tired of society that it is they who are ill, impotent, and in need of technical repair." Illich, *Medical Nemesis*, 9.

121. Geiger, "Medical Nemesis," BR1.

122. Illich, *Medical Nemesis*, 33.

123. Illich, *Medical Nemesis*, 236.

124. Illich, *Medical Nemesis*, 4.

125. Illich, *Medical Nemesis*, 62; As Illich argues, "Deprofessionalization of medicine means the unmasking of the myth according to which technical progress demands the solution of human problems by the application of scientific principles, the myth of benefit through an increase in the specialization of labor, through multiplication of arcane manipulations, and the myth that increasing dependence of people on the right of access to impersonal institutions is better than trust in one another." Illich, *Medical Nemesis*, 256.

126. Madar, "The People's Priest."

127. Geiger, "Medical Nemesis."

128. Geiger, "Medical Nemesis."

129. Geiger argues, "There are echoes here of Rousseau's Noble Sage: the paradise we have lost was the one within us; it was whatever enabled us, on our own, to make life feel whole and coherent, even if painful. We have traded it in for compulsory survival in a planned and engineered hell, an anesthetized existence in a world turned into a hospital ward, a 'managed maintenance of life on high levels of sub-lethal illness.'" Geiger, "Medical Nemesis."

130. In 1985, Jacob Needleman wrote, "[T]he part of the human psyche that is most centrally involved in the cure of illness, namely the attention or will, is not understood in the contemporary era . . . Nowadays, the only patients who discover will-power in themselves are those who, through mere chance or through their own exceptional character development, see with objective horror both their own situation and the total helplessness of their doctors, and, having no taste whatever for self-deception, find that there is no place to go but 'up'—

that is, inside themselves, where they chance to find the existence of a truly higher psycho-psychical energy that carries them through either what is called a 'miraculous' cure or an honorable death." Needleman, *The Way of the Physician*, 138.

131. Smith, "Limits to Medicine," 928.

132. Lowell S. Levin, "Self-Medication: The Social Perspective," in *Self-Medication: The New Era, A Symposium*. Stouffer's National Center Hotel, Washington, DC: Proprietary Association, March 31, 1981, 44.

133. See, for example, James C. Whorton, *Nature Cures: The History of Alternative Medicine in America* (Oxford: Oxford University Press, 2002), chapter 11; David Kopacz, *Re-humanizing Medicine: A Holistic Framework for Transforming Your Self, Your Practice, and the Culture of Medicine* (Winchester, UK: Ayni Books, 2014); See also Parachini, "Medical Iconoclast."

134. Cox, "Appreciation," 2002.

135. Susan M. Chambré, *Fighting for Our Lives: New York's AIDS Community and the Politics of Disease* (New Brunswick: Rutgers University Press, 2006), 33–34.

136. Allan Parachini, "Medical Iconoclast"; Irving Kenneth also expressed similar concerns in 1972, writing, "The change of medicine's commitment from a specific etiological model of disease to a multi-causal one and the greater acceptance of the concepts of comprehensive medicine, psychosomatics, etc., have enormously expanded that which is or can be relevant to the understanding, treatment and even prevention of disease. Thus it is no longer necessary for the patient merely to divulge the symptoms of his body but also the symptoms of daily living, his habits and his worries." Zola, "Medicine as an Institution," 493.

137. The interview playfully places "necessarily" in parentheticals. Parachini, "Medical Iconoclast."

138. See Madar, "People's Priest"; See also a summary of Illich provided by his publisher, Marion Boyars, "Ivan Illich," accessed June 20, 2016, http://www.marionboyars.co.uk/AUTHORS/Ivan%20Illich.html.

PART II THE SEEDS OF UNORTHODOXY

1. Barbara Ehrenreich and John Ehrenreich, "Health for Profit: The Big Business of Health," *Health-PAC Bulletin* (November 1969), 2; Barbara Ehrenreich, *The American Health Empire: Power, Profits, and Politics; A Report from the Health Policy Advisory Center* (New York: Random House, 1971).

2. For further discussion, see Gina M. Bright, *Plague-Making and the AIDS Epidemic: A Story of Discrimination* (New York: Palgrave Macmillan, 2012). For a discussion of those authors who do engage these points, see the introduction and chapters 4 and 5.

3. AIDS activist Mark Heywood, for example, has argued that, with AIDS, "for the first time in history, 'patients' demanded their rights, and did so in a manner that fundamentally challenged public health systems and public policy processes." See Mark Heywood, "The Unravelling of the Human Rights Response to HIV and AIDS and Why It Happened: An Activists' [sic] Perspective," AIDS Alliance, 2, accessed June 20, 2016, http://www.aidsalliance.org/assets/000/001/014/ESSAY1_MarkHeywood_original.pdf?1412944701

CHAPTER 4 EVERYDAY UNORTHODOXIES AND THE PEOPLE WITH AIDS COALITION (PWAC)

1. Peter Staley, for example, says of AIDS that, "It was the very first time in history where a patient group, from an illness or disease, showed up and demanded to be heard, to the bureaucrats in Washington." Peter Staley and David France, "'How to Survive a Plague': As ACT UP Turns 25, New Film Chronicles History of AIDS Activism in U.S.," by Amy Goodman, *Democracy Now!* (March 23, 2012), accessed July 10, 2016, http://www.democracynow.org/2012/3/23/how_to_survive_a_plague_as

2. A die-in is a form of protest where individuals lay in place, simulating their deaths.

3. Steven Epstein notes that PWA activism was staged at the level of the body. In *Impure Science*, he quotes an introduction PWA Jim Eigo gave during a conference presentation: "We in the communities most touched by AIDS have learned that the ultimate site of this struggle is the body . . . So here I am, my own and my only audiovisual aid. There will be no 'next slide.'" Steven Epstein, *Impure Science: AIDS, Activism, and the Politics of Knowledge* (Berkeley: University of California Press, 1996): 21.

4. James C. Scott, "Everyday Forms of Resistance," *Copenhagen Papers* 4, no. 1 (May 1989): 33–62, 33; Some authors critiqued the tendency for mass media to highlight public acts of protest over these everyday expressions of activism. In a 1990 article published in the PWAC's *Newsline*, Ed Sikov wrote, "It rankles me that the newspapers and magazines focus on ACT UP's media stunts to the exclusion of the day-to-day efforts of literally thousands of PWA Coalition and GMHC volunteers, then, in the same breath, criticizes ACT UP for being outrageous and drawing so much attention." Ed Sikov, "Have You Heard What They've Been Saying about You?" *PWAC Newsline* 55 (May 1990): 33–34.

5. As I discuss in the introduction, my description of everyday forms of resistance as expressions of activism is informed by feminist scholarship seeking to redefine the sphere of activism to include acts committed in the individual or personal sphere. See, for example, Naomi Abrahams, "Toward Reconceptualizing Political Action," *Sociological Inquiry* 62, no. 3 (July 1992): 327–347; Deborah G. Martin, Susan Hanson, and Danielle Fontaine, "What Counts as Activism: The Role of Individuals in Creating Change," *Women's Studies Quarterly* 35, no. 3/4 (Fall–Winter 2007): 78–94.

6. Michael Helquist observed, "For gay men, sex, that most powerful implement of attachment and arousal, is also an agent of communion, replacing an often hostile family and even shaping politics." Quoted in Dennis Altman, *AIDS in the Mind of America* (Garden City: Anchor, 1986), 7; See also George Chauncey, Jr., "Gay Men's Strategies of Everyday Resistance," in *Major Problems in the History of American Sexuality*, ed. Kathy Peiss (Boston: Houghton Mifflin Company, 2002): 356–366.

7. For example, Vicki Lynn Eaklor identifies the group as an AIDS service organization in the mold of GMHC, whereas Simon LeVay and Elisabeth Nonas describe it as a political action group similar to ACT UP. See Vicki L. Eaklor, *Queer America: A GLBT History of the 20th Century* (Westport: Greenwood, 2008), 177; Simon LeVay and Elisabeth Nonas, *City of Friends: A Portrait of the Gay and Lesbian Community in America* (Cambridge: MIT Press, 1995), 253.

8. In a speech at a Gay Pride Rally on June 25, 1988, Michael Callen referred to the decade as the "gay AIDies." See Michael Callen, ed., "Passive Genocide in the Reagan Aidies," in *Surviving and Thriving with AIDS: Collected Wisdom, Volume II* (New York: People with AIDS Coalition, 1988), 2:284.

9. Giordano described the sounds of living he heard outside the hospital where he was admitted in comparison to those coming from within the hospital. Tony J. Giordano, "Saturday Night," in *Unending Dialogue*, ed. Rachel Hadas (Boston: Faber and Faber, 1991).

10. Technically, the 1990 text *Surviving AIDS* is not a PWAC publication. It is an independent volume Callen produced after leaving the organization. However, given Callen's influence in the PWAC and the thematic similarities between it and the publications produced under the aegis of PWAC, I have included it here.

11. Whether or not the PWAC remained this open minded throughout its history is difficult to say. The group endured tremendous turnover among its leadership as individuals perished from AIDS. However, there is evidence of increased rigidity over time. For example, Callen, an outspoken critic of mainstream medicine, reported pushback from the board toward the end of his tenure. See, for example, a letter from Michael Callen to Bill Case, "Latest Newsline Crisis," July 30, 1989, folder 99, Michael Callen Papers, LGBT-NHA.
12. Jane Rosett, "A Tribute to Michael Callen," *PWAC Newsline*, 47 (September 1989): 5.
13. Susan Chambré, *Fighting for Our Lives: New York's AIDS Community and the Politics of Disease* (New Brunswick, NJ: Rutgers University Press, 2006).
14. Among the earliest groups formed were People with AIDS San Francisco, New York's Gay Men with AIDS, and New York's Wipe Out AIDS, the forerunner to HEAL. See Michael Callen and Dan Turner, "A History of the PWA Self-Empowerment Movement," in *Surviving and Thriving with AIDS: Collected Wisdom, Volume II*, ed. Michael Callen (New York: People with AIDS Coalition, 1988), 2:288–293.
15. PWArcs were people with AIDS-related complex, a prodromal syndrome initially used to differentiate individuals with HIV infection from those who had developed AIDS.
16. Callen and Turner, "A History of the PWA Self-Empowerment Movement."
17. The proceeding was the Fifth National Lesbian/Gay Health Conference, sponsored by the National Gay Health Education Foundation, American Association of Physicians for Human Rights, and the Gay and Lesbian Health Alliance of Denver.
18. Michael Callen and Dan Turner listed the following PWAs in attendance: Bobbi Campbell, Dan Turner and Bobby Reynolds from San Francisco; Phil Lanzaratta, Artie Felson, Michael Callen, Richard Berkowitz, Bill Burke, Bob Cecchi, Matthew Sarner and Tom Nasrallah from New York City; Gar Traynor from Los Angeles; a man named Elbert from Kansas City; an unnamed individual from Denver; and Michael Helquist, the partner of Mark Feldman, who had died of AIDS-related complications just prior to the conference. See Callen and Turner, "A History of the PWA Self-Empowerment Movement."
19. Advisory Committee of People with AIDS, "The Denver Principles: Statement from the Advisory Committee of People with AIDS," in *Surviving and Thriving with AIDS: Collected Wisdom, Volume II*, ed. Michael Callen (New York: People with AIDS Coalition, 1988), 2:294–295.
20. Callen and Turner, "A History of the PWA Self-Empowerment Movement," parenthetical in original.
21. Sean Strub, "What's Wrong with Our Movement," *POZ*, December 5, 2005. Excerpted from speech delivered December 1, 2005 at the National AIDS Memorial Grove in San Francisco. Strub is a long-term survivor with HIV, the founder of *POZ* magazine, and was a member of ACT UP.
22. Callen and Turner, "A History of the PWA Self-Empowerment Movement," 291.
23. "The Denver Principles (1983)," ACT UP NY, accessed April 20, 2016, http://www.actupny.org/documents/Denver.html; "The Denver Principles (1983)," UNAIDS, accessed April 20, 2016, http://data.unaids.org/pub/ExternalDocument/2007/gipa1983denverprinciples_en.pdf.
24. Two other individuals who did not attend the Denver Conference, Peter Nalbandian and John Berndt, also helped form PWA-New York. See Callen, "Introduction."
25. Callen, "Introduction."; See also Callen and Turner, "A History of the PWA Self-Empowerment Movement."
26. The naming of the New York-based PWA organizations is somewhat confusing. PWA-New York was the first group, which closed soon after launching to be succeeded by the PWA Coalition (PWAC). A successful organization with an impressive reach, the PWAC eventually

endured financial hardships and, by 1993, closed its doors, to be replaced by the People with AIDS Coalition of New York (PWAC/NY). This chapter focuses exclusively on the work of the PWAC (1985–1993).

27. Griffin Gold, the President of the PWAC, underscored this point: "A number of the Board would like more political action." Gold explained that "the Coalition can only allocate 20% of its budget for political advocacy, if it wishes to maintain its tax-exempt status." PWA Coalition Board of Directors Meeting Notes, October 21, 1987, box 65, folder 3, Board of Directors Minutes, Michael Callen Papers, LGBT-NHA.

28. Callen, "Latest Newsline Crisis"; Max Navarre, "Fighting the Victim Label," in *Surviving and Thriving with AIDS: Collected Wisdom, Volume II*, ed. Michael Callen (New York: People with AIDS Coalition, 1988), 2:21; Michael Callen, "Farewell," *PWAC Newsline* 47 (September 1989); Callen and Turner, "A History of the PWA Self-Empowerment Movement," 292.

29. Max Navarre, "AIDS in '88—An Editorial," *PWA Coalition Newsline* 30 (January 1988); Many PWAs living outside major cities noted that the *Newsline* was their primary source of information.

30. Nancy Tuana describes the women's health movement as, "an epistemological resistance movement geared at undermining the production of ignorance about women's health and women's bodies in order to critique and extricate women from oppressive systems often based on this ignorance, as well as creating liberatory knowledges." Nancy Tuana, "The Speculum of Ignorance: The Women's Health Movement and Epistemologies of Ignorance," *Hypatia* 21, no. 3 (2006): 1–19, 2.

31. "That moment" was the run-up to the Denver Conference.

32. Bruce Nussbaum, *Good Intentions: How Big Business and the Medical Establishment Are Corrupting the Fight Against AIDS* (New York: Penguin, 1990), 108.

33. Michael Callen, "People with AIDS-New York: A History," March 1984, box 6, Michael Callen Papers, LGBT-NHA.

34. Patricia Siplon has argued, "Probably the single most direct and dramatic translation from the women's health care movement to the self-empowerment AIDS movement occurred in the unveiling of the Denver Principles." Patricia D. Siplon, *AIDS and the Policy Struggle in the United States* (Washington, DC: Georgetown University Press, 2002), 33; Sean Strub made similar claims in his analyses of the principles. Sean Strub, "The Denver Principles Empowerment Index," *POZ*, April 21, 2010; Sean Strub, "Foreword," *POZ*, September 1, 2019.

35. Jones's work provides important context into Callen's life and activism, with a significant focus on the intersections between his activist work and creative endeavors and creative career as a musician and performer. Matthew J. Jones, *Love Don't Need a Reason: The Life and Music of Michael Callen* (Santa Barbara: Punctum Books, 2020), 84.

36. Michael Callen, *PWAC Newsline*, 6 (November 1985): 17; Callen would also remark that among the earliest supporters of the PWAC movement were feminists. Callen and Turner, "A History of the PWA Self-Empowerment Movement."

37. In an interview published in the *Newsline*, Fouratt argued, "The politics of AIDS as we've experienced them in the gay communities are very much affected by the positions that were put forth around Stonewall . . . To reduce the issues to a very simplistic level, the people that were active in the Gay Liberation Front did not see gay liberation as a single issue. We believed that only in a pretty radical transformation of the entire society would there come real freedom for lesbians and gay men to live their lives as they choose . . . GAA would be a single issue organization—concerned exclusively with gay rights. They didn't want to talk about feminism or racism, or classism or all those other issues that GLF was trying to bring together . . . For a lot of complicated reasons, GAA became the dominant philosophical and

political position. After all, if people thing [sic] the choice is between 'gay liberation as one big party' and 'gay liberation as a struggle to transform the whole society,' obviously the uncritical, if-it's-gay-it's-o.k. view is gonna be more attractive." Michael Callen, "Jim Fouratt: Unsung Hero," *PWAC Newsline* 18 (December 1986): 37–38; Fouratt helped to found Wipe Out AIDS, later renamed HEAL. I examine HEAL's history later in this volume.

38. Matthew J. Jones, *Love Don't Need a Reason.*

39. Joe Wright, "Only Your Calamity: The Beginnings of Activism by and for People with AIDS," *American Journal of Public Health* 103, no. 10 (October 2013): 1788–98, n63.

40. For examples of 1980s-era engagement with these ideas within the nursing profession, see Ellen Condliffe Lagemann, ed., *Nursing History: New Perspectives, New Possibilities* (New York: Teachers College Press, Columbia University, 1983); Peggy L. Chinn and Charlene Eldridge Wheeler, "Feminism and Nursing," *Nursing Outlook* 33, no. 2 (March–April 1985), 74–77; For more recent engagement with these ideas, see Teresa Chulach and Marilou Gagnon, "Working in a 'Third Space': A Closer Look at the Hybridity, Identity and Agency of Nurse Practitioners," *Nursing Inquiry* 21, no. 1 (March 2016): 52–63.

41. As Susan Chambré notes, "One caregiver commented that, 'GMHC gave me the bureaucratic cold shoulder because my lifemate hadn't been 'officially diagnosed' . . . [The] *PWA Coalition Newsline* was my lifeline, my sole source of information and human contact with other living, vibrant gay human beings wrestling with the implications of this vile epidemic and their own mortality." Susan Chambré, *Fighting for Our Lives*, 38.

42. Victor F. Zonana, "Bootstrap AIDS Research Giving Patients Active Role," *Los Angeles Times*, December 25, 1988.

43. Michael Callen, "People with AIDS-New York: A History."

44. Of Michael Callen, Joseph Sonnabend once commented, "[H]e embodied a sort of confrontational activism that I understand and respect—not the collaborationist kind. It starts with the importance of self-reliance and not depending on experts. I mean, you can't do without them, but you can't trust them either." Sean O. Strub, "The Good Doctor," *POZ*, July 1, 1998, 109.

45. This Harrington quote appears in Callen's archived notes from his publication of *Surviving AIDS*. In studies of PWA activism, relatively little attention is paid to those, like Callen, who identified as socialists. For an example of class-based analyses in AIDS activism scholarship, see Peter F. Cohen, "'All They Needed': AIDS, Consumption, and the Politics of Class." *Journal of the History of Sexuality* 8, no. 1 (July 1997): 86–115.

46. The *Medical Matters* section was inaugurated in May of 1989, but it essentially grouped under one section opinions that had appeared in the *Newsline* since its inception.

47. Michael Callen, "Newsline Policy on Medical Matters," *PWAC Newsline* 44 (May 1989): 53.

48. Michael Callen, *PWAC Newsline* 18 (December 1986): 32; Steven Epstein identified a similar phenomenon when he argued that AIDS activism resulted in "the multiplication of the successful pathways to the establishment of credibility and diversification of the personnel beyond the highly credentialed." Epstein, *Impure Science*, 3.

49. In the same piece, Herman argues, "Doctors are not the demigods that we were brought up to believe they are." Bob Herman, "How to Talk to Your Doctor," *PWAC Newsline* 17 (November 1986): 26–28; Herman was known for traveling to Paris to obtain the experimental drug HPA-23. He died of AIDS related complications in 1986. See Jeff Jarvis, "Desperate American AIDS Victims [sic] Journey to Paris, Hoping that a New Drug Can Stave off Death," *People*, August 12, 1985 and Sandy Rovner, "After Ten Years . . . Where We're Headed," *Washington Post*, June 19, 1990.

50. Gould argues, "One of the most significant aspects of social movements is that they are sites for nurturing counter-hegemonic affects, emotions, and norms about emotional display."

Deborah B. Gould, *Moving Politics: Emotion and ACT UP's Fight Against AIDS* (Chicago: University of Chicago Press, 2009), 41.

51. Michael Callen, "Survivors: Philip Lanzaratta," *PWAC Newsline* 8 (January 1986): 12–13.

52. Michael Callen, "Beating the Odds: More Thoughts on Surviving AIDS," *PWAC Newsline* 26 (September 1987): 28–29.

53. Callen estimated that 10 to 15 percent of PWAs lived long term, or longer than three years. In *Surviving AIDS,* he critiqued mainstream reporters for promulgating universal fatality narratives. Of one news outlet, he comments, "The editor underscores his contempt for the concept of an AIDS survivor by putting the word 'survivors' in quotes, as if to say 'of course, they're not *really* going to survive AIDS, but we'll call them survivors just to humor them.'" In other cases, he interviewed reporters from the *New York Times* and the *Wall Street Journal* who admitted that whitewashing AIDS as universally fatal had become standard journalistic practice. See Callen, *Surviving AIDS,* 53.

54. In another example, Callen tells of allowing a *Newsweek* photographer into his home to capture his image for a magazine spread on PWAs, only to have the correspondent reject him—and his body—for not having visible Kaposi sarcoma (KS) lesions. When the photographer arrived, he scoffed at Callen's appearance, shrieking, "Where are your lesions? I need someone with lesions," before storming out. Callen, *Surviving AIDS,* 56.

55. Max Navarre, "Fighting the Victim Label," *October,* January 24, 1987, 143.

56. Callen, *Surviving AIDS,* 10; Callen would also argue, "Admitting the possibility of survival means that people around us may have to suffer the disappointment of our hopes along with us in a new way. If death from AIDS is *not* inevitable, then each death is uniquely painful. And each struggle to survive is uniquely empowering." Callen, *Surviving AIDS,* 69.

57. Michael Callen, ed., "Surviving and Thriving with AIDS," in *Surviving and Thriving with AIDS: Collected Wisdom, Volume II* (New York: People with AIDS Coalition, 1988), 2:131. Previous version published in the *Village Voice,* May 3, 1988.

58. Sonnabend singles out Anthony Fauci, who argued that patients presenting with PCP as the first manifestation of AIDS should be expected to live thirty-six to forty weeks. "His statement demonstrated an astonishing discrepancy between the experience of many community physicians who treat AIDS patients on a day to day basis and those whose focus is primarily on research rather than patient management." Joseph Sonnabend, "More Thoughts on Preventing Pneumocystis Pneumonia," in *Surviving and Thriving with AIDS: Collected Wisdom, Volume II,* ed. Michael Callen (New York: People with AIDS Coalition, 1988), 2:65.

59. Sonnabend's critique of mainstream biomedical practice was emblematic of historic power struggles in the construction of biomedical knowledge. It furthermore mirrors historical debates between rationalists, who hung their hats on theory, and empiricists, who relied upon knowledge gained through experience (see Chapter 1 of this volume).

60. Max Navarre, "Playing for Keeps," *Surviving and Thriving with AIDS: Collected Wisdom, Volume II,* ed. Michael Callen (New York: People with AIDS Coalition, 1988): 197.

61. Callen, *Surviving AIDS,* 62; Cass Martin echoed Callen's comments in the *Newsline,* writing, "The expectation is that the moment you test HIV antibody positive, you are one of the living dead awaiting only the formality of your cremation. Sadly, most AIDS organizations are in collusion with this world-view as, in order to become respectable and acceptable to the bodies which fund them, they have made pacts not to have activist elements within their structure and, further, to publicly disengage them[selves] from such activity." Cass Martin, "The Necrophiliacs of AIDS" *Newsline* 75 (April 1992): 18. A similar essay later appeared in John Lauritsen and Ian Young, eds., *The AIDS Cult: Essays on the Gay Health Crisis* (Provincetown, Asklepios, 1997).

62. Callen, *Surviving AIDS,* 88; Callen would eventually field claims that he appeared too healthy to have AIDS and that he was an "AIDS carpetbagger." In a sensational article pub-

lished in the *Newsline*, he included an itemized list of his symptoms, a copy of a biopsy report, and a letter from his physician, Sonnabend. He wrote, "I am taking the absurd measure of publishing my biopsy report below, including a photo copy of the slide containing the KS tissue. For those still unconvinced, private viewings of my lesions can be arranged." Michael Callen, "ARE YOU NOW OR HAVE YOU EVER BEEN?" *Newsline* 40 (January 1989): 35; Duberman also discusses Callen's publication of his medical records. Martin Duberman, *Hold Tight Gently: Michael Callen, Essex Hemphill, and the Battlefield of AIDS* (New York: The New Press, 2016): 134.

63. Nathaniel Pier took to comparing AIDS research trials to Santa Claus, noting, "[Y]ou see them represented everywhere, but they do not really exist." Nathaniel Pier, "Open Letter to Mr. Jim Gottlieb (Chief of Staff for Representative T. Weiss), September 14, 1988," in *AIDS Patient Care* (February 1989): 4.

64. Marcus Boon and Kate Hunter, "Dr Joseph A Sonnabend Takes a Look: An Interview," *PWA Coalition Newsline* 72 (December 1991), 27.

65. Michael Callen, ed., "The Pros and Cons of Taking AZT: A Round Table Discussion: June 21, 1988," in *Surviving and Thriving with AIDS: Volume II* (New York: People with AIDS Coalition, 1988), 2:87.

66. Marty Robinson, "Institutional Stagnation Plus Prejudice Equals Death," *PWAC Newsline* 24 (June 1987): 31.

67. Bob Lederer, "Holistic Treatments: Where's the Research, Where's the Proof?" *PWAC Newline* 50 (December 1989): 35.

68. James's perspectives on AIDS treatment and AIDS treatment activism were nuanced. In presenting this article, I do not mean to suggest that all of James's perspectives can be reduced to the quoted passage (which appears to have come from his *AIDS Treatment News*). Indeed, as Duberman has noted, James would come to support AZT. What is of interest here is the fact that the *Newsline* author invoked James in this way to articulate a point that is roughly antimodern. Ibid. 36; for Duberman's discussion of James, see *Hold Tight Gently*, 130.

69. The author grants that some researchers, including Robert Gallo, may have been "execrable human beings," but they deserved respect nonetheless. Stewart Frankel, "Letter to the Editor," *PWAC Newsline* 21 (March 1987): 19.

70. Michael Callen, *PWAC Newsline* 21 (March 1987): 21, emphasis in original.

71. In particular, see Epstein, *Impure Science*, 256–258.

72. Callen, *Surviving AIDS*, 199; Callen expressed a similar sentiment in a 1987 *Newsline* article: "When one federal researcher passionately implored me to beg PWAs in treatment trials to stay off all other medications to insure [sic] the data from trials was 'clean,' I nearly rose from my chair and with equal passion said that it was not the obligation of PWAs to die for the cause of 'good' science; it was the obligation of scientists to design protocols large enough to take into account the reality that many PWAs are on many substances simultaneously." Michael Callen, "How to Die for the Greater Good for the Greater Number of People," *PWAC Newsline* 26 (September 1987): 29.

73. Max Navarre, "Newsline Editor Max Navarre Responds," in *Surviving and Thriving with AIDS Collected Wisdom, Volume II*, ed. Michael Callen (New York: People with AIDS Coalition, 1988), 91.

74. Wayne, "Lying and Cheating to Get in a Protocol," *PWAC Newsline* 45 (June 1989): 37–38. The author's surname was not printed; parentheticals in original.

75. Callen famously refused to print the term "AIDS virus" in the *Newsline*, actively editing contributors' letters to omit the expression.

76. In one example, Marita Sturken cites the 1993 Canadian film *Zero Patience* wherein Callen appears as "Miss HIV," an anthropomorphized version of HIV. Sturken states that Callen scolds other viruses who wish to claim cofactor status in causing AIDS, while lamenting that nobody understands her. In his cameo, Callen argues, "Despite all the research, despite billions of dollars, not one reputable scientist has proven absolutely and conclusively that I disabled people's immune systems." He furthermore ends his segment by singing, "Tell a story of a virus, of greed, ambition and fraud, a case of science gone bad." For Sturken's summary, see Marita Sturken, *Tangled Memories: The Vietnam War, the AIDS Epidemic, and the Politics of Remembering* (Berkeley: University of California Press, 1997), 251.

77. Seth C. Kalichman, *Denying AIDS: Conspiracy Theories, Pseudoscience, and Human Tragedy (Conspiracy Theories, Pseudoscience, and Human Tragedy)*, 175. Although Kalichman credits Duesberg with inspiring denialism, he calls HEAL, "one of the most active denialist organizations, still centered on holistic treatments while defying HIV as the cause of AIDS." Kalichman, *Denying AIDS*, 137.

78. As a matter of historical chronology, the claim is easily refuted, as PWA engagement with unorthodox etiological arguments predated Duesberg's commentary on HIV. In fact, the very first issue of the *PWAC Newsline*, published two years before Duesberg entered the debate, featured an article wherein Callen questioned the public's uncritical acceptance of the viral etiological theory. Callen wrote, "I do not believe that LAV/HTLV-III 'causes' AIDS. It may—or may not—play some role, but the notion that AIDS spreads like syphilis or gonorrhea or like a common cold is patently absurd. It has been my experience and my observation that AIDS is a complicated disease to develop. It seems clear to me that AIDS is certainly not a one-shot deal." See Michael Callen, "Media Watch," *PWAC Newsline* 1 (June 1985): 7; Duesberg's first article on the topic would not appear until 1987. See Peter Duesberg, "Retroviruses as Carcinogens and Pathogens: Expectations and Reality," *Cancer Research* 47, no. 5 (March 1987): 1199–1220; Duesberg likely developed his perspective in the years preceding 1987. However, his ideas did not become famously—and infamously—known until 1987. In 1986, at 49, he was elected to the National Academy of Sciences and awarded an NIH Outstanding Investigator Award. As a 2008 *Discover* article declared, "Since the 1987 article on HIV, Duesberg has become a pariah among scientists." Jeanne Lenzer, "AIDS 'Dissident' Seeks Redemption . . . and a Cure for Cancer," *Discover*, May 14, 2008.

79. Epstein found that the number of unsubstantiated claims made by scientists concerning the etiological role of HIV in AIDS increased greatly from 1984–1986. Furthermore, while authors would initially write into journals to protest the claim that a single virus was destroying individuals' immune systems, such letters largely stopped post–1984. In his analysis of this consolidation of scientific certainty, Epstein cites Paula Treichler, who argues, "By repeatedly citing each other's work, a small group of scientists quickly established a dense citation network, thus gaining early (if ultimately only partial) control over nomenclature, publication, invitation to conferences, and history." See Epstein, *Impure Science*, 81–84.

80. In one *PWAC Newsline* piece, Callen railed, "How, I ask myself, did we fall into the shorthand of calling HIV the 'AIDS virus' and when and how did the term 'HIV Disease" creep into usage? Doesn't anyone else remember how 'appropriately' skeptical the press was about Gallo's announcement about HTLV-III? *Everyone* seemed to smell the same rat . . . In the weeks surrounding Gallo's announcement, press accounts would cautiously refer to HTLV-III as the 'putative' AIDS virus. Reporters were generally careful to remind readers that the assertion that HTLV-III was 'the cause' of AIDS was a hypothesis which was yet to be proven. Then, suddenly, the qualifiers disappeared and the caution evaporated. HIV was decreed to be the cause of AIDS. Wait? Did we miss something?" Michael Callen, "Why I Do Not Believe that HIV is the Cause of AIDS," *PWAC Newsline*, 29 (December 1987): 35, emphasis in original.

81. In the late 1980s, Robert Gallo was accused of misappropriating a sample of LAV from French researchers and claiming to have isolated it himself. He denied these claims and later

NIH investigations cleared him of wrongdoing. See, for example, John Crewdson, "The Great AIDS Quest: Science under the Microscope," *Chicago Tribune*, November 19, 1989, Special Section; Gallo was a frequent target of both Callen and other PWAs, who found him to be dismissive of PWA activism. In one *PWAC Newsline* article, Callen tells of his efforts to ask Gallo to discuss other potential causes of AIDS. "When I persisted with my questions, he got nasty and said words to the effect that he didn't know what *I'd* done for people with AIDS, but *he* was busy saving lives and questions like mine were a waste of his valuable time. In other words, by questioning the religion of HIV, I'm killing people." Michael Callen, "Montreal AIDS Conference: A 'Major Stressor Event,'" *PWAC Newsline* 46 (July–August 1989): 44. Emphasis in original.

82. HTLV-III was an early term introduced by Robert Gallo to describe the causative agent of AIDS. A French team led by Luc Montagnier suggested the term LAV. Eventually, researchers acknowledged that the causative agent of AIDS was not a member of the HTLV family. Both teams furthermore agreed to discontinue the use of these chosen terms and instead refer to the virus as HIV.

83. In the same piece, Callen cites Sir Karl Popper's falsification principle, juxtaposing Popper's beliefs with mainstream AIDS research. Michael Callen, *Newsline* (September 1986), 24; In his personal papers, Callen reflects on attending a scientific conference: "I've come to a BAPTIST CONVENTION and asked to consider the possibility that god doesn't' exist." Handwritten Notes, Box 8, Community Research Initiative, 1989, Michael Callen Papers, LGBT-NHA. Emphasis in original.

84. Letter from Michael Callen to Neville Hodgkinson of the *Sunday Times* of London, July 17, 1993, box 8, folder 237, Michael Callen Papers, LGBT-NHA; In an article in his short-lived *AIDS Forum* publication, Callen argued, "Anyone unwilling to genuflect before the god of HIV . . . will most likely be denied research funding." *AIDS Forum*, 1, no. 1 (January 1989): 1, box 11, folder 320, Michael Callen Papers, LGBT-NHA.

85. LAV was an earlier name used to describe the virus, eventually renamed HIV.

86. Michael Callen, "Media Watch," *PWAC Newsline* 5 (October 1985): 10; Callen's concerns with AIDS's ability to foment panic harkens back to the first edition of the *Newsline*. In it, he criticized *New York Native* and *Advocate* articles recommending that people with AIDS air dry dishes and boil sheets that had come into contact with bodily fluids. In the second edition, he critiqued a now famous *Life Magazine* cover that had intoned, "Now No One is Safe from AIDS." Approximately two years later, he criticized ACT UP for attempting to promote the notion that AIDS was poised to spread into the general population. See Michael Callen, "Media Watch," PWAC *Newsline* 1 (June 1985): 7; Michael Callen, "Media Watch," *PWAC Newsline* 2 (July 1985): 3; Michael Callen, *PWAC Newsline* 23 (May 1987): 28.

87. Sonnabend argued, "The repeated infections with CMV, the reactivation of EBV, exposure to multiple allogeneic semens and infection with other sexually transmitted pathogens result in an *accumulation* of effects that interact either addictively or synergistically to result in a switch to a self-sustaining condition." He first formulated his theory in 1983. See Joseph A. Sonnabend, Steven S. Witkin, and David T. Purtilo, "A Multifactorial Model for the Development of AIDS in Homosexual Men," circa 1983, 5, box 11, folder 306, Michael Callen Papers, LGBT-NHA; Joseph A. Sonnabend, "Acquired Immunodeficiency Syndrome: Opportunistic Infections and Malignancies in Male Homosexuals," *Journal of the American Medical Association* 249, no. 17 (1983): 2370.

88. Callen explained, "You've got George Bush saying it's a disease of behavior, and that's what we believe it is. We're saying it neutrally; he's being moralistic." Anne-christine D'Adesky, "The Man Who Invented Safe Sex Returns," *Out*, Summer 1992, 33; Similarly, on coauthoring the first safer sex manual with Michael Callen and Richard Berkowitz, Sonnabend commented,

"[I]n those days, GMHC hated us because we spoke about promiscuity and used words like *sperm* and *rectum* in public." Strub, "The Good Doctor."

89. Raymond Keith Brown, *AIDS, Cancer and the Medical Establishment* (New York: Robert Speller and Sons, 1986): 131. Callen reviewed the book in Issue 13 (June–July 1986) of the *Newsline*. Emphasis on words "gay community" removed from original.

90. In addition to citing interviews with other PWAs in support of the multifactorial model, Callen referred to his own experience, chronicling the sexually transmitted diseases he had contracted prior to developing AIDS. He argued, "I remain convinced—based on my own experience and my conversations with other gay men with AIDS—that AIDS is a the [sic] result of a constant barrage of infections over a period of time. I guess I'm a rabid multifactorialist, I just don't buy this crap about one 'unlucky' sexual encounter causing AIDS." Michael Callen, "Media Watch," *PWAC Newsline*, 2 (July 1985): 3; See also Carola Burroughs, "AIDS and Cofactors: A Homeopathic Perspective," *PWAC Newsline* 74 (March 1992); "Out of the AIDS Grist: The Newsline Talks with Michael Callen," *PWAC Newsline* 75 (July 1992): 24; See also an interview between Michael Callen and Celia Farber of *SPIN* magazine, quoted in Joan Shenton, "Compassionate Celebrity," *Continuum Magazine* 4, no. 6 (June–July 1997).

91. In *Surviving AIDS*, Callen invoked chronic diseases to explain the multifactorial model, musing, "With heart disease, people understand that genetics, diet, exercise, and other factors conspire to determine whether or not one will suffer a stroke. But for some reason, most people abandon any notion that getting sick is a multifactorial process once an infectious agent is involved." Callen, *Surviving AIDS*, 13, n7; Similarly, he argued, "A multifactorial model suggests that multiple exposures to infectious and non-infectious immunosuppressive factors conspire, over time, to produce AIDS. A useful disease model would be heart disease: one wouldn't ask which particular pat of butter caused a heart attack. Clearly cholesterol builds up over time." Michael Callen, ed. "Can Women Transmit AIDS?" in *Surviving and Thriving with AIDS: Collected Wisdom, Volume II* (New York: People with AIDS Coalition, 1988), 226.

92. Elizabeth Fee and Daniel Fox, "Introduction: The Contemporary Historiography of AIDS," in *AIDS: The Making of a Chronic Disease*, Ed. Elizabeth Fee and Daniel Fox (Berkeley: University of California Press, 1991), 4.

93. In a 1983 letter sent to the editor of *New York Magazine*, Callen argued, "Society's irrational and insidious hatred of homosexuality has forced too many of us into the ghetto of the bathhouse circuit . . . That so many gay men continue to seek refuge from our homophobic society in such disease-polluted places is perhaps the saddest observation about AIDS that I can make." Letter from Michael Callen to Editor Ed Kosner of *New York Magazine* (June 15, 1983), Box 1, Folder 8, Joseph Sonnabend Papers, NYPL-MAD; Similarly, Sonnabend noted that his concerns with structural dimensions of illness were shaped by a young adulthood spent in South Africa during the rise of the pro-apartheid Afrikaner National Party. Anne Christine D'Adesky, "The Man Who Invented Safe Sex Returns," 33.

94. Callen, *Surviving AIDS*, 6.

95. Mr. Schick, "Letter to the Editor," *PWA Coalition Newsline* 37 (October 1988).

96. Callen attempted to differentiate between accepting responsibility and blaming oneself for being sick. See, for example, Callen, *Surviving AIDS*, 187; Luis Palacios-Jimenez made a similar distinction in a *Surviving and Thriving with AIDS* article, writing, "Learn about responsibility! I am responsible to my illness, but I'm not responsible for it." Luis Palacios-Jimenez, "Little Bits of Wisdom," in *Surviving and Thriving with AIDS: Collected Wisdom, Volume II*, ed. Michael Callen (New York: People with AIDS Coalition, 1988), 24.

97. See, for example, Jennifer Brier, "Locating Lesbian and Feminist Responses to AIDS, 1982–1984," *Women's Studies Quarterly* 35, no. 1–2 (Spring–Summer 2007): 234–248; This should not be taken to mean that Callen or Berkowitz condemned gay sex—or promiscuity—on moral grounds. To the contrary, they argued, "Neither of us has experienced a moment of guilt about our own promiscuous behavior . . . Neither of us has problems with our gayness or with sexuality; we have problems with disease." For a discussion of this topic, see Martin Duberman, *Hold Tight Gently: Michael Callen, Essex Hemphill, and the Battlefield of AIDS* (New York: The New Press, 2016), 59.

98. I do not mean to argue that Callen's views were thoroughly Illichian. Indeed, he sought to recapture the power of institutions for the good of PWAs while Illich railed against institutions. However, Callen knew of Illich's ideas: his archives cite Illich and he referred to the author in talks, such as one he gave at the American Public Health Association's Annual Meeting in 1986 titled, "Life in the Reagan AIDies." See http://michaelcallen.com/mikes-writing/life-in-the-reagan-aidies/

99. As Jennifer Brier argues, "By marking the healthcare industry as a manufacturer of ill health, Patton reasoned that community-based, feminist activism would produce the conditions for sexual health." Brier also analyzes Callen and Berkowitz's pamphlet. Jennifer Brier, "Locating Lesbian and Feminist Responses to AIDS, 1982–1984," *Women's Studies Quarterly* 35, no. 1–2 (Spring–Summer 2007): 244; See also Jennifer Brier, *Infectious Ideas: U.S. Political Responses to the AIDS Crisis* (Chapel Hill: University of North Carolina Press, 2009); David France described Callen and Berkowitz's work as "feminist critiques of the male ego." David France, *How to Survive a Plague* (New York City: Vintage Books, 2017), 98.

100. Robert Crawford has analyzed responsibility narratives both during the AIDS pandemic and earlier. See, for example, Robert Crawford, "You are Dangerous to Your Health: The Ideology and Politics of Victim Blaming," *International Journal of Health Services*, 7, no. 4 (1977): 663–80; Robert Crawford, "The Boundaries of the Self and the Unhealthy Other: Reflections on Health, Culture, and AIDS," *Social Science and Medicine*, 38 (1994): 1347–1365.

101. Callen's critique of the mainstream biomedical model should not be taken to mean that he was less critical of unorthodox ideas. In fact, he demanded "the very best science" in support of all etiological and therapeutic AIDS models. As I describe later in this chapter, his views were unorthodox insofar as he critiqued the character and competence of mainstream biomedical professionals and demanded the establishment of new systems informed by PWA perspectives. Furthermore, as Duberman has noted, in addition to supporting the multifactorial model, Callen thought Duesberg was "dead wrong about there being no infectious process" and critiqued Lauritsen's *The AIDS War* as a "tedious, flip reduction of complex and subtle statements." See Duberman, *Hold Tight Gently*, 99–100.

102. Interestingly, by Sonnabend's own admission, the multifactorial model was extremely difficult to test using standard double-blind study design.

103. For a discussion of the trials, see Epstein, *Impure Science*, 198.

104. Joseph Foulon, "Medically Speaking: Compound S," *PWAC Newsline* 12 (May 1986): 2. Compound S was an early name for AZT.

105. Paul Lande, "Letter to Michael Callen," *PWAC Newsline* 20 (February 1987): 14.

106. Navarre argued, "Certainly, the current fashion of prescribing AZT to virtually anyone with a few symptoms has contributed greatly to the trends towards AIDS-it is. The medical love affair with AZT is particularly alarming to those of us who remain unconvinced that HIV is 'the cause' of AIDS. Every time I hear HIV referred to as the 'AIDS virus,' my teeth start to grind." Max Navarre, "AIDS-it is," in *Surviving and Thriving with AIDS: Collected Wisdom, Volume II*, ed. Michael Callen (New York: People with AIDS Coalition, 1988), 45.

107. Max Navarre, "Some Thoughts on Experimental Drugs," *PWAC Newsline* 22 (April 1987): 18; The PWAC's critiques of AZT provoked conflict with other AIDS service organizations. The leader of Project Inform, for example, at one point issued thinly veiled critiques of the PWAC when he questioned the "New Yorkers who have so effectively convinced thousands of people around the country that AZT is a poison." Letter from Martin Delaney to Mathilde Krim, "Compound Q Frenzy," September 21, 1989, box 7, folder 210, Michael Callen Papers, LGBT-NHA.

108. Michael Callen, "AZT Results Announced," *PWAC Newsline* 16 (October 1986): 1.

109. Sonnabend's quote comes from the first edition of the *HEAL Quarterly* 1, no. 1 (Fall 1989): 3. Copies of all available *HEAL Quarterly* articles found in HEAL-A; Callen similarly critiqued the expectation among researchers that PWAs would take AZT long-term, arguing, "The idea that individuals should take chemotherapy every day for the rest of their lives is completely unprecedented." Callen, *Surviving AIDS*, 212.

110. Michael Callen, "Message from the Editor," *AIDS Forum* 1, no. 2 (1989): 1.

111. Callen noted, "First, I'm *not* on AZT . . . I think it's Drano in pill form and you couldn't pay me to take it. It's cytotoxic, which means it kills cells. It inhibits DNA synthesis, which is the basis of all life." Michael Callen, ed., "AIDS 201," in *Surviving and Thriving with AIDS: Collected Wisdom, Volume II* (New York, People with AIDS Coalition, 1988), 7.

112. Michael Callen, "Pros and Cons of Taking AZT," 78.

113. Callen also recounted physicians having angrily approached him, saying that their patients had refused to take AZT based on his suggestions. See Callen, "AIDS 201," 3; Michael Callen, "Newsline Policy on Medical Matters," 53.

114. Callen, *Surviving AIDS*, 27; Michael Callen, "Surviving and Thriving with AIDS," 130–139, 137.

115. Callen, *Surviving AIDS*, 110, 119.

116. Callen, *Surviving AIDS*, 111; Other articles similarly discussed the refusal of many long-term PWAs to take AZT. See, for example, Buzz Wolf, "A Long-Term Survivor Speaks Out," *PWAC Newsline* 46 (July–August 1989): 30; Marcus Boon and Kate Hunter, "Dr. Joseph Sonnabend Takes a Look," 30.

117. Duberman, *Hold Tight Gently*, 130.

118. Burroughs Wellcome Representative, "Letter to Michael Hirsch," *PWAC Newsline* 25 (July–August 1987): 13–14.

119. Cass Mann and Stuart Marshall, "HIV—Questions Not Answers," *Positively Healthy News* 3 (March 1989); Callen also argued that the GMHC's decision not to distribute the second volume of *Surviving and Thriving with AIDS* to its clients stemmed from its leaders' beliefs that the diversity of opinion it presented would confuse and overwhelm PWAs. Memo from Michael Callen to PWAC Board (January 16, 1989), box 6. GMHC (1989–1990), Michael Callen Papers, LGBT-NHA.

120. Michael Callen, "AIDS is a Gay Disease!" *PWAC Newsline* 42 (March 1989): 61. Emphasis in original.

121. Richard Grant, "Staying Alive," *Independent*, January 4, 1992.

122. Steve Rose. "Letter to the Editor," *PWAC Newsline* 44 (May 1989): 6.

123. Duberman, *Hold Tight Gently*, 128.

124. Larry Kramer voiced similar concerns. In a 1987 letter, he asked Dick Thompson of *Time* Magazine whether he was aware that "87% of all NIH protocols in existence and being planned for the next five years are still only for AZT?" He furthermore listed drugs that no NIH protocol was studying: Ampligen, AL 721, Colony Stimulating Factors, Ribavirin, Imuthiol, Antabuse, Foscarnet, DHPG, Fusidic Acid, and Carrisyn. Similarly, Callen argued that mainstream medicine's celebration of magic bullets forestalled research into aerosolized pentamidine, an agent he believed could treat *Pneumocystis carinii* pneumonia. Letter from Larry Kramer to Dick Thompson of Time Magazine (December 3, 1987), Box 4, CRI Press (1987–1988), Folder 105, Michael Callen Papers, LGBT-NHA.

125. John Lauritsen and Hank Wilson, *Death Rush: Poppers and AIDS* (Inland Book Co, 1986).

126. Lauritsen argued, "If 'AIDS' is caused largely by toxins, what is an appropriate treatment? Not still another drug, but freedom from toxins. Long-term survivors, almost without exception have avoided toxic chemotherapy (like AZT) and are repairing their bodies through a more healthy lifestyle, exercise, good nutrition, rest and stress reduction, and avoidance of harmful substances (including cigarettes, alcohol, heroin, cocaine, MDA, quaaludes, ethyl chloride, poppers and all other 'recreational drugs')." See John Lauritsen, "The Case Against AZT," *PWAC Newsline* 47 (September 1989): 58. Parentheticals in original.
127. This back and forth appeared in Issue 51 (January 1990) of the *Newsline*. Marc Colter penned the initial article critical of AZT; Rob Schick replied in support of the drug, prompting a rebuttal from John Lauritsen and a rejoinder by Rob Schick; By the late 1980s, Schick had become increasingly frustrated with those who attacked AZT, at one point writing, "Truth is, the people who say AZT is no good don't know science from a hole in the ground. They're the same ones who can't admit AIDS is caused by HIV. They won't face up to the harsh truth that they're in a fringe group which has been dangerously wrong all these years." See Rob Schick, "The Crazy Case Against AZT," 49 (November 1989): 35.
128. For a discussion of Callen's later reservations, see Duberman, *Hold Tight Gently*, 130–133, 230.
129. Jane Rosett, "A Tribute to Michael Callen," 5.
130. David Summers, "Acupuncture as an Alternative," *PWAC Newsline* 1 (June 1985): 5.
131. See, for example, Andrew T. Weil, *Health and Healing: The Philosophy of Integrative Medicine and Optimum Health* (Boston: Houghton Mifflin, 2004): 24.
132. Alan Burns, "H.E.A.L.," *PWAC Newsline* 17 (November 1986).
133. Peter Dvarackas, "Self Hypnosis: A Gift You Give to Yourself," in *Surviving and Thriving with AIDS: Collected Wisdom, Volume II*, ed. Michael Callen (New York: People with AIDS Coalition, 1988), 119.
134. See, for example, Burroughs, "AIDS and Cofactors," 74; Michael Ellner, "Letter to the Editor," *PWAC Newsline* 53 (1990): 9.
135. Tom Herman, "Homeopathy and AIDS," *Newsline*, 44 (May 1989).
136. In his draft notes for *Surviving AIDS*, Callen quotes George M. Engel, who argued, "An important aspect of many concepts for disease has been the tendency to ascribe disease to a 'bad' influence, usually something external which gets into the body. This theme characterizes most primitive and prescientific views of disease and has reappeared repeatedly in various guises in the scientific era." See notes, box 7, folder 195, "Surviving AIDS," 1988, Michael Callen Papers, LGBT-NHA.
137. In 1988, for example, Michael Ellner penned a letter supportive of Callen's editorship of the *Newsline*. "I am writing to support Michael Callen's skepticism regarding HIV as the 'cause of' AIDS . . . It is my opinion that it is implausible that HIV causes AIDS even if it's proved that there's a germ factor in AIDS. Modern medical research has yet to prove a *single* cause in any illness—and yet we are to believe HIV causes this very complex syndrome. Multifactorial views apply to all disease and quite frankly the *germ* view has never held water." Michael Ellner, "Letter to the Editor," *Newsline* 37 (October 1988): 11–12. Emphasis in original.
138. As Carola Burroughs writes, "From a holistic health perspective, and particularly from the standpoint of homeopathic theory, nearly all disease is multifactorial, because it involves the interaction of elements which are hereditary, environmental, and behavioral." Burroughs, "AIDS and Cofactors," *Newsline* 79 (March 1992), 17.
139. Alex Idavoy, "Holistics 101: An Alternative Beginning," *PWAC Newsline* 74 (March 1992): 33; ACT UP also formed a committee that examined alternative and holistic treatments for AIDS. Though never its main focus, this committee's work intersects themes explored in this volume. Speaking of the ability for AIDS to motivate a holistic reconceptualization of health

and disease, ACT UP member and PWA Jon Greenberg wrote, ". . . AIDS breaks down the intellectual and spiritual barriers leaving one open not only to ideas but also spiritual insights, many of which some of us have spent years trying to keep out with cleverly constructed intellectual and spiritual walls." Jon Greenberg, "The Metaphysics of AIDS," 1992–1993, excerpt reproduced at https://scalar.usc.edu/nehvectors/levine/media/Jon-Greenberg-Political-funeral-flyer.pdf

140. Alan Burns, "H.E.A.L."

141. Michael Hirsch, "Holistic Health Care for AIDS," in *Surviving and Thriving with AIDS, Volume II*, ed. Michael Callen (New York: People with AIDS Coalition, 1988), 122.

142. Bob Lederer, "Holistic Treatments."

143. Peter Dvarackas, "Surviving AIDS with the Wisdom of the East," in *Surviving and Thriving with AIDS, Volume II*, ed. Michael Callen (New York: People with AIDS Coalition, 1988), 124–128.

144. Alex Idavoy, "Holistics 101."

145. For example, a 1988 *Newsline* contributor argued, "While conventional medicine continues to search for a 'magic bullet' and ignores or rejects alternative treatments as 'quackery,' holistic medicine teaches us that the true source of magic is within our own bodies already, waiting to be tapped." Carola Burroughs, "Mechanisms of Holistic Healing," *PWAC Newsline* 39 (December 1988).

146. The author, Michael Hirsch, elsewhere argued that holistic methods allowed PWAs to, "[take] a more active role in the treatment of their medical condition by adopting sound nutritional practices, by employing methods to reduce both generalized and illness-related stress, by examining and re-directing negative thought patterns, and by releasing depressing and dis-empowering emotions such as fear and internalized homophobia." Michael Hirsch, "Holistic Health Care," in *Surviving and Thriving with AIDS, Vol II*, ed. Michael Callen (New York: People with AIDS Coalition, 1988) 122; See also letter from Michael Hirsch in response to Paul Lande, *PWAC Newsline* 8 (January 1986): 8.

147. *PWAC Newsline*, 11 (April 1986): 17.

148. This framing may have been the result of a *Newsline* editorial policy cautioning individuals against celebrating "chauvinistic" healing systems that purported to solve all problems PWAs encountered. See, for example, "Alternative Therapies: Managing Editors' Note," *Newsline* 10 (March 1986); Some contributors furthermore expressed concern with the hope PWAs invested in alternative treatments. In one *Newsline* piece, Max Navarre worried that his friends and colleagues had turned one alternative egg lipid agent, AL721, into a symbol of self-empowerment: ". . . I think because of this home grown quality, egg lipids have themselves emerged as a symbol of self-empowerment. We have confused the product with the motivation behind the product's availability. And how shocking when self-empowerment fails. When the home grown treatment is as fallible as that offered by the big boys, [where] does one turn?" Max Navarre, "Editorial," *PWAC Newsline* 25 (July–August 1987).

149. Michael Hirsch, "Holistic Health Care for AIDS," 123.

150. These texts provoked controversy for, among other things, arguing that individuals living with cancer could affect their disease by visualizing "their white-blood cells as armies attacking and annihilating their tumors." See Louis Weisberg, "'Incurable' Patients Work at Healing Themselves," *The Philadelphia Inquirer*, June 12, 1988, L1; Bernie Siegel, *Love, Medicine and Miracles* (New York: HarperCollins, 1988); O. Carl Simonton, Stephanie Matthews-Simonton, and James L. Creighton, *Getting Well Again: A Step-by-Step Self-Help Guide to Overcoming Cancer for Patients and Their Families* (Los Angeles: TarcherPerigree, 1978); these positions are reminiscent of philosophies harkening back to the nineteenth-century irregular healer Phineas Quimby, who was inspired by mesmerists. Quimby advocated a visualization approach to healing cancer. See James C. Whorton, *Nature Cures: The History of Alternative Medicine in America* (Oxford, Oxford University Press, 2002), 279.

151. Weisberg, "'Incurable' Patients"; Sally Fisher argues, "If we see illness as a warning signal that there is something not working about our lives or as a symptom of a deeper issue, then we can aid and nurture our healing progress. If one has cancer, it is necessary to release the past and allow the resentments to dissolve in order to heal and prevent further complications." Sally Fisher, "Creating a Climate for Health," "AIDS Mastery and Visualization Workshop," box 2, folder 4, PWAC Archives, NYPL-MAD.

152. Steven James, "Visualization in Healing," *Newsline* 20 (February 1987): 38. Emphasis in original; Elsewhere, James argues, "Personal power is probably the key factor in healing, and to me having personal power means developing the singleness and strength of purpose, of vision, and of will to transcend circumstances which, outwardly, might seem overwhelming. It requires not only an assertion of faith, but hard work and perseverance." Steven James, "Reflections on Healing, Honesty and Personal Power," in *Surviving and Thriving with AIDS: Hints for the Newly Diagnosed, Volume I*, ed. Michael Callen (New York: People with AIDS Coalition, 1987).

153. Dvarackas, "Self Hypnosis," 118–119.

154. In *Surviving and Thriving with AIDS: Collected Wisdom*, Hirsch reflected on the value of holistic health models: "While AIDS/ARC has introduced an inordinate amount of grief and loss into our lives, at the same time, a more holistic approach to our personhood and our physical health has afforded man the opportunity to create a deeper sense of self love, a profound renewal of personal spirituality, and a new-found commitment to such essential humanistic values as brotherly love and charity. For many, a more holistic look at oneself and one's health has provided these persons with the drive and the inner resources to keep forging ahead in their struggle to *live* with AIDS." Hirsch, "Holistic Health Care for AIDS," 123.

155. Paul Lande, for example, wrote, "Louise Hay is a businesswoman! She is no Messiah or magician, except perhaps in making you part with your money . . . It is frightening to see her rapidly becoming a cult hero . . ." "On Louise Hay, Messiahs, Charlatans & Rationality," *Newsline* 7 (December 1985); In response to Lande's letter, Tom Cunningham defended Hay as a "consciousness catalyst." *Newsline* 8 (January 1986); Max Navarre also criticized Land's piece and lauded Michael Hirsch for making alternative therapies known to PWAs. Max Navarre, "Letter," *Newsline* 8 (January 1986).

156. See Duberman, *Hold Tight Gently*, 163.

157. Weisberg, "'Incurable' Patients."

158. Callen, *Surviving AIDS*, 99.

159. For further discussion of Callen's perspective on research, treatment, and health activism, see Duberman's *Hold Tight Gently*, particularly chapter 4.

160. James, "Holistic Approaches to AIDS," internal parentheses removed.

161. Identified in *Surviving AIDS* as Ron (no last name given), 159.

162. Identified in *Surviving AIDS* as Gary Mackler, 175.

163. Callen, *Surviving AIDS*, 75. Callen's reference to homeopathic doses of naltrexone (Vivitrol) is interesting, as it was a mainstream medication that, when employed in this manner, was viewed as both unorthodox and holistic. For a discussion of the drug, see Neenyah Ostrom, "Enhancing Immunity," *New York Native*, September 18, 1989.

164. "My doctor figures that such lifestyle changes may not hurt," Peck writes, "but are not very significant as long as I carry deadly HIV in my body." Larry Peck, "My Doctor and My Chiropractor," *Newsline* 38 (November 1988): 37–38; cases wherein PWAs used holistic treatment modalities alongside unapproved pharmacologic treatments (e.g., those procured from other countries) are particularly interesting, as they demonstrate that the currents I have

identified as sustaining unorthodox health activism do not always work synergistically. To take an unapproved, and perhaps not yet rigorously tested, pharmaceutical drug exposes oneself to toxicity. Such agents could generate opposition on antiheroic grounds.

165. Callen would note, "To be frank, we wish we didn't have to form PWA Health Group. It's a monumental pain in the ass, a logistical nightmare and a situation which exposes both Tom [Hannan] and me to great personal financial risk. In the best of all possible worlds, the federal government, Praxis Pharmaceuticals (which manufacturers another egg lecithin substance known as AL 721) or health food stores would make this non-toxic food substance available to anyone who wanted it. But for a variety of complicated political reasons, to our knowledge, there are no immediate plans to make egg lecithin extract available to those who desire it except for the efforts of PWA Health Group (and two similar ventures out on the West Coast)." Michael Callen, "PWA Health Group Update," *PWAC Newsline* 23 (May 1987): 11.

166. Such language no doubt resonated with some readers of the *Newsline*. However, it is important to acknowledge that it also likely served a legal function, allowing the PWAC to endeavor to skirt federal laws governing the procurement of unapproved drugs. "PWA Health Group Statement of Purpose," September 1988, PWA Health Group, Michael Callen Papers, LGBT-NHA.

167. Callen would also teach PWAs how to make the egg lipid mixture at home in a video wherein he appears dressed as Julia Child; so worried were group leaders that the federal government would identify PWAs through postal records of households receiving dextran sulfate that they discussed the creation of a "matchmaking" program, whereby individuals who did not have AIDS or ARC could volunteer to receive drugs on behalf of PWAs. They compared the suggestion to non-Jewish Dutch people who, during World War II, wore yellow stars to dilute the significance of Nazi-imposed rules targeting Jewish communities. See Questionnaire, PWA Health Group, Michael Callen Papers, LGBT-NHA.

168. The CRI was inspired and informed by community-based cancer research initiatives on the West Coast in addition to the Community Constituency Consortium, which helped to facilitate community-based AIDS research on the West Coast.

169. One workshop flyer read, "The Visualization Workshop puts us in touch with our self-worth, love and power. It allows us to re-align habitual behavior patterns into dynamic expressions of choice. Visualization is the opportunity to step into our Vision and be Healed." "AIDS Mastery and Visualization Workshop," box 2, folder 4, PWAC Coalition Archives, NYPL; Discussion of the PWA Health Group and Northern Lights Alternatives sharing office space found in "Meeting, April 14, 1988," PWA Health Group, Michael Callen Papers, LGBT-NHA.

170. Jane Rosett, "A Tribute to Michael Callen," *PWAC Newsline* 47 (September 1989).

171. Michael Callen, "An Open Letter to Readers of the PWA Newsline," *PWAC Newsline*, 20 (February 1987).

172. Callen, "Latest *Newsline* Crisis."; The PWAC registered some success in outreach, including forming support groups for Spanish-speaking PWAs, people of color, and women.

CHAPTER 5 PATIENT, HEAL THYSELF

1. *Information Packet*, Undated, HEAL Archive. In many formulations of group literature, the term "complementary" appears in parentheses alongside the word "alternative."

2. See, for example, Susan Chambré, *Fighting for Our Lives: New York's AIDS Community and the Politics of Disease* (New Brunswick: Rutgers University Press, 2006).

3. See, for example, Seth Kalichman, *Denying AIDS: Conspiracy Theories, Pseudoscience, and Human Tragedy* (New York: Copernicus Press, 2009).

4. Interviews with Michael Ellner were conducted in November of 2009 in conjunction with coursework completed under the mentorship of Mary Marshall Clark, Director of Columbia University's Center for Oral History Research ("Oral History, Methods and Theory," OHMA 4015G, Call Number: 81598).

5. These interviews focus specifically on the history of ACT UP but are useful, since several early HEAL leaders eventually became active in ACT UP. See ACT UP Oral History Project, a program of MIX, the New York Lesbian & Gay Experimental Film Festival.

6. Eugene Fedorko, "Interview 144," interview by Sarah Schulman, August 25, 2012, 7, ACT UP-OHP.

7. Fedorko, "Interview 144."

8. Larry Kramer, "1,112 and Counting," *New York Native* 59, March 14–27, 1983.

9. Michael Callen, "Jim Fouratt: Unsung Hero," *PWAC Newsline* 18 (December 1986): 36; In his ACT UP interview, Fouratt also argued, "The only message you got was death . . . there was no hope at all." Jim Fouratt, "Interview 066," interview by Sarah Schulman, November 28, 2006, 36, ACT UP-OHP.

10. See, for example, Thomas L. Long, *AIDS and American Apocalypticism* (Albany: State University of New York Press, 2005).

11. Gould describes the emotional habitus of a group as "the socially constituted, prevailing ways of feeling and emoting, as well as the embodied, axiomatic understandings and norms about feelings and their expression." Deborah Gould, *Moving Politics: Emotion and ACT UP's Fight Against AIDS* (Chicago: University of Chicago, 2009), 10; Fouratt would argue that HEAL first formed to challenge universal fatality narratives with discourse centered about hope. "[W]e tried to set up a group that gave some sort of hope . . . You've got to have hope. You just can't deal with death." Fouratt, "Interview 066."; some sources place the founding of Wipe out AIDS in 1981, though its name presumably dates to 1982, the year the CDC first used the term *AIDS*.

12. Fouratt, "Interview 066," 35–36.

13. One 1985 advertisement in the *PWAC Newsline* explained, "HEAL (Health Education AIDS Liaison) is a group whose goal is to provide support and information regarding natural ways of self-recovery . . . In its efforts to explore the natural methods of health improvement and maintenance, HEAL has sponsored presentations that have included acupuncture, homeopathy, herbology, meditation, visualization techniques, polarity therapy, shiat-su therapy, iridiology, and the proper medicinal use of macrobiotics. Many people in the group, but not all, are attempting to follow macrobiotic principles." *PWAC Newsline* 7 (December 1985): 19–20.

14. Fedorko, "Interview 144," 7–8.

15. Michael Ellner, interview by Matthew Kelly, November 2, 2009.

16. "Medicine: When to Use It," *HEAL Comprehensive Information Packet*, HEAL-A. This informational packet is undated but was likely penned in the mid-1980s.

17. The article continues, "[H]olistic medicine simply insists that the *whole* patient be considered, including physical, spiritual and mind issues, and that drugs should not be administered unless proven safe and necessary." Alan Burns, "H.E.A.L.," *PWAC Newsline* (1986): 21.

18. In the Burns article, Cunningham is quoted as stating, "I just can't stand this victim mentality—you know, 'AIDS victim,' . . . You never see 'cancer victim' or 'heart victim'—the government, the medical establishment, and the media have built a conspiracy of hopelessness around this disease. It infuriates me."

19. The first entry on Callen's list recognized that long-term PWAs actively experimented with alternative healing approaches. The second entry specified, "Most or all had used approaches such as shiatsu massage, acupuncture, or visualization. A clear majority were

involved with groups such as Louise Hay, or AIDS Mastery or Metaphysical Alliance." Michael Callen, "7 Very Important Qualities," *HEAL Quarterly* 1, no. 1 (Fall 1989), HEAL-A. This article additionally appeared in HEAL's Information Packet, circa 1994, on file at UT-TFRBL.

20. Letter from William Case, executive director of PWAC to Frank Russo, executive director of HEAL, June 27, 1988, HEAL-A; Similarly, a letter from the PWAC's Deputy Executive Director observed, "The importance of your programs is exemplified by the daily requests we receive, on our Hotline, for services such as you offer." Letter from Christopher L. Babick, deputy executive director of PWAC, to Gene Fedorka [sic], president of HEAL, June 24, 1988, HEAL-A.

21. Letter from Bruce Woods Patterson, MSW, hotline coordinator, to HEAL, July 31, 1992, HEAL-A.

22. Letter from Don Troise, director of department of health AIDS hotline, Bureau of Laboratories, to Michael Ellner of HEAL, March 1, 1991, HEAL-A.

23. ARC stood for AIDS-related complex, a prodromal syndrome used to differentiate individuals with HIV infection from those who had developed AIDS.

24. HEAL Information Packet, circa 1994, 1, UT-TFRBL.

25. Letter from HEAL Member, February 8, 1989, HEAL-A. Sender's name redacted.

26. HEAL Information Packet, 1.

27. One can dedicate a full volume to exploring the *Native's* reporting on unorthodox AIDS theories through the late 1980s. One reader, for example, would write to the newspaper's editor in 1987, commenting, "I find nothing wrong with the reports in the *Native* on alternative theories and treatment for AIDS. However, the presentation of [editor] Ortleb's pet theories is shockingly irresponsible, yellow journalism at its worst, the ravings of a lunatic." "Letters," *New York Native*, April 6, 1987, 6.

28. Fedorko, "Interview 144," 8.

29. Michael Callen, ed. "The Pros and Cons of Taking AZT: A Round Table Discussion: June 21, 1988," in *Surviving and Thriving with AIDS Collected Wisdom, Volume II* (New York: People with AIDS Coalition, 1988): 72.

30. Fedorko argued that Burroughs Wellcome was guilty of "whipping up all these doctors to prescribe AZT and giving them these lovely soirées with these fancy canapés." Fedorko, "Interview 144," 28.

31. As a measure of this sentiment, one of the characters in the play *Angels in America* refers to the drug as "poison." The first half of the piece, *Millennium Approaches*, was workshopped in 1990, premiered in 1991, and was awarded the Pulitzer Prize for Drama in 1993. Tony Kushner, *Angels in America: A Gay Fantasia on National Themes* (New York: TCG, 2006), 271.

32. Bob Lederer, "Curb Your Dogma," *POZ*, June 1, 1995. This article was included in one of HEAL's Comprehensive Information Packet (circa 1996), along with a letter written in response by Ellner, challenging several of Lederer's critiques. HEAL-A.

33. Fedorko, "Interview 144," 10.

34. For Fedorko's comments, see Fedorko, "Interview 144," 18–19; Fouratt argued, "Every time a new drug would come down the pike ACT UP's Treatment and Data would get all excited and people would get all excited. And for someone like me who thinks about side effects, and long term, and quality of living, and all that sort of stuff that's as important as taking the new drug. ACT UP got the inside path to access to that drug. And Keith [Haring] and Ethyl [Eichelberger] both got it. And they got it in large dosages when they found out later that that was lethal. And Ethyl Eichelberger committed suicide and Keith died. Now am I saying that ACT UP caused that? Or ACT UP's Treatment and Data people caused that? No, I don't say that, but I think that it has to be said that that is what happens when you don't step back a moment and say, what are we putting into our bodies? . . . When a person is desperate and you've got Larry Kramer screaming, 'Drugs into bodies! Drugs into bodies! If you don't want to do this, then you're not helping!' And all that sort of stuff. And the doctors who don't believe in giving choice to their client . . . who say, 'You take this, you take AZT or you're not my patient.' This is awful." Fouratt, "Interview 066", 54.

35. Fedorko, "Interview 144," 9.

36. Fedorko, "Interview 144," 19.

37. Fedorko commented, "[He] was a representative of the homocracy and white AIDS establishment and political pandering." The "homocrat" is a term for gay men who make a living representing gay causes. Fedorko, "Interview 144," 10; In a 1986 interview conducted by Michael Callen and published in the *PWAC Newsline*, Fouratt argued that professional AIDS service organizations were the successors to the Gay Activists Alliance (GAA), an organization founded in 1969 by individuals concerned with the Gay Liberation Front's radical activism. For Fouratt, the GAA's reticence to challenge pervasive social inequities such as racism and classism yielded a simplistic "If it's gay, it's ok" organizational philosophy. He critiqued this perspective, arguing that the gay lifestyle was itself shaped by societal oppression, and would level similar charges against orthodox AIDS organizations through the 1980s. See Michael Callen, "Interview by Michael Callen with Jim Fouratt," *PWAC Newsline* 18 (December 1986): 37–38, and Fouratt, "Interview 066"; For a discussion of the divide between "professional" and "radical" activists, see Benjamin H. Shepard, "The Queer/Gay Assimilationist Split: The Suits versus the Sluts," *Monthly Review* 53, no. 1 (May 2001).

38. Homeopathy, for example, has been referred to as the "aristocracy of quackery" and "the quackery of the drawing room." James C. Whorton, *Nature Cures: The History of Alternative Medicine in America* (Oxford: Oxford University Press, 2002), 68; A 2010 study published in *Pain Medicine* furthermore argued that alternative medicine therapies usually attract individuals with higher education levels and income. S. Khady Ndao-Brumblay and Carmen R. Green, "Predictors of Complementary and Alternative Medicine Use in Chronic Pain Patients," *Pain Medicine* 11, no. 1 (January 2010): 16–24.

39. "Introduction," *HEAL Comprehensive Information Packet*, circa 1996. HEAL-A.

40. Undated, untitled document from HEAL Archive, HEAL-A.

41. Lederer, "Curb Your Dogma"; Similarly, in a filmed HEAL television program recorded in 1993, HEAL member James Scutero argued, "Basically, if you want to live, fire your doctor." See Michael Ellner, "Preventing Illness/Preventing Health: Prophylaxis and the Medical Windfall," HEAL Videos, 1993, Video Transcripts on Alternative Theories of AIDS, prepared for Michael Ellner and HEAL by Mark Gabrish Conlan, HEAL-A.

42. See, for example, Peter Duesberg, *Inventing the AIDS Virus* (Washington, DC: Regnery, 1996).

43. Kalichman, *Denying AIDS*, 138–141.

44. Joseph E. Davis, "Introduction: Holism against Reductionism," in *To Fix or to Heal: Patient Care, Public Health, and the Limits of Biomedicine*, eds. Joseph E. Davis and Ana Marta Gonzalez (New York: New York University Press, 2016): 2–3. Parenthetical removed.

45. Davis, "Introduction"; See also Howard S. Berliner and J. Warren Salmon, "The Holistic Alternative to Scientific Medicine: History and Analysis," *International Journal of Health Services* 10, no. 1 (1980).

46. The president of the American Holistic Health Association, for example, has referred to health holism as "an ancient approach to health." Suzan Walter, "Holistic Health," *The Illustrated Encyclopedia of Body-Mind Disciplines* (New York: The Rosen Publishing Group, 1999), Reproduced at http://ahha.org/selfhelp-articles/holistic-health/; Another leading alternative health informational organization erroneously claims that both allopathic and homeopathic medicine are ancient and opposing systems. See Tim O'Shea, "Conventional Medicine vs. Holistic: A World of Difference," *Cancer Tutor*, December 22, 2016, accessed January 12, 2017, https://www.cancertutor.com/conventional-medicine-vs-holistic-a-world-of-difference/.

47. As a critical analysis of health holism published in 1989 noted, the movement argued that human disease was far more complicated than linear "cause and effect" relationships suggested, resulting from the complex interaction of myriad variables. See Kristine Beyerman Alster, *The Holistic Health Movement* (Tuscaloosa: University of Alabama Press, 1989): 61.

48. Holistic health activism through the second half of the twentieth century dealt heavily with cancer treatments, with the 1950s witnessing the rise of the Hoxsey herbal tonic, the 1960s the rise of Krebiozen, and the 1970s laetrile and the Therapeutic Touch.

49. Elizabeth Fee and Daniel Fox chronicle this transformation. Elizabeth Fee and Daniel Fox, eds., *AIDS: The Making of a Chronic Disease* (Berkeley: University of California Press, 1991); See also Steven G. Deeks, Sharon R. Lewin, and Diane V. Havlir, "The End of AIDS: HIV Infection as a Chronic Disease," *Lancet* 382, no. 9903 (November 2013): 1525–1533.

50. Joe Wright, "Remembering the Early Days of 'Gay Cancer,'" All Things Considered, National Public Radio, May 8, 2006; See also Dennis Altman, *AIDS in the Mind of America* (Garden City: Anchor, 1986), 35.

51. Gallo initially identified "human T-cell leukemia virus" as the cause of AIDS. He later changed the name to "human T-cell lymphotrophic virus" before the name HIV was adopted as a compromise between French and U.S. researchers. See Steve Connor, "The Virus Reveals the Naked Truth," *New Scientist* 12 (February 1987): 55–58.

52. "What is a Chronic Disease? Important Things to Know about Chronic Diseases for Persons with Disabilities," Illinois Disability and Health Program, Illinois Department of Health, accessed September 25, 2016, http://www.idph.state.il.us/idhp/idhp_ChronicDisease.htm.

53. "About Chronic Diseases," National Health Council, Rev 7/29/2014, accessed Sep 26, 2016, http://www.nationalhealthcouncil.org/sites/default/files/NHC_Files/Pdf_Files/About ChronicDisease.pdf.

54. James H. Thrall, "Prevalence and Costs of Chronic Disease in a Health Care System Structured for Treatment of Acute Illness," *Radiology* 235, no. 1 (2005): 9–12.

55. Some supporters of alternative and holistic approaches to AIDS directly invoked the language of chronicity in their activism. Niro Markoff Asistent's 1991 alternative health volume begins with the acclamation, "[M]ore and more people are realizing that AIDS is a chronic condition, and a major opportunity for personal and planetary transformation." Niro Markoff Asistent, *Why I Survive AIDS* (New York: Simon and Shuster, 1991), 4.

56. Andrew Cort, "HIV and the Cause of AIDS," *HEAL Bulletin* 1, no. 2 (Winter 1990), HEAL-A; Cort's acclamation lends credence to an analysis James S. Gordon would make of health holism in 1988: "At a time when narrow perspectives and single solutions appear inadequate to our problems," Gordon observed, "holism has emerged as an alternative, a catchall for our hopes." James S. Gordon, *Holistic Medicine* (New York: Chelsea House Publishing, 1988); See also "Test Your HIV I.Q. (The Alternative AIDS Test)," *HEAL Quarterly* 1, no. 1 (Fall 1989), HEAL-A. Also located in box 6, AZT (1988–1990), folder 193, Michael Callen Papers, LGBT-NA

57. Similar appeals to individuals' sense of personal responsibility appear throughout the archive. A 1988 *HEAL Newsletter* article penned by Dr. Raymond K. Brown, author of *AIDS, Cancer and the Medical Establishment* (New York: Robert Speller and Sons, 1986), argued that PWAs who survived the longest were "those taking an active role in shaping their health program, rather than passively waiting for their doctor's next instruction."; Several HEAL information packets produced through the 1990s warned PWAs not to place all of their faith in mainstream doctors, arguing, "You must learn to count on yourself! Your greatest help will

come from personal responsibility and self-empowerment."; In the first edition of the *HEAL Quarterly*, Michael Wayne Miles co-opts the language of mainstream biomedicine to advocate holistic self-empowerment: "Self-empowerment is becoming aware of your options, alternatives and choices you have in your life and your health. You get involved and take responsibility. Because you believe in yourself and your ability to take care of yourself, this is your magic bullet." See Raymond K. Brown, *HEAL Newsletter* 1, no. 2 (March 1988): 2, HEAL-A; "Introduction," *HEAL Comprehensive Information Packet*, circa 1996, HEAL-A; Michael Wayne Miles, "Self-Empowerment is the Magic Bullet," *HEAL Quarterly* 1, no. 1 (Fall 1989): 3, HEAL-A.

58. *SPIN* magazine claimed that early in the epidemic, Gallo rejected multifactorial models, arguing that HIV "kills like a truck" while dismissing talk of cofactors as "cock and horseshit." "Gallo Rethinks HIV," *SPIN*, July 1988, 97.

59. Michael L. Culbert, "AIDS—Facing Fear, Fancy, and Fact," HEAL Information Packet, circa 1993, UT-TFRBL.

60. Ellner, interview by Matthew Kelly.

61. F. R. Buianouckas, "AIDS: The Syndrome in a Nutshell" (April 1988), HEAL-A.

62. Ellner, interview by Matthew Kelly.

63. Other HEAL publications would echo these views. A 1995 article titled "Condomania," for example, argued, "Does terrorizing the population do harm? You bet it does! Think what is happening here. It is one thing to tell our daughters not to get pregnant until they are married and ready for children. But we are teaching our children (and everyone else) that 'intimacy means death' . . . We are telling them that they may die a horrible death unless they intrude on the lovemaking process by using some artificial means to prevent their body fluids from intermingling, even though for many that is an important part of the sexual experience." Peter W. Plumley, "Condomania," *HEAL Bulletin, Special Edition*, 1995, HEAL-A.

64. "AIDS Psychology: Interview with Michael Ellner and John Lauritsen," *Tony Brown's Journal*, aired January 30, 1994, Video Transcripts on Alternative Theories of AIDS, prepared for Michael Ellner and HEAL by Mark Gabrish Conlan, HEAL-A.

65. John Lauritsen and Hank Wilson, *Death Rush: Poppers & AIDS* (Inland Book Co., 1986).

66. John Lauritsen, "Looking Back on Berlin," *HEAL Bulletin* (Fall–Winter 1993), HEAL-A; John Lauritsen, "The Risk—AIDS Hypothesis," HEAL Comprehensive Information Packet HEAL-A, reprinted from *Reappraising AIDS* 3, no. 8 (August 1995).

67. "AIDS Psychology: Interview with Michael Ellner and John Lauritsen."

68. Ellner, interview by Matthew Kelly.

69. An opponent of the HIV etiological model, Willner injected himself with the blood of an individual diagnosed with HIV, declaring "I will repeat the process of sticking myself with the blood of an HIV positive person on television in every city of the world until this genocide stops." See "Doctor Injects Himself with HIV+ Blood," *POZ*, February 1, 1995; For Willner's discussion of recreational drug use among gay communities, see Robert E. Willner, "A Call for the Truth about AIDS: A White Paper on the Viral-AIDS Hypothesis" (January–February 1995), 9, HEAL-A.

70. Willner, "A Call for the Truth about AIDS," 8.

71. "Is AIDS a New Disease?" HEAL Info Pages, circa mid-1990s, HEAL-A.

72. See, for example, John Lauritsen, "The Risk—AIDS Hypothesis."; Lese Dunton, "Getting beyond AIDS," *New York Native* 246, January 4, 1988, 19–22, republished in HEAL Information Packet, UT-TFRBL.

73. F. R. Buianouckas, "AIDS: The Syndrome in a Nutshell" (April 1988), 7, HEAL-A.

74. In their 1980 article, Howard S. Berliner and J. Warren Salmon defined this level of engagement as "health as praxis." Berliner and Salmon, "The Holistic Alternative," 142.

75. Lese Dunton, "Getting beyond AIDS."
76. "AIDS Psychology: Interview with Michael Ellner and John Lauritsen."
77. Gina Kolata, "Federal Delay in Lowering Standard for Doses of AIDS Drug is Assailed," *New York Times*, December 27, 1989, A19; Gina Kolata, "U.S. Halves Dosage for AIDS Drug," *New York Times*, January 17, 1990, B6; See also Ann C. Collier, et al., "A Pilot Study of Low-Dose Zidovudine in Human Immunodeficiency Virus Infection," *New England Journal of Medicine* 323 (October 1990): 1015–1021.
78. As Ellner argued, "[Burroughs Wellcome] sat on those studies and these people were lied to . . . The battle cry was, 'We don't care if they kill us, we want access to life-saving drugs just in case' . . . Desperate people make desperate decisions, and these people were very desperate. Being an outsider and not being directly at risk, I could watch the consequences of AZT and I was among four or five people tops who were protesting it at the time. And all of us were shouted down, and that was about when HEAL began to fall from grace. And that's when people started to accuse us of being political." Ellner, interview by Matthew Kelly.
79. Ellner explained, "I had had rooms full of people say they thought preventive antibiotics made them sick in the first place. And now they were being told if you take them, you won't get PCP pneumonia and the drugs were Bactrim and aerosol pentamidine and it was like insanity. Well, every AIDS group was pushing them vigorously as this was the thing to do. And because I was leading the meetings, I was able to say anything I wanted. And so I challenged it." Ellner, interview by Matthew Kelly.
80. "Preventing Illness/Preventing Health: Prophylaxis and the Medical Windfall," Michael Ellner, HEAL Videos, 1993, Video Transcripts on Alternative Theories of AIDS, prepared for Michael Ellner and HEAL by Mark Gabrish Conlan. HEAL-A.
81. The source is a column appearing in an alternative medicine publication that positively reviewed a dissident text featuring articles by Michael Ellner, John Lauritsen, Casper Schmidt and others. Elizabeth A. Ely, "Read at Your Peril," Review of *The AIDS Cult*, *Townsend Letter for Doctors & Patients* (January 1998).
82. In discussing one PWA member of HEAL, Ellner argued, "Unfortunately, he took the early preventative antibiotics and they killed him in my opinion, which really pushed my resolve to challenge it. In other words, members of HEAL did take the treatment and it was not a pleasant thing to watch. They did believe that it was the answer." Ellner, interview by Matthew Kelly.
83. Bob Lederer, "Curb Your Dogma." Parenthetical removed; Fedorko's resignation from HEAL has been described as a direct result of Ellner's attacks on prophylactic responses to AIDS. In a 1996 *POZ* article, he is quoted as saying, "I see more and more new cases of PCP that likely could have been prevented with prophylactic measures. These are people uneducated about AIDS, many from susceptible minority populations. They listen to HEAL's messages and just end up getting PCP." Amy Feehan, "Breathe Deeply and Hold," *POZ*, May 1, 1996.
84. DiFerdinando, who was, by this point, HEAL's executive director, also argued, "The alternative community is well aware that the microbe theory of disease has more of a political, economic and emotional function than a medical one and, particularly [since] catalytic books like Ivan Illich's *Medical Nemesis*, had long since rejected it. But then with the advent of 'infectious AIDS', they all suddenly jumped right back into the 'deadly virus' roller coaster. All of a sudden its [sic] the new exception, and viruses are in vogue again because our government scientists, corporate media and conventional medical community say so." See Tom DiFerdinando, "This is a Challenge" (September 12, 1997), HEAL-A.
85. Michael H. Cohen, *Beyond Complementary Medicine: Legal and Ethical Perspectives on Health Care and Human Evolution* (Ann Arbor: University of Michigan Press, 2003): 12.

86. The song captures the speaker's frustration with a guru who invokes the oil of Aphrodite and the "dust of the grand wazoo" and claims to be able to cure disease. Confronting the guru, the speaker remarks, "And I said look here brother / Who you jiving with that cosmik debris? / Now what kind of a guru are you, anyway? / Look here brother, don't waste your time on me." See Frank Zappa, "Cosmik Debris," recorded March 1974, track 5 on Apostrophe ('); Various authors have linked New Age therapeutics with hippies. See, for example, Karen de Witt, "Health Officials Give Holism a Checkup," New York Times, April 25, 1978, 43.

87. The International Monetary Fund notes, "The term 'globalization' began to be used more commonly in the 1980s, reflecting technological advances that made it easier and quicker to complete international transactions—both trade and financial flows. It refers to an extension beyond national borders of the same market forces that have operated for centuries at all levels of human economic activity—village markets, urban industries, or financial centers." International Monetary Fund Staff, "Globalization: A Brief Overview," *International Monetary Fund Issues Brief* 2, no. 8 (May 2008).

88. Fritjob Capra, *The Turning Point* (Toronto: Bantam Books, 1988), 15–16; Capra had earned acclaim as the author of 1975's *The Tao of Physics*. See also "Books," accessed August 28, 2016, http://www.fritjofcapra.net/books/.

89. They included the 1989 *HEAL Quarterly* column "Change Your Health by Changing Your Thoughts," *HEAL Quarterly* 1, no. 1 (Fall 1989), HEAL-A; "The Turning Point: A Creative Healing Workshop" with Dr. Andrew Cort and Michael Ellner, undated. HEAL-A; an advertisement for a seminar titled "Tapping Your Psychospiritual Possibilities: Understanding and Using the Healing Powers of the Human Mind," HEAL-A; and "Hypnoimmunotherapy and AIDS," by Michael Ellner, undated, HEAL-A.

90. One HEAL informational packet includes a *New York Native* article written by a PWA who used guided meditation, Louise Hay, and visualization tapes. Dunton, "Getting beyond AIDS."

91. Hay established widespread notoriety by the late 1980s. Her 1988 text *You Can Heal Yourself* sold over thirty-five million copies, and she appeared on programs such as the *Oprah Winfrey Show*. Mark Oppenheimer, "The Queen of the New Age," *New York Times Magazine*, May 4, 2008; However, her claims generated significant controversy, with online message boards decrying her therapeutic approach as chicanery and quackery. See, for example, "Louise Hay is a Dangerous Quack," *Spirituality Is No Excuse*, January 24, 2014, accessed September 20, 2016, https://spiritualityisnoexcuse.wordpress.com/2014/01/24/louise-hay-is-a-dangerous-quack/, and "Quack Watch," discussion thread on *POZ Forums*, February 28, 2015, accessed September 20, 2016, http://forums.poz.com/index.php?topic=57962.0.

92. For a discussion of social medicine, see Dorothy Porter, "How Did Social Medicine Evolve, and Where is It Heading?" *PloS Medicine* 3, no. 10 (2006): e399.

93. Margaret Meade, "One Vote for this Age of Anxiety," *New York Times*, May 20, 1956, 227; See also R. B. Goodwin and M. B. Stein, "Generalized Anxiety Disorder and Peptic Ulcer Disease Among Adults in the United States," *Psychosomatic Medicine* 64, no. 6 (2002): 862–6.

94. For a discussion of neurasthenia, see Julie Beck, "'Americanitis': The Disease of Living Too Fast," *The Atlantic*, March 11, 2016.

95. On Auden's homosexuality, see Paul Fussell, "The Poet Himself," *New York Times*, October 4, 1981, reviewing Humphrey Carpenter *W. H. Auden: A Biography* (Boston: Houghton Mifflin Co, 1981).

96. Of note, despite his claim that AIDS dissidence "begins and ends with Peter Duesberg," Kalichman does cite Schmidt's early article as predating Duesberg. See Kalichman, *Denying AIDS*, 25–26.

97. We have very little information regarding Schmidt's life, though we know that he died of AIDS-related conditions in 1994. His experience in South Africa may have been similar to Sonnabend's, who attended medical school when the pro-apartheid Afrikaner Party came to power. Years later, Sonnabend noted that the experience had left him "unable to join groups of any kind. I'm totally suspicious of the demagoguery . . . I'm distrustful of not speaking to the simplicity of one's original motivation . . ." See Anne-Christine d'Adesky, "The Man Who Invented Safer Sex Returns," *Out*, Summer 1992, 31.

98. Casper G. Schmidt, "The Group-Fantasy Origins of AIDS" in *The AIDS Cult: Essays on the Gay Health Crisis*, eds. John Lauritsen and Ian Young (Provincetown: Asklepios, 1997). Originally published in *The Journal of Psychohistory*, 32 (1984).

99. Schmidt, "The Group-Fantasy," 12. Parenthetical omitted.

100. Schmidt, "The Group-Fantasy," 41, 50–51.

101. For epidemiological support, Schmidt cites the work of Canadian researcher Francois Sirois, *Mass Psychogenic Illness: A Social Psychological Analysis*, eds. Michael J. Colligan, James W. Pennebaker and Lawrence R. Murphy (Hillside, NJ: Lawrence Erlbaum, 1982); For anthropological support, he cites the work of Bronislaw Malinowski, who studied the Melanesian people of the Trobriand Islands in New Guinea. Bronislaw Malinowski, *Crime and Custom in Savage Society* (London: Kegan Paul, Trench, Trubner, 1926).

102. Ian Young claims that Schmidt remained committed to his group hysteria AIDS paradigm until his death. Ian Young, "The Psychohistorical Origins of AIDS: An Interview with Casper Schmidt," in *The AIDS Cult: Essays on the Gay Health Crisis*, eds. John Lauritsen and Ian Young (Provincetown: Asklepios, 1997). Originally published in *The Journal of Psychohistory*, Summer 1984.

103. Foucault published *Discipline and Punish* in French in 1975 and in English in 1977. Bourdieu published *La Distinction* in French in 1979 and in English in 1984.

104. Lauritsen argued that gay men's use of recreational drugs was a product of symbolic violence, with oppression forcing gay men to engage in underground practices and conservative hatred teaching them that their lives did not matter. Schmidt would touch upon these topics in the arena of sex, arguing that social shaming caused gay men to remove themselves from groups and engage in a "libidinization of the retaliatory fury with inappropriate sexual excitement." See Lauritsen, "The Risk—AIDS Hypothesis," and Schmidt, "The Group-Fantasy," 34.

105. One HEAL publication states, "AIDS is the result of many co-factors in one's life. Co-factors can include nutrition, multiple infections, self-image, spirituality, will to live, substance abuse, exercise, rest, stress and much more." Michael Wayne Miles, "Self-Empowerment is the Magic Bullet," *HEAL Quarterly* 1, no. 1 (Fall 1989), HEAL-A; Similarly, a HEAL information packet argues, "There is much evidence that ARC and AIDS are multifactorial problems and that HIV may simply be a co-factor: other germs, histories of drug abuse, other chronic infections, poor nutrition, environmental poisoning and intense, chronic stress may each be equally important as a cause and equally necessary to treat." In its list of factors underlying AIDS, the same source includes, "histories of medical and 'recreational' drug abuse, chronic infections, chronically poor nutrition, environmental poisoning and intense, chronic stress." HEAL Information Packet, undated, UT-TFRBL, 3.

106. Ellner also argued, "[I]t was impossible not to be impressed by the hysteria in the early '80s. Everywhere I turned, I was getting, 'Always fatal, always fatal, always fatal.'" Ellner, interview by Matthew Kelly.

107. Michael Ellner, "Don't be Scared to Death," HEAL Information Packet, undated. UT-TFRBL.

108. Students of the history of medicine will identify shades of Mesmerism in Ellner's theories. Indeed, hypnotherapy traces its origins to late eighteenth and early nineteenth-century

German physician Franz Mesmer's belief system. In at least one instance, HEAL literature directly invokes Mesmer. See Tom DiFerdinando, "Psychosocial Tension and the Lure of the AIDS Zone," presented at First International Meeting of Integral Psychosomatic Medicine, Sao Paolo, Brazil (May 3, 2006), HEAL-A.

109. DiFerdinando, "Psychosocial Tension," 4.

110. Ellner continued, "I believe that anytime a person accepts information (regardless of the source) without evaluating it, that person is open to cultural self-hypnosis and all the associated hypnobehaviors (trance logic, positive and negative hallucinations, etc.)" Michael Ellner, "'Cultural Hypnosis' and Questioning the HI-Virus," *HEAL Quarterly* 1, no. 3. (1991), reprinted for ACT UP's National People of Color AIDS Activist Conference, March 24, 1991, HEAL-A; Many later pieces of HEAL literature prominently featured bolded "HIV=AIDS=DEATH" logos.

111. Michael Ellner, "Psychological Genocide: The Push for AIDS Testing," 1990, HEAL-A; Ellner, "'Cultural Hypnosis' and Questioning the HI-Virus."

112. Tom DiFerdinando, "Dirty Words: The AIDS Fraud in Context," HEAL Basic Information Packet, undated, HEAL-A.

113. Rev. Dr. Michael Ellner, "Protective Stupidity: Epidemic Hysteria, Mass Hypnosis and Escaping from the AIDS Zone," circa 2000, HEAL-A.

114. Cort continues, "When health care is concerned only with combating disease and symptoms, it allows us to engage in the dangerous illusion that we can keep doing everything wrong (to ourselves, to each other, to the planet) and that we will somehow 'get away with it.' As long as scientists find a cure for heart disease, we can keep on eating badly. As long as scientists find a cure for cancer, we can continue to pollute the environment." Andrew Cort, *Our Healing Birthright: Taking Responsibility for Ourselves and Our Planet* (Rochester, VT: Inner Traditions, 1991): xiv. This text received a favorable review in an undated *HEAL Quarterly* article, HEAL-A.

115. Geiger, H. Jack, "Medical Nemesis: the 20th Century's Leading Luddite Turns to Medicine," *New York Times*, May 2, 1976.

116. Ellner did not necessarily welcome the dissident label affixed to HEAL's later work. Describing the group's efforts to define their movement, he recalled, "[W]e were looking at different words and we were thinking of 'rethinkers.' We were thinking of 'critics.' We were thinking of 'analysts.' I've always been one who doesn't like labels, but if you want to call me a dissident, I'd much prefer that to being called a denialist, which is an ugly, unfair term." Ellner, interview by Matthew Kelly.

117. For mention of HEAL chapters in Arizona, Australia, Argentina, Canada, Detroit, England, Minnesota, and New Hampshire, see Christine Maggiore, *What if Everything You Thought You Knew about AIDS Was Wrong?* 4th ed. (Studio City, CA: American Foundation for AIDS Alternatives, 2000); for HEAL chapters in Florida and Oregon, see "Re. Survey," email message from chrism@cogent.net to cory@direct.ca (October 1998), HEAL-A; for the Seattle group, see "HEAL Seattle Group Now Forming," HEAL/Seattle 2, no. 1 (Spring 1995), HEAL-A; for the New Hampshire group, see also "Notice from Dr. M. Dennis Paul, President, HEAL of New Hampshire" (April 19, 1995), HEAL-A; for the Vermont chapter, see *PWAC Newsline* 37 (October 1988).

118. See, for example, Michael Ellner, "The HIV/AIDS Dispute moves to Harlem," *Continuum* 5, no. 5; Michael Ellner, "Tricked Again: Political Visions and Latex Law Suits in New York," *Continuum* 5, no. 3; Ellner and DiFernando would additionally applaud the *Sunday Times* of London, *SPIN, New York Native, Tony Brown's Journal*, Earl Caldwell of the *New York Daily News, Penthouse, National League for Nursing*, Joan Shenton, and Meditel. See Michael Ellner and Tom DiFerdinando, "Deconstructing AIDS: The Advanced Iatrogenic Disease Syndrome," *HEAL Bulletin* (Spring–Summer 1994), HEAL-A.

119. One advertisement for the "HEAL this Week" television program noted that it aired every Friday on Channel 17 of Manhattan/Paragon Cable. It also describes HEAL as "the only major AIDS organization not bought off by pharmaceutical, corporate or government interests." HEAL-A.

120. Duesberg, for example, argued that HIV failed to satisfy Koch's postulates, a point that has been refuted by mainstream scientists myriad times. See Peter Duesberg, "HIV is Not the Cause of AIDS," *Science* 241 (July 1988): 514–517.

121. Ellner, interview by Matthew Kelly.

122. Josh Getlin, "AIDS and Minorities: Fear, Ignorance Cited: Toll Is Especially Severe Among Blacks, Latinos; Leaders Ask Funds for Information Programs," *Los Angeles Times*, August 10, 1987.

123. Lena Williams, "Rights Group Urges Blacks to Take a Larger Role on AIDS," *New York Times*, May 30, 1987; Sheryl Gay Stolberg, "Epidemic of Silence: Eyes Shut, Black America Is Being Ravaged by AIDS," *New York Times*, June 29, 1998.

124. In many cases, these collaborations were facilitated by individuals who claimed membership in multiple communities.

125. HHS Letter to HEAL, 1989, HEAL-A; at least one educational social worker member of HEAL also began holding workshops for parents of children diagnosed with AIDS. These events convinced some families to explore holistic treatment alternatives for their children's conditions." Personal correspondence with group members, April 10, 2010.

126. Cliff Goodman, "The Fall of the House of AZT: An Afro-Centric View," *Comprehensive Information Packet*, 1991, HEAL-A.

127. Cliff Kali Goodman, "Heal Happenings: October 13th" *HEAL Quarterly* (Fall–Winter 1992): 3. HEAL-A.

128. Cliff Kali Goodman, "The Fall of the House of AZT." Parenthetical in original.

129. Several other HEAL representatives spoke, including Tom DiFerdinando, Barnett Weiss (both from HEAL New York) and Roberto Giraldo (an advisor for HEAL New York and President of the Group for the Scientific Reappraisal of the HIV/AIDS Hypothesis). Cliff Goodman died in 1992. Michael Ellner, "The HIV/AIDS Dispute," 30.

130. Video footage of speaker presentations have been preserved by the dissident vaccine organization Vaccines Are Dangerous; Ellner's comments parallel an article published in *Essence* magazine in 1990, which begins with telling of the agenda for a fictitious secret governmental meeting: "'We can use this virus to eliminate certain populations,' [the scientist] explains. 'We thought we'd try homosexuals first—nobody cares what happens to them, anyway, they'll be little outcry. And if the virus proves effective—we can move on to other populations. Like the Black underclass. That'll help cut down on the dollars you have to spend on welfare . . . A few years later, in San Francisco, New York, Miami, and Los Angeles, gay men begin to sicken and die. A few years after that, poor Blacks also succumb to the same puzzling symptoms. The genocide project has begun." Karen Grisby Bates, "AIDS: Is It Genocide?" *Essence*, 21, September 1990.

131. Maggiore later drew national headlines for her refusal to give antiretrovirals to her child, who was HIV positive. The baby died in 2005. Maggiore died in 2006.

132. David France, "Challenging the Conventional Stance on AIDS," *New York Times*, December 22, 1998, F6.

133. Charles L. Ortleb, "Editorial AIDSGate: The Nurse Rivers Syndrome," *New York Native*, July 29–August 11, 1985, 6–7.

134. Martin P. Levine, "Bad Blood: The Health Commissioner, the Tuskegee Experiment, and AIDS Policy," *New York Native*, February 16, 1987, 13–16.

135. Sean Lawrence, "Into Africa, for Ntozake Shange," *Christopher Street*, 115.58, 1987.
136. "AIDS vs. All of Us," *Amsterdam News*, November 28, 1987, 12.
137. "AIDS vs. All of Us."
138. During this time, despite disagreements regarding some of the ideas the publications endorsed, HEAL supported them. When ACT UP called for a boycott of the *Native*, HEAL urged its members to buy two copies.
139. Tony Brown, "Blacks and Gays Need Each Other," *Los Angeles Sentinel*, March 23, 1989, A7; As noted earlier, Michael Ellner also appeared on Tony Brown's television program.
140. David Gilbert, *AIDS Conspiracy Theories: Tracking the Real Genocide* (Arm the Spirit, 1997).
141. Gilbert, *AIDS Conspiracy Theories.*

CONCLUSION

1. David Rosner and Susan Reverby, eds., *Health Care in America: Essays in Social History* (Philadelphia: Temple University Press, 1979).
2. Roy Porter, "The Patient's View: Doing Medical History from Below," *Theory and Society* 14, no. 2 (1985): 175–198.
3. As Roberta Bivins has argued, "At least until the advent of social history, histories of alternative medicines also struggled to overcome the frequent conflation of these practices with 'quackery'—a conflation profoundly influenced by the dismissive hostility of established medicine to systems that were simultaneously cosmologically heretical and economically competitive." See Roberta Bivins, "Histories of Heterodoxy," in *The Oxford Handbook of the History of Medicine*, ed. Mark Jackson (Oxford: Oxford University Press, 2011).
4. Patricia Barnes et al., "Complementary and Alternative Medicine Use Among Adults: United States," *Advance Data from Vital and Health Statistics*, U.S. Department of Health and Human Services (May 27, 2004); David Eisenberg et al. "Trends in Alternative Medicine Use in the United States, 1990–1997," *Journal of the American Medical Association* 280, no. 18 (1998): 1569–1575; Institute of Medicine, Committee on the Use of Complementary and Alternative Medicine by the American Public, *Complementary and Alternative Medicine in the United States* (Washington, DC: National Academies Press, 2005), 34.
5. Steven Epstein describes Foucault's microphysics of power as, "the dispersal of fluxes of power throughout all the cracks and crevices of the social system; the omnipresence of resistance at every site; and the propagation of knowledge, practices, meanings, and identities out of the deployment of power." Steven Epstein, *Impure Science: AIDS, Activism, and the Politics of Knowledge* (Berkeley: University of California Press, 1996), 4.
6. This complex expression of self-empowerment was anticipated by Michel Foucault in his enumeration of movements that "are an opposition to the effects of power which are linked with knowledge, competence, and qualification: struggles against the privileges of knowledge. But they are also an opposition against secrecy, deformation, and mystifying representations imposed on people." See Michel Foucault, "The Subject and Power," *Critical Inquiry* 8, no. 4 (1982): 777–795. This article was published mere weeks before the CDC used the term "AIDS" for the first time.
7. In making this point, I do not mean to suggest that PWAs' actions in any way required atonement, but rather that some individuals' discussions of responsibility discourse suggest translations between causal and moral responsibility narratives. Furthermore, I do not suggest that all PWAs would describe their actions in this way.
8. This should not be taken to mean that only only members of privileged socioeconomic classes embrace unorthodox healing systems. The members of HEAL, for example, included many

individuals who viewed themselves as less socioeconomically privileged than those in leadership roles within GMHC. Furthermore, the PWAC's *Newsline*, a rich resource advocating unorthodox etiological and therapeutic models, was circulated within communities of socioeconomically underprivileged individuals. Copies, for example, made their way to U.S. prisons which, in turn, prompted the publication's editors to create a column featuring the correspondence the group received from prisoners with AIDS.

9. Other examples of the borderland model can be found among members of the African American community living outside New York. In 1985, DC area African American Bishop Rainey Cheeks, who identifies as HIV positive, formed Us Helping Us, a group committed to embracing holistic approached to AIDS. "If I get shot, don't call an herbalist—get my ass to a hospital," he commented in a 2001 *POZ* interview. "Then, when I'm stitched back up, I'll have my green tea. It's all about finding a balance in your life." Walter Armstrong, "Bishop Rainey Cheeks," *POZ*, December 1, 2001, internal quotation mark omitted. Duberman describes Us Helping Us as featuring "internal cleansing, fasting, meditation, the intake of oxygen, and the harnessing of sexual energy . . . to aid in the healing process." Duberman 292. Sabrina Chase has furthermore documented engagement with alternative healing practices among Latinx communities living with HIV/AIDS. Sabrina Chase, *Surviving HIV/AIDS in the Inner City: How Resourceful Latinas Beat the Odds* (Rutgers University Press, 2011); See also Justin Abraham Linds, "Ferments and the AIDS Virus: Interspecies Counter-Conduct in the History of AIDS," *Medical Humanities* 45, no. 4 (August 2019): 435–442, 435.

10. Although my analysis focuses on lessons of relevance to orthodox health professionals, it applies to any individual whose practice is bounded by a set of professional standards, assumptions, values, and systems of knowledge production.

11. James Harvey Young, for example, recounts conflicts between early leaders of the National Institute of Health's Office of Alternative Medicine (later the National Center for Complementary and Alternative Medicine and then the National Center for Complementary and Integrative Medicine) who challenged mainstream efforts to embrace alternative healing modalities by subjecting them to double-blind clinical review. See James Harvey Young, "The Development of the Office of Alternative Medicine in the National Institutes of Health, 1991–1996," *Bulletin of the History of Medicine* 72, no. 2 (1998): 279–298.

12. For discussions of public health campaigns focused on reducing tobacco use, see Cati G. Brown-Johnson and Judith J. Prochaska, "Shame-Based Appeals in a Tobacco Control Public Health Campaign: Potential Harms and Benefits," *Tobacco Control* 24, no. 5 (2015): 419–420; Hannah R. Farrimond and Helene Joffe, "Pollution, Peril and Poverty: A British Study of the Stigmatization of Smokers," *Journal of Community and Applied Social Psychology* 16, no. 6 (October 2006): 481–49; for campaigns focused on reducing obesity, see Rebecca Puhl, *Shame Campaigns: Do They Work?* Obesity Action, accessed December 12, 2016, http://www.obesityaction.org/educational-resources/resource-articles-2/weight-bias/shame-campaigns-do-they-work; Rebecca Puhl, J. L. Peterson, and J. Luedicke, "Fighting Obesity or Obese Persons? Public Reactions to Obesity-Related Health Messages," *International Journal of Obesity* 37, no. 6 (June 2013): 774–782; for campaigns focused on reducing alcohol consumption, see Emily Bell et al., "It's a Shame! Stigma against Fetal Alcohol Spectrum Disorder: Examining the Ethical Implications for Public Health Practices and Policies," *Public Health Ethics* 9, no. 1 (April 2016): 65–77; see also Ron Bayer, "Stigma and the Ethics of Public Health: Not Can We but Should We," *Social Science and Medicine* 67, no. 3 (August 2008): 463–472; Leah Berkenwald, "Shame and Blame: Facing the Unintended Consequences of Health Messaging," *Huffington Post Blog*, March 24, 2012, accessed December 12, 2016, http://www.huffingtonpost.com/leah-berkenwald/shame-and-blame-facing-th_1_b_1223659.html; Gina Kolata, "The Shame of Fat Shaming," *New York Times*, October 1, 2016.

13. Azhar Hussain et al. "The Anti-vaccination Movement: A Regression in Modern Medicine," *Cureus* 10, no. 7 (2018): e2919; Philip Ball "Anti-vaccine Movement Could Undermine Efforts to End Coronavirus Pandemic, Researchers Warn," *Nature* 581 (2020): 251.
14. Essex argued, "The biggest disaster imposed on us was Duesberg with his statements that HIV did not cause AIDS . . . I think Duesberg played the biggest role in giving [former South African President Thabo Mbeki] a convenient excuse to avoid supplying drugs." Susan Brink, "Fake Cures for AIDS Have a Long and Dreadful History," *NPR* (August 17, 2014), accessed April 5, 2022. https://www.npr.org/sections/goatsandsoda/2014/07/15/331677282/fake-cures-for-aids-have-a-long-and-dreadful-history
15. Meredith Y. Smith et al., "Zidovudine Adherence in Persons with AIDS: The Relation of Patient Beliefs about Medication to Self-Termination of Therapy," *Journal of General Internal Medicine* 12, no. 4 (1997): 216–223. Within the quoted passage, the authors cite the following studies: S. Catt, J. Stygall, and J. Catalan, "Health Beliefs of HIV Asymptomatic Individuals about Taking Zidovudine (ZDV)," VIII International Conference on AIDS Amsterdam, The Netherlands, 1992; G. Todak, R. Kertzner, R. H. Remien, et al., "Psychosocial Factors in the Decision to Decline Zidovudine (ZDV) Treatment in HIV Seropositive Gay Men," VII International Conference on AIDS, San Francisco, CA, 1991; J. E. Samuels et al., "Zidovudine Therapy in an Inner City Population," *Journal of the Acquired Immune Deficiency Syndrome* 3 (1990): 877–82; B. B. O'Connor, J. S. Lazar, and W. H. Anderson, "Ethnographic Study of HIV Alternative Therapies," VIII International Conference on AIDS, Amsterdam, The Netherlands, 1992; J. H. Samet, et al., "Compliance with Zidovudine Therapy in Patients Infected with Human Immunodeficiency Virus, Type 1: A Cross-Sectional Study in a Municipal Hospital Clinic," *American Journal of Medicine* 92 (1992): 495–502. Parenthetical removed.
16. Bob Carver, "A New Song in Plague Time," *a hundred LEGENDS* (Northern Lights Alternatives and the Design Industries Foundation for AIDS, 1989). The volume is a collection of art, photographs, poetry, prose, music, and other media created by 127 people with AIDS.
17. Arizona Homeopathic and Integrative Medical Association, "Homeopathy and COVID-19," July 12, 2020, https://arizonahomeopathic.org/homeopathy-and-covid-19/; 7Song, "An Herbalist's Notes on the COVID-19 Virus," Northeast School of Botanic Medicine," March 6, 2022, accessed June 1, 2022, https://www.americanherbalistsguild.com/sites/americanherbalistsguild.com/files/7song-herbalistnotescovid-19.pdf. Vibhu Paudyal et al., "Complementary and Alternative Medicines Use in COVID-19: A Global Perspective on Practice, Policy and Research," *Research in Social and Administrative Pharmacy* 18, no. 3 (March 2022): 2524–2528.
18. Linda Nordling, "Unproven Herbal Remedy against COVID-19 Could Fuel Drug-Resistant Malaria, Scientists Warn," *Science*, May 6, 2020.
19. Naomi Oreskes, "The Reason Some Republicans Mistrust Science: Their Leaders Tell Them To," *Scientific American*, June 1, 2021.
20. Michael Gerson, "Too Many Americans are Still in Covid Denial," *Washington Post*, May 20, 2022.
21. Peter J. Hotez, "The Antiscience Movement is Escalating, Going Global and Killing Thousands," *Scientific American*, March 29, 2021.
22. In 2020, *Nature* published a piece outlining ways Trump was perceived to have meddled in pandemic science. Giuliana Viglione, "Four Ways Trumps Has Meddled in Pandemic Science," *Nature*, November 3, 2020.
23. Jacob Carter et al., "Presidential Recommendations for 2020: A Blueprint for Defending Science and Protecting the Public," Union of Concerned Scientists, January 29 2020.
24. Kiera Butler, "Anti-Vaxxers Have a Dangerous Theory Called 'Natural Immunity.' Now It's Going Mainstream," *Mother Jones*, May 12, 2020.

25. Physicians Daniel W. Erickson and Artin Massih have critiqued this claim, arguing, "Sheltering in place decreases your immune system. And then as we all come out of shelter in place with a lower immune system and start trading viruses, bacteria—what do you think is going to happen? Disease is going to spike." Quoted in Barry Brownstein, "COVID-19 Lockdowns May Destroy Our Immune System," *Intellectual Takeout*, April 29, 2020, accessed June 1, 2021, https://www.intellectualtakeout.org/covid-19-lockdowns-may-destroy-our-immune-systems/?fbclid=IwAR3DTEJabeH_b2epo6T1ue8zQD9X-7aXAriKJtqpM-rAnKYLvRMGctMXf8E

26. Winston Peters, "'Sorry Sunshine, Wrong Place.' New Zealand Deputy PM Tells Off Conspiracy Theorist," *The Guardian*, October 15, 2020. Some authors further allege that COVID-19 does not exist and is instead the creation of "global elites" intent on curtailing individual freedom. Roland Imhoff and Pia Lamberty, "A Bioweapon or a Hoax? The Link Between Distinct Conspiracy Beliefs about the Coronavirus Disease (COVID-19) Outbreak and Pandemic Behavior," *Social Psychology and Personality Science* (July 2020): 1–9.

27. One theory, since refuted by researchers, suggests that SARS-CoV-2 was intentionally designed to include genes from HIV. See Mohamad S. Hakim, "SARS-CoV-2, Covid-19, and the Debunking of Conspiracy Theories," *Reviews in Medical Virology* 31, no. 6 (November 2021): e2222.

28. Some authors have identified other links between 1980s and 1990s–era AIDS activism and policies governing the testing of COVID-19 treatments. Marie-Amélie George, "The Fight Against AIDS Has Shaped How Potential Covid-19 Drugs Will Reach Patients," *Washington Post*, April 29, 2020.

29. For a discussion of many of these topics, see Cass Sunstein, *#Republic: Divided Democracy in the Age of Social Media* (Princeton: Princeton University Press, 2017).

30. Julie Jiang, Xiang Ren, and Emilio Ferrara, "Social Media Polarization and Echo Chambers in the Context of COVID-19: Case Study," *JMIRx Med* 2, no. 3 (July–September 2021): e29570.

31. A. Westervelt, "How the Fossil Fuel Industry Got the Media to Think Climate Change Was Debatable," *Washington Post*, January 10, 2019.

32. Richard Hofstadter, "The Paranoid Style in American Politics," *Harper's Magazine*, November 1964.

33. Pew Research Center, "Public and Scientists' Views on Science and Society," January 29, 2015, accessed January 14, 2017, see page 37. http://www.pewinternet.org/files/2015/01/PI_ScienceandSociety_Report_012915.pdf.

34. Mark Lynas, "Even in 2015, the Public Doesn't Trust Scientists," *Washington Post*, January 30, 2015, accessed December 27, 2016, https://www.washingtonpost.com/posteverything/wp/2015/01/30/even-in-2015-the-public-doesnt-trust-scientists/.

BIBLIOGRAPHY

ARCHIVES

ACT UP Oral History Project (ACT UP-OHP)
Cornell University Library Rare and Manuscript Collection (CUL-RMC)
Health Education AIDS Liaison Archive (HEAL-A)
Health Education AIDS Liaison Newsletter Articles (see HEAL-A, UT-TFRBL)
Interviews with Michael Ellner (performed by Matthew Kelly)
Lesbian, Gay, Bisexual and Transgender Community Center National History Archive (LGBT-NHA)
New York Public Library Manuscripts and Archives Division (NYPL-MAD)
New York Public Library, Science Industry and Business Branch (NYPL-SIB)
People with AIDS Coalition Newsline Articles (see CUL-RMC, LGBT-NHA, NYPL-MAD, NYPL-SIB)
University of Toronto Thomas Fisher Rare Book Library (UT-TFRBL)

SELECT SCHOLARLY ARTICLES, CHAPTERS, DISSERTATIONS, AND MONOGRAPHS

Abrahams, Naomi. "Towards Reconceptualizing Political Action." *Sociological Inquiry* 62, no. 3 (July 1992): 327–347.

Advisory Committee of People with AIDS. "The Denver Principles: Statement from the Advisory Committee of People with AIDS." In *Surviving and Thriving with AIDS: Collected Wisdom, Volume II*, edited by Michael Callen. New York: People with AIDS Coalition, 1988.

Alster, Kristine Beyerman. *The Holistic Health Movement*. Tuscaloosa: University of Alabama Press, 1989.

Altman, Dennis. *AIDS in the Mind of America*. Garden City: Anchor, 1986.

Altman, Dennis. "Legitimation through Disaster: AIDS and the Gay Movement." In *AIDS, The Burdens of History*, edited by Elizabeth Fee and Daniel Fox. Berkeley: University of California Press, 1988.

Anzaldúa, Gloria. *Borderlands: La Frontera, The New Mestiza*. San Francisco: Aunt Lute Books, 1987.

Ashby, T. A. "Editorial." *Maryland Medical Journal* (December 12, 1885).

Auden, W. H. *The Age of Anxiety*. Princeton: Princeton University Press, 2011.

Ayanian, John and Donald Berwick. "Do Physicians Have a Bias toward Action?: A Classic Study Revisited." *Medical Decision Making* 11, no. 3 (July–September 1991): 154–158.

Baker, Robert. "Explaining the Birth of Bioethics, 1947–1999." In *Before Bioethics: A History of American Medical Ethics from the Colonial Period to the Bioethics Revolution*, 274–318. Oxford: Oxford University, 2013.

Bakwin, Harry. "Pseudodoxia Pediatrica." *New England Journal of Medicine* 232 (June 1945): 691–697.

Ball, Philip. "Anti-vaccine Movement Could Undermine Efforts to End Coronavirus Pandemic, Researchers Warn." *Nature* 581 (2020): 251.

Balmer, Randall. "C. Everett Koop and the Religious Right." *Christian Century*, March 6, 2013.

Barnes, Patricia M., Eve Powell-Griner, Kim McFann, and Richard L. Nahin. "Complementary and Alternative Medicine Use among Adults: United States." U.S. Department of Health and Human Services DHHS Publication No. (PHS) 2004–1250. *Advance Data from Vital and Health Statistics* 343, May 2004.

Barnet, Robert J. "Ivan Illich and the Nemesis of Medicine." *Medicine, Health Care and Philosophy* 6 (October 2003): 273–286.

Bayer, Ronald. "HIV Exceptionalism Revisited." *AIDS & Public Policy Journal* 9, no. 1 (1994): 16.

———. *Private Acts, Social Consequences: AIDS and the Politics of Public Health*. New York: Free Press, 1989.

———. "Public Health Policy and the AIDS Epidemic: An End to HIV Exceptionalism?" *New England Journal of Medicine* 324 (May 1991): 1500–1504.

———. "Stigma and the Ethics of Public Health: Not Can We but Should We." *Social Science and Medicine* 67, no. 3 (August 2008): 463–472.

Bayer, Ronald and Gerald Oppenheimer. *AIDS Doctors: Voices from the Epidemic; An Oral History*. New York: Oxford University Press, 2002.

Bell, Emily, Gail Andrew, Nina Di Pietro, Albert E. Chudley, James N. Reynolds, and Eric Racine. "It's a Shame! Stigma against Fetal Alcohol Spectrum Disorder: Examining the Ethical Implications for Public Health Practices and Policies." *Public Health Ethics* 9, no. 1 (April 2016): 65–77.

Bequaert Holmes, Helen and Laura M. Purdy, eds. *Feminist Perspectives in Medical Ethics*. Bloomington: Indiana University Press, 1992.

Bergman, Jeanne. "The Cult of HIV Denialism." *Achieve: A Quarterly Journal on HIV Prevention, Treatment and Politics* (Spring 2010): 16–18.

Berliner, Howard S. and J. Warren Salmon. "The Holistic Alternative to Scientific Medicine: History and Analysis." *International Journal of Health Services* 10, no. 1 (1980).

Berman, Edgar. *The Solid Gold Stethoscope*. New York: Macmillan, 1976.

Bivins, Roberta. *Alternative Medicine?: A History*. Oxford: Oxford University Press, 2007.

———. "Histories of Heterodoxy." In *The Oxford Handbook of the History of Medicine*, edited by Mark Jackson. Oxford: Oxford University Press, 2011.

Bix, Amy Sue. "Engendering Alternatives." In *The Politics of Healing: Histories of Alternative Medicine in Twentieth-Century North America*, edited by Robert D Johnston. New York: Routledge, 2004.

Black, David. *The Plague Years: A Chronicle of AIDS, the Epidemic of Our Times*. New York: Simon and Schuster, 1986.

Bocock, Robert. *Consumption*. New York: Routledge, 1993.

Bohm, Peter E. "Drug Addiction." In *Adult Psychopathology*, edited by Francis J. Turner. New York: Free Press, 1984.

Boston Women's Health Collective. *Women and Their Bodies: A Course*. Boston: Boston Women's Health Collective, 1970.

Bouchelle, E. F. "Practical Remarks on Congestive Fever." *Southern Medical and Surgical Journal* (June 1847): 355–360.

Bourdieu, Pierre. *In Other Words: Essays toward a Reflexive Sociology*. Redwood City, CA: Stanford University Press, 1990.

Boxill, Roger. *Shaw and the Doctors*. New York: Basic Books, 1969.

Brandt, Allan M. "AIDS in Historical Perspective: Four Lessons from the History of Sexually Transmitted Diseases." *American Journal of Public Health* 78, no. 4 (1988): 367–371.

Brandt, Allan M. and Martha Gardner. "Antagonism and Accommodation: Interpreting the Relationship between Public Health and Medicine in the United States during the 20th Century." *American Journal of Public Health* 90, no. 5 (2000): 707–715.

Brecher, Edward M. and Consumer Reports Editors. *Licit and Illicit Drugs: The Consumers Union Report on Narcotics, Stimulants, Depressants, Inhalants, Hallucinogens, and Marijuana—Including Caffeine, Nicotine and Alcohol.* Boston: Little Brown, 1973.

Brewin, Thurstan B. "Fraternizing with Fringe Medicine." *British Journal of General Practice* 44, no. 383 (June 1994): 243–244.

———. "Logic and Magic in Mainstream and Fringe Medicine." *Journal of the Royal Society of Medicine* 86, no. 12 (December 1993): 721–723.

Brier, Jennifer. *Infectious Ideas: U.S. Political Responses to the AIDS Crisis.* Chapel Hill: University of North Carolina Press, 2009.

———. "Locating Lesbian and Feminist Responses to AIDS, 1982–1984." *Women's Studies Quarterly* 35, no. 1–2 (Spring–Summer 2007): 234–248.

Bright, Gina M. *Plague-Making and the AIDS Epidemic: A Story of Discrimination.* New York: Palgrave Macmillan, 2012.

Brown, E. Richard. *Rockefeller Medicine Men: Medicine and Capitalism in America.* Berkeley: University of California Press, 1979.

Brown, Michael P. *RePlacing Citizenship: AIDS Activism and Radical Democracy.* New York: The Guilford Press, 1997.

Brown, Raymond Keith. *AIDS, Cancer and the Medical Establishment.* New York: Robert Speller and Sons, 1986.

Brown-Johnson, Cati G. and Judith J. Prochaska. "Shame-Based Appeals in a Tobacco Control Public Health Campaign: Potential Harms and Benefits." *Tobacco Control* 24, no. 5 (2015): 419–420.

Burnham, John C. "America's Golden Age: What Happened to It?" *Science* 215, no. 4539 (March 1982): 1474–1479.

Butler, Kurt. *Consumer's Guide to Alternative Medicine.* New York: Prometheus Books, 1992.

Callahan, Daniel. "Bioethics and Policy—a History." In *From Birth to Death and Bench to Clinic: The Hastings Center Bioethics Briefing Book for Journalists, Policymakers, and Campaigns,* edited by Mary Crowley. Garrison, NY: The Hastings Center, 2008, ix–x.

Callahan, Gerald N. *Infection: The Uninvited Universe.* New York: St. Martin's Press, 2006.

Callen, Michael, ed. "AIDS 201." In *Surviving and Thriving with AIDS: Collected Wisdom, Volume II.* New York: People with AIDS Coalition, 1988.

———. "Introduction." In *Surviving and Thriving with AIDS: Hints for the Newly Diagnosed, Volume I.* New York: People with AIDS Coalition, 1987.

———. "Life in the Reagan AIDies." American Public Health Association's Annual Meeting, 1986. Accessed July 1, 2022. http://michaelcallen.com/mikes-writing/life-in-the-reagan-aidies/.

———. "Passive Genocide in the Reagan Aidies." In *Surviving and Thriving with AIDS: Collected Wisdom, Volume II.* New York: People with AIDS Coalition, 1988.

———. *Surviving AIDS.* New York: Harper Collins, 1990.

———. "Surviving and Thriving with AIDS." In *Surviving and Thriving with AIDS: Collected Wisdom, Volume II.* New York: People with AIDS Coalition, 1988, 2:131.

———. *Surviving and Thriving with AIDS: Hints for the Newly Diagnosed, Volume I.* New York: People with AIDS Coalition, 1987.

———. "The Pros and Cons of Taking AZT: A Round Table Discussion: June 21, 1988." In *Surviving and Thriving with AIDS: Collected Wisdom, Volume II.* New York: People with AIDS Coalition, 1988.

Callen, Michael and Dan Turner. "A History of the PWA Self-Empowerment Movement." In *Surviving and Thriving with AIDS: Collected Wisdom, Volume II*, edited by Michael Callen. New York: People with AIDS Coalition, 1988.

Caplan, Arthur L. "'Who Lost China?' A Foreshadowing of Today's Ideological Disputes in Bioethics." *Hastings Center Report* 35, no. 3 (May–June 2005): 12–13.

Caplan, Eric. *Mind Games: American Culture and the Birth of Psychotherapy*. Berkeley: University of California Press, 1998.

Capra, Fritjof. *The Turning Point*. Toronto: Bantam Books, 1988.

Carson, Rachel. *Silent Spring*. Boston: Houghton Mifflin Company, 1962.

Carter, Jacob, Taryn MacKinney, Genna Reed, and Gretchen Goldman. "Presidential Recommendations for 2020: A Blueprint for Defending Science and Protecting the Public." Union of Concerned Scientists, January 29, 2020.

Carter, Richard. *The Doctor Business*. Garden City: Doubleday, 1958.

Carver, Bob Jr. "A New Song in Plague Time." In *a hundred LEGENDS*. Northern Lights Alternatives, 1986.

Cayleff, Susan E. *Wash and be Healed: The Water-Cure Movement and Women's Health*. Philadelphia: Temple University Press, 1991.

Chakrabarty, Dipesh. "Minority Histories, Subaltern Pasts." *Postcolonial Studies* 1, no. 1 (1998): 15–29.

Chambré, Susan M. *Fighting for Our Lives: New York's AIDS Community and the Politics of Disease*. New Brunswick: Rutgers University Press, 2006.

Chase, Sabrina. *Surviving HIV/AIDS in the Inner City: How Resourceful Latinas Beat the Odds*. New Brunswick: Rutgers University Press, 2011.

Chauncey, George Jr. "Gay Men's Strategies of Everyday Resistance." In *Major Problems in the History of American Sexuality*, edited by Kathy Peiss. Boston: Houghton Mifflin Company, 2002.

Chinn, Peggy L. and Charlene Eldridge Wheeler. "Feminism and Nursing." *Nursing Outlook* 33, no. 2 (March–April 1985): 74–77.

Chulach, Theresa and Marilou Gagnon. "Working in a 'Third Space': A Closer Look at the Hybridity, Identity and Agency of Nurse Practitioners." *Nursing Inquiry* 21, no. 1 (March 2016): 52–63.

Cohen, Michael H. *Beyond Complementary Medicine: Legal and Ethical Perspectives on Health Care and Human Evolution*. Ann Arbor: University of Michigan Press, 2003.

Cohen, Peter F. "'All They Needed': AIDS, Consumption, and the Politics of Class." *Journal of the History of Sexuality* 8, no. 1 (July 1997): 86–115.

Colgrove, James. "The McKeown Thesis Statement: A Historical Controversy and Its Enduring Influence." *American Journal of Public Health* 92, no. 5 (2002): 725–729.

———. *State of Immunity: The Politics of Vaccination in Twentieth Century America*. Berkeley: University of California Press, 2006.

Collier, Ann C., Samuel Bozzette, Robert W. Coombs, Dennis M. Causey, David A. Schoenfeld, Stephen A. Spector, Carla B. Pettinelli, Glen Davies, Douglad D. Richman, John M. Leedom, et al. "A Pilot Study of Low-Dose Zidovudine in Human Immunodeficiency Virus Infection." *New England Journal of Medicine* 323 (October 1990): 1015–1021.

"Confessions of a Chiropractor." *Journal of the American Medical Association* 68, no. 9 (1917): 732.

Connor, Steve. "The Virus Reveals the Naked Truth." *New Scientist* 12 (February 1987): 55–58.

"Conquering the Chronic Disease." *Science News* 116, no. 17 (October 1979): 277–278.

Conrad, Peter. "The Social Production of Disease and Illness." In *The Sociology of Health and Illness, Critical Perspectives*, edited by Peter Conrad. Waltham, MA: Worth Publishers, 2009.

Cooper, E. L., ed. *Stress, Immunity and Aging*. New York: Marcel Dekker, 1984.

Cort, Andrew. *Our Healing Birthright: Taking Responsibility for Ourselves and Our Planet*. Rochester, VT: Inner Traditions, 1991.

Costa. *Between Two Stools*. London: Remington and Company, 1883.

Cox, Henry. "Appreciation: A Prophet, a Teacher, a Realistic Dreamer." *National Catholic Reporter*, December 20, 2002.

Culyba, Rebecca. "Classification and the Social Construction of Disease in Medical Systems: A Historical Comparison of Syphilis and HIV/AIDS in the United States." PhD diss. Northwestern University, 2008.

Crawford, Robert. "Healthism and the Medicalization of Everyday Life." *International Journal of Health Services* 10, no. 3 (1980): 365–388.

———. "Individual Responsibility and Health Politics in the 1970s." In *Health Care in America: Essays in Social History*, edited by Susan M. Reverby and David Rosner, 247–268. Philadelphia: Temple University Press, 1979.

———. "The Boundaries of the Self and the Unhealthy Other: Reflections on Health, Culture, and AIDS." *Social Science and Medicine* 38 (1994): 1347–1365.

———. "You are Dangerous to Your Health: The Ideology and Politics of Victim Blaming." *International Journal of Health Services* 7, no. 4 (1977): 663–680.

Crimp, Douglass, ed. *AIDS: Cultural Analysis, Cultural Activism*. Cambridge: MIT Press, 1988.

Crosby, Alfred. *America's Forgotten Pandemic: The Influenza of 1918*. 2nd ed. Cambridge: Cambridge University Press, 2003.

Cumming, William Fullerton. *Notes of a Wanderer, in Search of Health through Italy, Egypt, Greece, Turkey up the Danube, and Down the Rhine, Volume I*. London: Saunders and Otley, 1839.

Curtiss, Romaine J. "Medical Empiricism, Homeopathy and Codes." *Western Lancet* XII, no. 8 (1883): 351–359.

Daniels, J. Reese. "A Noble Profession: A Retort to Our Critics within the Bar." *American Bar Association Journal* 43 (February 1957): 119.

Davidovitch, Nadav. "Negotiating Dissent." In *The Politics of Healing: Histories of Alternative Medicine in Twentieth Century North America*, edited by Robert D. Johnston, New York: Routledge, 2004.

Davis, Joseph E. "Introduction: Holism against Reductionism." In *To Fix or to Heal: Patient Care, Public Health, and the Limits of Biomedicine*, edited by Joseph E. Davis and Ana Marta Gonzalez. New York: New York University Press, 2016.

Deeks, Steven G., Sharon R. Lewin, and Diane V Havlir. "The End of AIDS: HIV Infection as a Chronic Disease." *Lancet* 382, no. 9903 (November 2013): 1525–1533.

"The Denver Principles (1983)." ACT UP NY. Accessed April 20, 2016. http://www.actupny.org/documents/Denver.html.

"The Denver Principles (1983)." UNAIDS. Accessed April 20, 2016. http://data.unaids.org/pub/ExternalDocument/2007/gipa1983denverprinciples_en.pdf.

DiFerdinando, Tom. "Psychosocial Tension and the Lure of the AIDS Zone." Presented at First International Meeting of Integral Psychosomatic Medicine, Sao Paolo, Brazil (May 3, 2006).

Duberman, Martin. *Hold Tight Gently: Michael Callen, Essex Hemphill, and the Battlefield of AIDS*. New York: The New Press, 2016.

Dubos, René. *Man, Medicine, and Environment*. New York: The New American Library, 1968.

———. *So Human an Animal: How We Are Shaped by Surroundings and Events*. New York: Scribner, 1968.

Duesberg, Peter. "HIV is Not the Cause of AIDS." *Science* 241 (July 1988): 514–517.

———. *Inventing the AIDS Virus*. Washington, DC: Regnery, 1996.

———. "Retroviruses as Carcinogens and Pathogens: Expectations and Reality." *Cancer Research* 47, no. 5 (March 1987): 1199–1220.

Dvarackas, Peter. "Self Hypnosis: A Gift You Give to Yourself." In *Surviving and Thriving with AIDS: Collected Wisdom, Volume II*, edited by Michael Callen. New York: People with AIDS Coalition, 1988.

———. "Surviving AIDS with the Wisdom of the East." In *Surviving and Thriving with AIDS: Collected Wisdom, Volume II*, edited by Michael Callen. New York: People with AIDS Coalition, 1988.

Dzur, Albert W. *Democratic Professionalism: Citizen Participation and the Reconstruction of Professional Ethics, Identity and Practice*. University Park, PA: Pennsylvania State University, 2008.

Eaklor, Vicki L. *Queer America: A GLBT History of the 20th Century*. Westport: Greenwood, 2008.

"Editorial." *The American Medical Journal* XXV, no. 12 (1897): 567–570.

Ehrenreich, Barbara. *The American Health Empire: Power, Profits, and Politics; A Report from the Health Policy Advisory Center*. New York: Random House, 1971.

Ehrenreich, Barbara and John Ehrenreich. "Health for Profit: The Big Business of Health." *Health-PAC Bulletin* (November 1969): 2.

Ehrenreich, John, ed. "Introduction: The Cultural Crisis in Modern Medicine." In *The Cultural Crisis of Modern Medicine*. New York: Monthly Review Press, 1978.

Eisenberg, David, Roger B. Davis, Susan L. Ettner, Scott Appel, Sonja Wilkey, Maria Van Rompay, and Ronald C. Kessler. "Trends in Alternative Medicine Use in the United States, 1990–1997: Results of a Follow-up National Survey." *Journal of the American Medical Association* 280, no. 18 (1998): 1569–1575.

Eley, Geoff. "Dilemmas and Challenges of Social History since the 1960s: What Comes after the Cultural Turn?" *South African Historical Journal* 60, no. 3 (2008): 310–322.

Ely, Elizabeth A. "Read at Your Peril." *Townsend Letter for Doctors & Patients* (January 1998).

Engel, George L. "A Unified Concept of Health and Disease." *Perspectives in Biology and Medicine* 3, no. 4 (1960): 459–485.

———. "The Need for a New Medical Model: A Challenge for Biomedicine." *Science* 196, 4286 (1977): 129–136.

Epstein, Cynthia Fuchs. "The Multiple Realities of Sameness and Difference: Ideology and Practice." *Journal of Social Issues* 53, no. 2 (1997): 259–278.

Epstein, Steven. "Activism, Drug Regulation, and the Politics of Therapeutic Evaluation in the AIDS Era: A Case Study of ddC and the 'Surrogate Markers' Debate." *Social Studies of Science* 27 (1997): 691–726.

———. *Impure Science: AIDS, Activism, and the Politics of Knowledge*. Berkeley: University of California Press, 1996.

Evans, John H. *The History and Future of Bioethics: A Sociological View*. Oxford: Oxford University Press, 2014.

Farrimond, Hannah R. and Helene Joffe. "Pollution, Peril and Poverty: A British Study of the Stigmatization of Smokers." *Journal of Community and Applied Social Psychology* 16, no. 6 (October 2006): 481–49.

Fee, Elizabeth and Daniel Fox, eds. *AIDS: The Burdens of History*. Berkeley: University of California Press, 1988.

———. "Introduction: The Contemporary Historiography of AIDS." In *AIDS: The Making of a Chronic Disease*. Berkeley: University of California Press, 1991.

Firestone, John M. *Trends in Prescription Drug Prices*. Washington, DC: American Enterprise Institute for Public Policy Research, 1970.

Fogel, Robert William. *The Fourth Great Awakening and the Future of Egalitarianism*. Chicago: University of Chicago Press, 2002.

Forman, Maury and David Horsey, eds. *Cartooning AIDS Around the World*. Dubuque, IA: Kendall Hunt, 1992.

Flannery, Michael A. "The Early Botanical Medical Movement as a Reflection of Life, Liberty, and Literacy in Jacksonian America." *Journal of the Medical Library Association*. 90, no. 4 (October 2002): 442–454.

Foucault, Michel. *Discipline and Punish: The Birth of the Prison*. London: Tavistock, 1977.

———. "La Fonction Politique de l'intellectuel." In *Dits et Écrits*, Vol. II: 1976–1988, edited by Daniel Defert and Francois Ewald, 112. Paris: Gallimard, 2001.

———. "The Crisis of Medicine or the Crisis of Antimedicine?" Translated by Edgar C. Knowlton, Jr., William J. King, and Clare O'Farrell. Lecture at Rio de Janeiro State University, Rio de Janeiro, Brazil, October 1974.

———. "The Subject and Power." *Critical Inquiry* 8, no. 4 (1982): 777–795.

France, David. *How to Survive a Plague*. New York: Vintage Books, 2017.

Frank, Arthur W. and Therese Jones. "Bioethics and the Later Foucault." *Journal of Medical Humanities* 24, no. 3/4 (December 2003): 179–186.

Freidson, Eliot, L. *Profession of Medicine: A Study of the Sociology of Applied Knowledge*. New York: Dodd, Mead and Company, 1975.

Friedan, Betty. *The Feminine Mystique*. New York: W. W. Norton and Co., 1963.

Fuller, Robert C. *Alternative Medicine and American Religious Life*. Oxford: Oxford University Press, 1989.

———. *Mesmerism and the American Cure of Souls*. Philadelphia: University of Pennsylvania Press, 1982.

Funkhouser, G. Ray. "The Issues of the Sixties: An Exploratory Study in the Dynamics of Public Opinion." *The Public Opinion Quarterly* 37, no. 1 (1973): 62–75.

Galdston, Iago, ed. *Beyond the Germ Theory: The Roles of Deprivation and Stress in Health and Disease*. New York: Health Education Council, 1954.

Gamson, William A. and Howard Schuman. "Some Undercurrents in the Prestige of Physicians." *American Journal of Sociology* 68, no. 4 (January 1963): 463–470.

Gevitz, Norman, ed. *Other Healers: Unorthodox Medicine in America*. Baltimore: Johns Hopkins University Press, 1988.

Gilbert, David. *AIDS Conspiracy Theories: Tracking the Real Genocide*. Arm the Spirit, 1997.

Goldsmith, Jeff. "The Paradigm Shift: Transforming from an Acute to Chronic Care Model." *Decisions in Imaging Economics* (1990): 13–19.

Goldstein, Michael S. *Alternative Health Care: Medicine, Miracle, or Mirage?* Philadelphia: Temple University Press, 1999.

Goodwin, R. B. and M. B. Stein. "Generalized Anxiety Disorder and Peptic Ulcer Disease Among Adults in the United States." *Psychosomatic Medicine* 64, no. 6 (2002): 862–6.

Gordon, James S. *Holistic Medicine*. New York: Chelsea House Publishing, 1988.

———. "Holistic Medicine: Advances and Shortcomings." *Journal of Western Medicine* 136, no. 6 (June 1982): 546–551.

Gould, Deborah B. *Moving Politics: Emotion and ACT UP's Fight Against AIDS*. Chicago: University of Chicago Press, 2009.

Greene, Jeremy A. and Scott H. Podolsky. "Reform, Regulation and Pharmaceuticals—The Kefauver-Harris Amendments at 50." *New England Journal of Medicine* 367, no. 16 (October 2012): 1481–1483.

Grmek, Mirko D. *History of AIDS: Emergence and Origin of a Modern Pandemic*. Princeton: Princeton University Press, 1993.

Gurin, Joel. "The Changing Medical Model." *The University of California San Francisco Magazine* 1, no. 2 (1978).

Hadas, Rachel, ed. *Unending Dialogue.* Boston: Faber and Faber, 1991.

Hadler, Nortin M. *Worried Sick: A Prescription for Health in an Overtreated America.* Chapel Hill: University of North Carolina Press, 2008.

Hakim, Mohamad S. "SARS-CoV-2, Covid-19, and the Debunking of Conspiracy Theories." *Reviews in Medical Virology* 31, no. 6 (November 2021): e2222.

Haller, John S. Jr. *The History of American Homeopathy: From Rational Medicine to Holistic Health Care.* New Brunswick: Rutgers University Press, 2013.

———. *Kindly Medicine: History of Physio-Medicalism in America, 1836–1911.* Kent, OH: Kent State University Press, 1997.

———. *Medical Protestants: The Eclectics in American Medicine, 1825–1939.* Carbondale: Southern Illinois University, 1994.

———. *The People's Doctors: Samuel Thomson and the American Botanical Movement: 1790–1860.* Carbondale, IL: Southern Illinois University Press, 2001.

Hannaway, Caroline. "Commentary on Workshop 1: Before AIDS: An Overview of Previous U.S. Epidemics to Clarify the Administrative, Scientific, and Social Responses to Mass Disease." In *AIDS and the Historian: Proceedings of a Conference at the National Institutes of Health 20–21 March 1989,* edited by Victoria A. Harden and Guenter B. Risse, 1–32. NIH Publication no. 91-1584 (March 1991).

Harrington, Mark. "AIDS Activists and People with AIDS." In *Tactical Biopolitics: Art, Activism and Technoscience,* edited by Beatriz da Costa and Kavita Philip, 323–340. Cambridge: MIT Press, 2008.

Harrington, Michael. *The Other America: Poverty in the Unites States.* New York: Macmillan Publishers, 1962.

Harris, Craig G. in *Brother to Brother: New Writings by Black Gay Men,* edited by Essex Hemphill. Boston: Alyson Publications, 1991.

Harris, Richard. *A Sacred Trust.* New York: New American Library, 1966.

Hartch, Todd. *The Prophet of Cuernavaca: Ivan Illich and the Crisis of the West.* Oxford: Oxford University Press, 2015.

Hernandez, Kelly Lytle. "Borderlands and the Future History of the American West." *Western Historical Quarterly* 42, no. 3 (Fall 2011): 325–330.

Herzberg, D. L. '"The Pill You Love Can Turn on You': Feminism, Tranquilizers, and the Valium Panic of the 1970s." *American Quarterly* 58, no. 1 (March 2006): 79–103.

Hess, David J. "CAM Cancer Therapies in Twentieth Century North America." In *The Politics of Healing: Histories of Alternative Medicine in Twentieth Century North America,* edited by Robert D. Johnston. New York: Routledge, 2004.

Hirsch, Michael. "Holistic Health Care for AIDS." In *Surviving and Thriving with AIDS: Collected Wisdom, Volume II,* edited by Michael Callen. New York: People with AIDS Coalition, 1988.

Hofstadter, Richard. "The Paranoid Style in American Politics." *Harper's Magazine,* November, 1964.

Hollinger, David A. "Science as a Weapon in *Kulturkampfe* in the United States during and after World War II." *Isis* 86, no. 3 (1995): 440–54.

Holmes, Oliver Wendell. *Medical Essays: 1842–1882.* Boston: Houghton, Mifflin and Company, 1883.

Hotez, Peter J. "The Antiscience Movement is Escalating, Going Global and Killing Thousands." *Scientific American* (March 29, 2021).

Hussain, Azhar, Syed Ali, Madiha Ahmed, and Sheharyar Hussain. "The Anti-vaccination Movement: A Regression in Modern Medicine." *Cureus* 10, no. 7 (2018): e2919.

Illich, Ivan. *Medical Nemesis: The Expropriation of Health*. New York: Pantheon, 1976.

———. "A Plea for Body History (Twelve Years after Medical Nemesis)." *Bulletin of Science, Technology and Society* 6 (1986): 19–22.

Imber, Jonathan B. *Trusting Doctors: The Decline of Moral Authority in American Medicine*. Princeton: Princeton University Press, 2008.

Imhoff, Roland and Pia Lamberty. "A Bioweapon or a Hoax? The Link Between Distinct Conspiracy Beliefs about the Coronavirus Disease (COVID-19) Outbreak and Pandemic Behavior." *Social Psychology and Personality Science* (July 2020): 1–9.

Ingelfinger, F. J. "Deprofessionalizing the Profession." *New England Journal of Medicine* 294, no. 6 (February 1976): 334–335.

Inlander, Charles B., Lowell S. Levin, and Ed Weiner. *Medicine on Trial: The Appalling Story of Ineptitude, Malfeasance, Neglect and Arrogance*. New York: Prentice Hall Press, 1988.

Institute of Medicine. Committee on the Use of Complementary and Alternative Medicine by the American Public, *Complementary and Alternative Medicine in the United States*. Washington, DC: National Academies Press, 2005.

Institute of Medicine. *The Future of the Public's Health*. Washington, DC, 2003.

International Monetary Fund Staff. "Globalization: A Brief Overview." *International Monetary Fund Issues Brief* 2, no. 8 (May 2008).

Jackson, Charles O. "A Difficult Pill to Swallow." *Reviews in American History* 9, no. 4 (December 1981): 516–520.

Jackson, Mark. *The Age of Stress: Science and the Search for Stability*. Oxford: Oxford University Press, 2013.

James, John S. "AIDS, AL 721, and Lecithin." *AIDS Treatment News* 8 (July 18, 1986).

James, Steven. "Reflections on Healing, Honesty and Personal Power." In *Surviving and Thriving with AIDS: Hints for the Newly Diagnosed, Volume I*, edited by Michael Callen. New York: People with AIDS Coalition, 1987.

Jennings, Bruce. "Biopower and the Liberationist Romance." *Hastings Center Report* 40, no. 4 (July–August 2010): 16–20.

Jiang, Julie, Xiang Ren, and Emilio Ferrara. "Social Media Polarization and Echo Chambers in the Context of COVID-19: Case Study." *JMIRx Med* 2, no. 3 (July–September 2021): e29570.

Johnson, Walter. "On Agency." *Journal of Social History* 37, no. 1, Special Issue (2003): 113–124.

Johnston, R. D., ed. *The Politics of Healing: Histories of Alternative Medicine in Twentieth Century North America*. New York: Routledge, 2004.

Jones, Matthew J. *Love Don't Need a Reason: The Life and Music of Michael Callen*. Santa Barbara: Punctum Books, 2020.

Jonsen, Albert R. "Beating up Bioethics." *Hastings Center Report* 31, no. 5 (September–October 2001): 40–45.

———. *The Birth of Bioethics*. Oxford: Oxford University Press, 2003.

———. "A History of Bioethics as Discipline and Discourse." In *Bioethics: An Introduction to the History, Methods, and Practice*. 3rd ed. Edited by Nancy S. Jecker, Albert R. Jonsen, and Robert A. Pearlman. Toronto: Jones and Bartlett Learning, 2012.

Journal of New Drugs 3 (1963): 149.

Kalichman, Seth C. *Denying AIDS: Conspiracy Theories, Pseudoscience, and Human Tragedy*. New York: Copernicus Press, 2009.

Kaempffert, Waldemar. "The Case for Planned Research." *American Mercury* 57 (1943): 557, quoted in John C. Burnham. "American Medicine's Golden Age: What Happened to It?" *Science* 215, no. 4539 (March 1982): 1474–1479.

Kaufman, Joel. *Over the Counter Pills That Don't Work*. New York: Pantheon Books, 1983.

Kaufman, Martin. *Homeopathy in America: The Rise and Fall of a Medical Heresy*. Baltimore: Johns Hopkins University Press, 1971.

Kellogg, C. W. "Calomel, Its Uses and Abuses." Read at Meeting of the San Joaquin Valley Medical Society, March 11, 1902. *Occidental Medical Times*. XVI, 4 (1902).

King, Lester S. "Shaw and the Doctors." *Journal of the American Medical Association* 209, no. 10 (September 1969): 1531.

Kirp, David L. *Learning by Heart: AIDS and Schoolchildren in America's Communities*. New Brunswick: Rutgers University Press, 1990.

Kirschmann, Anne Taylor. *A Vital Force: Women in American Homeopathy*. New Brunswick: NJ: Rutgers University Press, 2004.

Klerman, Gerald L. "Policy Issues on Provision of Mental Health Services in Primary Care Settings: A Federal View." In *Mental Health Services in General Health Care, Volume I: Conference Report*. Washington, DC: National Academy of Sciences, 1979, 31–40.

Kline, Wendy. *Bodies of Knowledge: Sexuality, Reproduction, and Women's Health in the Second Wave*. Chicago: University of Chicago Press, 2010.

Knowles, John H. "The Responsibility of the Individual." *Daedalus* 106, no. 1 (Winter 1977): 57–80.

Kopacz, David. *Re-humanizing Medicine: A Holistic Framework for Transforming Your Self, Your Practice, and the Culture of Medicine*. Winchester, UK: Ayni Books, 2014.

Kotlowsky, Dean. "The Knowles Affair: Nixon's Self-Inflicted Wound." *Presidential Studies Quarterly* 30, no. 3. (2000): 443–463.

Kruger, Steven F. "Medieval/Postmodern: HIV/AIDS and the Temporality of Crisis." In *Queering the Middle Ages*, edited by Glenn Burger and Steven F. Kruger. Minneapolis: University of Minnesota Press, 2001.

Kushner, Tony. *Angels in America: A Gay Fantasia on National Themes*. New York: TCG, 2006.

Lagemann, Ellen Condliffe, ed. *Nursing History: New Perspectives, New Possibilities*. New York: Teachers College Press, Columbia University, 1983.

Lander, Louise. *Defective Medicine: Risk, Anger, and the Malpractice Crisis*. New York: Farrar, Straus, and Giroux, 1978.

Lasagna, Louis C., ed. "Introduction." In *Controversies in Therapeutics*. Philadelphia: W.B. Saunders, 1980.

Lauritsen, John and Hank Wilson. *Death Rush: Poppers and AIDS*. New York: Inland Book Co, 1986.

Lauritsen, John and Ian Young, eds. *The AIDS Cult: Essays on the Gay Health Crisis*. Provincetown: Asklepios, 1997.

Lears, T. J. Jackson. *No Place of Grace: Antimodernism and the Transformation of American Culture, 1880–1920*. Chicago: University of Chicago Press, 1994.

Lee, Philip R. "America is an Overmedicated Society." In *Controversies in Therapeutics*, edited by Louis C. Lasagna. Philadelphia: W. B. Saunders, 1980.

Lee, Philip R. and Milton Silverman. *Pills, Profits, and Politics*. Berkeley: University of California Press, 1974.

Leonard, Ralph B. Monty. "The Calomel Rebellion." *Southern Medical Journal*, 8, no. 5 (1987): 638.

Lerner, Barron H. "From Careless Consumptives to Recalcitrant Patients: The Historical Construction of Noncompliance." *Social Science and Medicine* 45, no. 9 (1997): 1423–1431.

LeVay, Simon and Elisabeth Nonas. *City of Friends: A Portrait of the Gay and Lesbian Community in America*. Cambridge: MIT Press, 1995.

Leven, Maurice. *The Incomes of Physicians: An Economic and Statistical Analysis* (Chicago: University of Chicago Press, 1932): 50, quoted in William Weinfeld. "Income of Physicians, 1929–1949." *Survey of Current Business* (U.S. Department of Commerce, 1951), 14.

Levin, Lowell S. "Self-Medication: The Social Perspective." In *Self-Medication: The New Era, A Symposium*. Stouffer's National Center Hotel, Washington, DC: Proprietary Association, March 31, 1981, 44.

Levinson, C. J. "The Doctor's Case Against the Pill." *JAMA* 272, no. 2 (July 1996): 165–166.

Linds, Justin Abraham. "Ferments and the AIDS Virus: Interspecies Counter-Conduct in the History of AIDS." *Medical Humanities* 45, no. 4 (August 2019): 435–442.

Long, Thomas Lawrence. *AIDS and American Apocalypticism: The Cultural Semiotics of an Epidemic*. Albany: State University of New York Press, 2012.

Macklin, Ruth. "The New Conservatives in Bioethics: Who Are They and What Do They Seek?" *Hastings Center Reports* 36, no. 1 (January–February 2006): 34–43.

Macnair, A. L. "Benzodiazepines: Use, Overuse, Misuse, Abuse?" *The Lancet* 301, 7812 (June 1973): 1101–1102.

Madar, Chase. "The People's Priest." *American Conservative* 9, no. 2 (February 2010): 24–26.

Maggiore, Christine. *What if Everything You Thought You Knew about AIDS Was Wrong?* 4th 4th ed. Studio City, CA: American Foundation for AIDS Alternatives, 2000.

Mahapatra, Jayanta. *Relationship*. New York: The Greenfield Review Press, 1980.

Mann, Cass and Stuart Marshall. "HIV—Questions Not Answers." *Positively Healthy News* 3 (March 1989).

Marcellus, Jane. "Nervous Women and Noble Savages: The Romanticized 'Other' in Nineteenth-Century US Patent Medicine Advertising." *Journal of Popular Culture* 41, no. 5 (September 2008): 784–808.

Markoff Asistent, Niro. *Why I Survive AIDS*. New York: Simon and Shuster, 1991.

Martin, Deborah G., Susan Hanson, and Danielle Fontaine. "What Counts as Activism?: The Role of Individuals in Creating Change." *Women's Studies Quarterly* 35, no. 3/4 (Fall–Winter 2007): 78–94.

McCullagh and C. Behan. "Bias in Historical Description, Interpretation and Explanation." *History and Theory* 39, no. 1 (2000): 39–66.

McKeown, Robert E. "The Epidemiologic Transition: Changing Patterns of Mortality and Population Dynamics." *American Journal of Lifestyle Magazine* 3, no. 1 Suppl. (July 2009): 19S–26S.

McKinnie, Michael. "A Sympathy for Art: The Sentimental Economies of New Labour's Arts Policy." In *Blairism and the War of Persuasion: Labour's Passive Revolution*, edited by R. Johnson and D. L. Steinberg. London: Lawrence and Wishart, 2004.

Mikulski, Barbara. "Challenge I." In *Census Bureau Conference on Issues in Federal Statistical Needs Relating to Women: Research Papers Based on the 1978 Conference with Agency Responses*, edited by Barbara B. Reagan. Washington, DC: U.S. Department of Commerce Bureau of the Census, 1979.

Mills, Sara. *Michel Foucault*. New York: Routledge, 2003.

Mintz, Morton. *By Prescription Only: A Report on the Roles of the United States Food and Drug Administration. . . .* Boston: Beacon Press, 1967.

Mishler, Elliot G. "Viewpoint: Critical Perspectives on the Biomedical Model." In *Social Contexts of Health, Illness and Patient Care*. Cambridge: University of Cambridge, 1981.

Moberg, Carol L. "Friend of the Good Earth: René Dubos (1901–1982)." In *Launching the Antibiotic Era*, edited by Carol L. Moberg and Zanvil A. Cohn. New York: Rockefeller University Press, 1990.

Mohr, J. C. "American Medical Malpractice Litigation in Historical Perspective." *Journal of the American Medical Association* 283, no. 13 (April 2000): 1731–1737.

Morgan, John P. "The Politics of Medication." In *Controversies in Therapeutics*, edited by Louis C. Lasagna. Philadelphia: W. B. Saunders, 1980.

Muller, Charlotte. "The Overmedicated Society: Forces in the Marketplace for Medical Care." *Science* 176, no. 4034 (May 1972): 488–492.

Mullin, Tom. "Turbulent Time for Fluids." *New Scientist* (November 11, 1989): 53–55.

Murray, Stuart J. and Dave Holmes. "Introduction: Towards a Critical Bioethics." In *Critical Interventions in the Ethics of Healthcare*, edited by Stuart J. Murray and Dave Holmes. Farnham, England: Ashgate, 2009.

Murray, William. *Rough Notes on Remedies*, 4th ed. London: HK Lewis, 1901.

Naraindas, Harish, Johannes Quack and William S. Sax, eds. *Asymmetrical Conversations: Contestations, Circumventions, and the Blurring of Therapeutic Boundaries*. New York: Berghahn, 2014.

Navarre, Max. "AIDS-it is." In *Surviving and Thriving with AIDS: Collected Wisdom, Volume II*, edited by Michael Callen. New York: People with AIDS Coalition, 1988.

———. "Fighting the Victim Label." In *Surviving and Thriving with AIDS: Collected Wisdom, Volume II*, edited by Michael Callen. New York: People with AIDS Coalition, 1988.

———. "Newsline Editor Max Navarre Responds." In *Surviving and Thriving with AIDS: Collected Wisdom, Volume II*, edited by Michael Callen. New York: People with AIDS Coalition, 1988.

Ndao-Brumblay, S. Khady and Carmen R. Green, "Predictors of Complementary and Alternative Medicine Use in Chronic Pain Patients." *Pain Medicine* 11, no. 1 (January 2010): 16–24.

Needleman, Jacob. *The Way of the Physician*. New York: Harper & Row, 1985.

Nichols, John Benjamin. "Medical Sectarianism." *Journal of the American Medical Association* IX, no. 5 (1913): 331–337.

Nissenbaum, Stephen. *Sex, Diet and Debility in Jacksonian America: Sylvester Graham and Health Reform*. Chicago: The Dorsey Press, 1980.

Norsigian, J. "Our Bodies Ourselves and the Women's Health Movement in the United States: Some Reflections." *American Journal of Public Health* 109, no. 6 (May 2019): 844–846.

Nussbaum, Bruce. *Good Intentions: How Big Business and the Medical Establishment Are Corrupting the Fight Against AIDS*. New York: Penguin, 1990.

Olmsted, Dan and Mark Blaxill. *The Age of Autism: Mercury, Medicine, and a Man-Made Epidemic*. New York: St. Martin's Griffin, 2011.

Otis, Laura. *Membranes: Metaphors of Invasion in Nineteenth-Century Literature, Science, and Politics*. Baltimore: Johns Hopkins University Press, 1999.

Overall, Christine. "Reflections of a Sceptical Bioethicist." In *Philosophical Perspectives on Bioethics*, edited by. L. Wayne Sumner and Joseph Boyle, 166–167. Toronto: University of Toronto Press, 1996.

Palacios-Jimenez, Luis. "Little Bits of Wisdom." In *Surviving and Thriving with AIDS: Collected Wisdom, Volume II*, edited by Michael Callen. New York: People with AIDS Coalition, 1988.

Parvez, Bernard H. and S. Parvez. *Advances in Experimental Medicine: A Centenary Tribute to Claude Bernard*. New York: Elsevier/North-Holland Biomedical Press, 1989.

Paudyal, Vibhu, Shusen Sun, Rabia Hussain, Mohammed H. Abutaleb, and Eric Wesley Hedima. "Complementary and Alternative Medicines Use in COVID-19: A Global Perspective on Practice, Policy and Research." *Research in Social and Administrative Pharmacy* 18, no. 3 (March 2022): 2524–2528.

Pellegrino, Edmund. "Prescribing and Drug Ingestion: Symbols and Substances." Paper presented at the American Association for the Advancement of Science Annual Meeting, Boston, MA, February 18–24, 1976.

Pew Research Center. "Public and Scientists' Views on Science and Society." January 29, 2015. Accessed January 14, 2017. http://www.pewinternet.org/files/2015/01/PI_ScienceandSociety_Report_012915.pdf.

Pier, Nathaniel. "Open Letter to Mr. Jim Gottlieb (Chief of Staff for Representative T. Weiss), September 14, 1988." In *AIDS Patient Care* (February 1989): 4.

Piot, Peter and Ebrahim Shah. "Prevention and Control of Chronic Diseases." *British Medical Journal* 341 (November 2010): c4865.

Planned Parenthood. "The Birth Control Pill: A History." Accessed July 10, 2022. https://www.plannedparenthood.org/files/1514/3518/7100/Pill_History_FactSheet.pdf.

Poland, Jeffrey. *Metapsychology Online Review* 12, no. 35 (2008). http://metapsychology.mentalhelp.net/poc/view_doc.php?type=book&id=4438.

Porter, Dorothy. "How Did Social Medicine Evolve, and Where Is It Heading?" *PloS Medicine* 3, no. 10 (2006): e399.

Porter, Roy. "The Patient's View: Doing Medical History from Below." *Theory and Society* 14, no. 2 (March 1985): 175–198.

———. "Thomas Gisborne: Physicians, Christians and Gentlemen." In *Doctors and Ethics: The Earlier Historical Setting of Professional Ethics*, edited by Andrew Wear, Johanna Geyer-Kordesch, and Roger French. Atlanta: Rodopi, 1993.

Powles, John. "On the Limitations of Modern Medicine." *Science, Medicine and Man* 1, no. 1 (1973): 1–30.

"Proceedings of the Meeting." *Report of the Third Meeting of the British Association for the Advancement of Science*. London: John Murray, 1834.

Puhl, Rebecca. *Shame Campaigns: Do They Work?* Obesity Action. Accessed December 12, 2016. http://www.obesityaction.org/educational-resources/resource-articles-2/weight-bias/shame-campaigns-do-they-work.

Puhl, Rebecca, J. L. Peterson, and J. Luedicke. "Fighting Obesity or Obese Persons? Public Reactions to Obesity-Related Health Messages." *International Journal of Obesity* 37, no. 6 (June 2013): 774–782.

Quirke, Viviane and Jean-Paul Gaudillière. "The Era of Biomedicine: Science, Medicine, and Public Health in Britain and France after the Second World War." *Medical History* 52, no. 4 (October 2008): 441–452.

Rasmussen, Nicolas. "America's First Amphetamine Epidemic 1929–1971." *American Journal of Public Health* 98, no. 6 (June 2008): 974–985.

Rawlinson, Mary C. "Introduction." *The International Journal of Feminist Bioethics* 1, no. 1 (Spring 2008): 1.

"Retrospective," *The Medical Times: A Monthly Journal of Medicine, Surgery and the Collateral Sciences* (1909).

Reverby, Susan M. "Feminism & Health." *Health and History* 4, no. 1 (2002): 5–19.

Risse, Guenter B. "Epidemics and History: Ecological Perspectives and Social Responses." In *AIDS: the Burdens of History*, edited by Elizabeth Fee and Daniel Fox, 66. Berkeley: University of California Press, 1988.

Rogers, Naomi. *An Alternative Path: The Making and Remaking of Hahnemann Medical College and Hospital of Philadelphia*. New Brunswick: Rutgers University Press, 1998.

Rosenberg, Charles E. *Explaining Epidemics: And Other Studies in the History of Medicine*. Cambridge: Cambridge University Press, 1992.

———. *No Other Gods: On Science and American Social Thought*. Baltimore: Johns Hopkins University Press, 1997.

———. *Our Present Complaint: American Medicine, Then and Now*. Baltimore: Johns Hopkins, 2007.

———. "The Tyranny of Diagnosis: Specific Entities and Individual Experience." *The Milbank Quarterly* 80, no. 2 (June 2002): 237–260.

Rosenbrock, Rolf, F. Dubois-Arber, M. Moers, P. Pinell, D. Schaeffer, and M. Setbon. "The Normalization of AIDS in Western European Countries." *Social Science & Medicine* 50, no. 11 (June 2000): 1607–1629.

Rosner, David and Susan M. Reverby, eds. "Beyond the Great Doctors." In *Health Care in America: Essays in Social History*. Philadelphia: Temple University Press, 1979.

Ross, Loretta J. and Rickie Solinger. *Reproductive Justice: A History*. Oakland: University of California Press, 2017.

Rothman, David. *Strangers at the Bedside: A History of How Law and Bioethics Transformed Medical Decision Making*. New York: Basic Books, 1992.

Rothstein, William. *American Physicians in the Nineteenth Century: From Sects to Science*. Baltimore: Johns Hopkins University Press, 1972.

Rowe, Ed. *Homosexual Politics: Road to Ruin for America*. Washington, DC: Church League of America, 1984.

Sarason, Seymour Bernard. *Caring and Compassion in Clinical Practice*. London: Jason Aronson, 1977.

Seaman, Barbara. *The Doctor's Case Against the Pill*. Alameda: Hunter House, 1995.

Schmidt, Casper G. "The Group-Fantasy Origins of AIDS" in *The AIDS Cult: Essays on the Gay Health Crisis*, edited by John Lauritsen and Ian Young. Provincetown: Asklepios, 1997. Originally published in *The Journal of Psychohistory*, 32 (1984).

Scott, James C. "Everyday Forms of Resistance." *Copenhagen Papers* 4, no. 1 (May 1989): 33–62.

Scott, Joan. "Women's History." In *New Perspectives on Historical Writing*, edited by Peter Burke. University Park: Penn State University Press, 1992.

Sexton, John. "The Hollowness of Radical Bioethics." *The New Atlantis: A Journal of Technology and Society* 40 (Fall 2013): 89–103.

Shepard, Benjamin H. "The Queer/Gay Assimilationist Split: The Suits versus the Sluts." *Monthly Review* 53, no. 1 (May 2001).

Sherwin, Susan. *No Longer Patient: Feminist Ethics and Health Care*. Philadelphia: Temple University Press, 1992.

Shryock, Richard H. "Empiricism Versus Rationalism in American Medicine." *Proceedings of the American Antiquarian Society* 79, no. 1 (1969): 99–150.

Siegel, Bernie. *Love, Medicine and Miracles*. New York: Harper Collins, 1988.

Simonton, O. Carl. Stephanie Matthews-Simonton, and James L. Creighton, *Getting Well Again: A Step-By-Step Self-Help Guide to Overcoming Cancer for Patients and Their Families*. Los Angeles: TarcherPerigree, 1978.

Siplon, Patricia D. *AIDS and the Policy Struggle in the United States*. Washington, DC: Georgetown University Press, 2002.

Smith, Julia and Alan Whiteside. "The History of AIDS Exceptionalism." *The Journal of the International AIDS Society* 13, no. 47 (December 2010): 1758–2652.

Smith, Meredith Y., Bruce D. Rapkin, Anne Morrison, and Sandra Kammerman. "Zidovudine Adherence in Persons with AIDS: The Relation of Patient Beliefs about Medication to Self-Termination of Therapy." *Journal of General Internal Medicine* 12, no. 4 (1997): 216–223.

Smith, Richard. "Limits to Medicine. Medical Nemesis: The Expropriation of Health." *The Journal of Epidemiology and Community Health* 57, no. 12 (2004): 928.

Smith, Wesley J. *Culture of Death: The Assault on Medical Ethics in America*. San Francisco: Encounter Books, 2000.

Somers, Herman and Anne Somers. "The Paradox of Medical Progress." *New England Journal of Medicine* 266 (June 1962): 1253–1258.

Sonnabend, Joseph C. "Acquired Immunodeficiency Syndrome: Opportunistic Infections and Malignancies in Male Homosexuals." *Journal of the American Medical Association* 249, no. 17 (1983): 2370–2374.

———. "More Thoughts on Preventing Pneumocystis Pneumonia." In *Surviving and Thriving with AIDS: Collected Wisdom, Volume II*, edited by Michael Callen. New York: People with AIDS Coalition, 1988, 2:65.

Sontag, Susan. *Illness as Metaphor*. New York: Farrar, Straus and Giroux, 1978.

———. *Illness as Metaphor and AIDS and Its Metaphors*. New York: Picador, 2001.

Spangler, David. "Old Voyage, New Voyagers: The Maturing of Planetary Culture." In *The New Times Network*, compiled by Adams, Robert. London: Routledge & Kegan Paul, 1982.

Speaker, Susan Lynn. "Too Many Pills: Patients, Physicians, and the Myth of Overmedication in America, 1955–1980." PhD. diss. University of Pennsylvania, 1992.

Starr, Paul. "The Politics of Therapeutic Nihilism." *Hastings Center Report* 6, no. 5 (1976): 24–30.

———. *The Social Transformation of American Medicine*. New York: Basic Books, 1982.

Stevens, M. L. Tina. *Bioethics in America: Origins and Cultural Politics*. Baltimore: Johns Hopkins University Press, 2000.

———. Letters, *Hastings Center Report* (January–February 2002): 5.

Stevens, Rosemary. *American Medicine and the Public Interest*. New Haven, CT: Yale University Press, 1971.

Streitmatter, Rodger. *From 'Perverts' to 'Fab Five': the Media's Changing Depiction of Gay Men and Lesbians*. New York: Routledge, 2009.

Stribling, B.F.W. "Fogyism." In *Poems for the Old and Young*. Beardstown, IL: L. U. Reavis, 1857.

Strong, Philip. "The Pestilential Apocalypse: Modern, Postmodern and Early Modern Observations." In *Meddling with Mythology: AIDS and the Social Construction of Knowledge*, edited by Rosaline S. Barbour and Guro Huby. New York: Routledge, 1998.

Sturken, Marita. *Tangled Memories: The Vietnam War, the AIDS Epidemic, and the Politics of Remembering*. Berkeley: University of California Press, 1997.

Sumner, L. W. and Joseph Boyle. *Philosophical Perspectives on Bioethics*. Toronto: University of Toronto Press, 1996.

Sunstein, Cass. *#Republic: Divided Democracy in the Age of Social Media*. Princeton: Princeton University Press, 2017.

Swidler, Ann. "Culture in Action: Symbols and Strategies." *American Sociological Review* 51, no. 2 (April 1986): 273–286.

Szasz, Thomas. *The Medicalization of Everyday Life*. Syracuse, NY: Syracuse University Press, 2007.

———. *The Myth of Mental Illness*. New York: Harper & Row, 1961.

Tapper, Elliot B. "Doctors on Display: The Evolution of Television's Doctors." *Baylor University Medical Center Proceedings* 23, no. 4 (October 2010): 393–399.

Taylor, J. M. "Antiseptic Surgery in Country Practice." *The Medical and Surgical Reporter* LIX, no. 23 (1888): 704–707.

Temin, Peter. *Taking Your Medicine: Drug Regulation in the United States*. Cambridge: Harvard University Press, 1980.

Tesh, Sylvia Noble. "Disease Causality and Politics." *Journal of Health Politics, Policy and Law* 6, no. 3 (1981): 379–380.

———. *Hidden Arguments: Political Ideology and Disease Prevention Policy*. New Brunswick: Rutgers, 1996.

Thomas, Lewis. "On Magic in Medicine." *New England Journal of Medicine* 299, no. 9 (August 1978): 461–463.

Thomason, Jacqueline. "AIDS Organizations, U.S." In *Encyclopedia of Lesbian and Gay Histories and Cultures, Volume II*, edited by George E. Haggerty. New York: Garland Publishing, Taylor & Francis Group, 2000.

Thoreau, Henry David. *Walden and Civil Disobedience*. New York: Signet Classics, 1999.

Thorson, Robert M. *Walden's Shore*. Cambridge: Harvard University Press, 2015.

Thrall, James H. "Prevalence and Costs of Chronic Disease in a Health Care System Structured for Treatment of Acute Illness." *Radiology* 235, no. 1 (2005): 9–12.

Tomes, Nancy. "Epidemic Entertainments: Disease and Popular Culture in Early-Twentieth-Century America." *American Literary History* 14, no. 4 (Winter 2002): 625–652.

———. *The Gospel of Germs: Men, Women and the Microbe in American Life*. Cambridge: Harvard University Press, 1999.

———. "The Private Side of Public Health: Sanitary Science, Domestic Hygiene, and the Germ Theory, 1870–1900." In *Sickness and Health in America: Readings in the History of Medicine and Public Health*, edited by Judith Walzer Leavitt and Ronald L. Numbers. Madison: University of Wisconsin Press, 1997.

Tomycz, N. D. "A Profession Selling Out: Lamenting the Paradigm Shift in Physician Advertising." *Journal of Medical Ethics* 32, no. 1 (January 2006): 26–28.

Tong, Rosemarie Putnam. *Feminist Approaches to Bioethics: Theoretical Reflections and Practical Applications*. Abingdon, England: Routledge, 1996.

Trager, Oliver, ed. *AIDS: Plague or Panic?* New York: Facts on File, 1988.

Treichler, Paula. *How to Have Theory in an Epidemic: Cultural Chronicles of AIDS*. Durham: Duke University Press, 1999.

Tuana, Nancy. "The Speculum of Ignorance: The Women's Health Movement and Epistemologies of Ignorance." *Hypatia* 21, no. 3 (2006): 1–19.

Twain, Mark. *Huck Finn and Tom Sawyer among the Indians*. Berkeley: University of California Press, 2011.

———. "Remarks on Osteopathy." In *Mark Twain Speaking*, edited by Paul Fatout. Iowa City: University of Iowa Press, 1978.

Tyrer, Peter. "The Benzodiazepines Bonanza." *The Lancet* 304, no. 7882 (September 1974): 709–710.

U.S. Department of Justice. *Report of the Tort Policy Working Group on the Causes, Extent and Policy Implications of the Current Crisis in Insurance Availability and Affordability* February 1986.

Van Epps, Heather L. "René Dubos: Unearthing Antibiotics." *Journal of Experimental Medicine* 203, no. 2 (2006): 259.

Vass, Antony A. *AIDS: A Plague in Us; A Social Perspective*. Cambridge: Venus Academica, 1986.

Walter, Suzan. "Holistic Health." In *The Illustrated Encyclopedia of Body-Mind Disciplines*. New York: Rosen Publishing Group, 1999.

Wardwell, Walter, I. "The Reduction of Strain in a Marginal Social Role." *American Journal of Sociology* 61, no. 1 (July 1955): 16–25.

Warner, Margaret Humphreys. "Vindicating the Minister's Medical Role: Cotton Mather's Concept of the *Nishmath-Chajim* and the Spiritualization of Medicine." *Journal of the History of Medicine* 36, no. 3 (1981): 278–295.

Weil, Andrew T. *Health and Healing: The Philosophy of Integrative Medicine and Optimum Health*. Boston: Houghton Mifflin, 2004.

Weston, Anthony. "On the Body in Medical Self-Care and Holistic Medicine." In *The Body in Medical Thought and Practice*, edited by Drew Leder. Dordrecht: Kluwer Academic Publishers, 1992.

———. "Toward a Social Critique of Bioethics." *Journal of Social Philosophy* 22, no. 2 (Fall 1991): 109–118.

Wiegmann, Wendy. "Habitus, Symbolic Violence, and Reflexivity: Applying Bourdieu's Theories to Social Work." *Journal of Sociology and Social Welfare* 44, no. 4 (December 2017): 95–116.

Williams, Rhys H. "The Cultural Contexts of Collective Action: Constraints, Opportunities and the Symbolic Life of Social Movements." In *The Blackwell Companion to Social Movements*, edited by David A. Snow, Sarah A. Soule, and Hanspeter Kriesi. Malden, MA: Blackwell Publishing, 2004.

Whooley, Owen. *Knowledge in the Time of Cholera*. Chicago: University of Chicago Press, 2013.

Whorton, James C. *Nature Cures: The History of Alternative Medicine in America*. Oxford: Oxford University Press, 2002.

Wolf, Susan. *Feminism and Bioethics: Beyond Reproduction*. Oxford: Oxford University Press, 1996.

Wolfe, Sidney M., Christopher M. Coley, and the Health Research Group. *Pills That Don't Work: A Consumers' and Doctors' Guide to over 600 Prescription Drugs That Lack Evidence of Effectiveness*. New York: Farrar Straus Giroux, 1981.

Woolf, Virginia. *A Room of One's Own*. Oxford: Oxford University Press, 1998.

Wright, Joe. "Only Your Calamity: The Beginnings of Activism by and for People with AIDS." *American Journal of Public Health* 103, no. 10 (October 2013): 1788–98.

Yadavendu, Vijay Kumar. *Shifting Paradigms in Public Health: From Holism to Individualism*. New York: Springer, 2013.

Young, Ian. "The Psychohistorical Origins of AIDS: An Interview with Casper Schmidt." In *The AIDS Cult: Essays on the Gay Health Crisis*, edited by John Lauritsen and Ian Young. Provincetown: Asklepios, 1997.

Young, James Harvey. "The Development of the Office of Alternative Medicine in the National Institutes of Health, 1991–1996." *Bulletin of the History of Medicine* 72, no. 2 (1998): 279–298.

Youngner, Stuart J. and Robert Arnold. "Who Will Watch the Watchers?" *Hastings Center Report* 32, no. 3 (May–June 2002): 21–22.

Zola, Irving Kenneth. "Medicine as an Institution of Social Control." *The Sociological Review* 20, no. 4 (April 1972): 487–504.

INDEX

Abrahams, Naomi, 5
Ackerknecht, Erwin, 168n27
activism, defined, 5
ACT UP (AIDS Coalition to Unleash Power), 117; AIDS exceptionalism and, 41; AZT and, 106–107; boycott of the *Native,* 209n138; Callen on, 191n86; challenging AIDS dissidence, 139; criticism of, 184n4; Denver Principles and, 89; "drugs into bodies" campaigns and, 157n8; Fedorko on, 123; HEAL leaders and, 199n5; holistic health and, 195–196n139; protests, 1–2; PWAC compared to, 87, 89; study of, 82
ACT UP Oral History Project, 117
ACT UP Treatment and Data Committee, 106–107, 122, 200–201n34
acupuncture, 110, 119
"Acupuncture as an Alternative," 108
acyclovir, 112
Addiction Research Foundation, 65
Advocate (newspaper), 191n86
aerosolized pentamidine (NebuPent), 105
African American communities: AIDS dissidence and, 138–139; borderland mode and, 210n9; everyday forms of resistance and, 145; HEAL and, 137–138; pediatric AIDS and AIDS cases in, 137
African American leaders, HEAL's outreach initiatives and, 137, 138
African American media, collaboration with gay media, 138–140
agency, multifactorial model of AIDS etiology and individual, 102–103
AIDS: conspiracy theories about, 140; described as plague, 38, 40, 119; development of underground groups and, 86–87; editorial cartoonists' images of, 38–39; historical memory and, 37–38; infectious disease narratives and, 51; labeled "gay cancer," 23, 102; located within history, 38–41; media whitewashing of, 188n53; medication prophylaxis for, 129–130; progress narrative for, 40; public response to, 41–42; role of mind in treatment of, 131; seeking answers in history of infectious diseases, 15–16; study of, 36–37; study of past epidemics and, 40–41, 168n23
AIDS, Cancer and the Medical Establishment (Brown), 101
AIDS activism: everyday forms of resistance and, 2, 4, 5, 145; on individual scale, 86; popular images of, 1; role of patient activist in, 3. *See also* unorthodox AIDS activism
AIDS activists: debates between accomodationist and radical, 91; public protests by, 85–86
AIDS denialism/AIDS dissidence, 124; dismissed as radical expressions of the fringe, 6–7; HEAL and, 136–137, 138–139; preventable deaths and, 148. *See also* Duesberg, Peter
AIDS etiology, 163n50; array of, 121; biopsychosocial model, 132–134; Callen and, 27, 99, 100–103, 190n78, 190n80, 191n84, 191n88, 192n90–91; cause of, 11; emphasis on viral, 121; Epstein on, 190n79; HEAL and, 124, 127, 131–137; history of repeated infections and, 101–103, 127, 191n87; PWAC and, 99–103; rejecting role for HIV in, 3; religion and, 34; Sonnabend on, 191n87; unorthodox health activism and, 144. *See also* multifactorial model of AIDS etiology
AIDS exceptionalism, 40–42
AIDS fatalism, 119
AIDS history, divided into infectious era and chronic disease era, 125–126
AIDS Hotline, 121
"AIDS in Historical Perspective" (Brandt), 39
AIDS Mastery workshops, 110–111, 131, 144, 148, 200n19
AIDS Network, 90
AIDS Project Los Angeles, 95
AIDS research, 189n63, 189n72; criticism by PWAs of, 96–99; HIV as target of, 103; insistence on gathering "clean/pure" data, 98, 99; PWAC and criticism of, 96–99

AIDS service organizations, 82; criticized for promoting fatality narrative, 95; relationship with HEAL, 118. *See also* ACT UP (AIDS Coalition to Unleash Power); Gay Men's Health Crisis (GMHC)
AIDS: The Burdens of History (Fee & Fox), 39
AIDS: The Making of a Chronic Disease (Fee & Fox), 102
AIDS Treatment News, 6
AIDS War, The (Lauritsen), 193n101
AIDS Watchdog Group (Boston), 105–106
AIDS Zone, Ellner and, 134–135
AL-721, 113, 196n146, 198n165
alcohol consumption, public health campaigns on, 147, 210n12
allopathic medicine, 201–202n46
allopaths, homeopaths characterization of, 25
aloe, in R.A.C. pills, 162n21
alternative health approaches, long-term PWAs and, 199–200n19
alternative health movements: attacks on heroic medicine by, 21–22; focus on institutions of, 18; health holism and, 49; Illich and, 78; PWAC contributors' embrace of, 107–114; religious/spiritual practices and, 31–35; study of, 17–18
alternative therapies; cancer and, 22–23; for COVID-19, 149; health holism: for AIDS, 105, 106, 112; rates of use by Americans, 19. *See also* complementary medicine
American Association for the Advancement of Science, 66
American Foundation for Homeopathy, 28
American Holistic Health Association, 201n46
American Magazine, 69
American Medical Association (AMA), 25; birth control pill and, 176n37; campaign against social medicine, 180n99; lifting ban on physician advertising, 70–71; Medicare legislation and, 72; political campaigns, 68, 72
American Medical Journal of St. Louis, 26
American National Association of Science Writers' Science-in-Society Award, 166n3
amphetamines, 63, 64
Amsterdam News (newspaper), 43, 139, 140
amyl nitrate inhalants ("poppers"), 128
Anderson, Edward, 167n13
Angel of Bethesday (Mather), 33
Angels in America (Kushner), 200n31
Anthony, Susan B., 31
anti-authoritarianism: bioethics and, 53–54; critique of pharmaceutical corporations and, 106; history of medicine in the U.S. and, 27–30; Illich and, 77; social response to COVID-19 pandemic and, 150
antibiotic prophylaxis, Ellner on, 129, 204n78, 204n82, 204n83
antibiotic revolution, 42
antibiotics, gay men's exposure to, 128
anticontagionist measures, 168n27
antidepressants, 64
antidogmatism, critique of pharmaceutical corporations and, 106
antigenic stress, proposed as cause of AIDS, 127–128
antiheroism, AZT, 104
anti-intellectualism: social response to COVID-19 pandemic and, 150; Thomsonian medicine and, 27
antimodern discourse, COVID-19 and, 150
antimodern sentiment: history of medicine in the U.S. and, 30–35; roots of, 165n63
antipsychiatry movement, 72
antiretrovirals, 16, 86, 103, 105, 122, 134; didanosine, 109, 122, 134; NIH and, 104, 194n124; refusing, 138, 148, 208n131. *See also* azidothymidine (AZT; Retrovir)
anti-vaxxers, 147–148
anxiety: disease and, 132; fatality narratives and, 134; psychotropic drugs and, 63
Anzaldúa, Gloria, 18
applied social theory, Schmidt and, 133
Arena, The (journal), 28
assembly line, clinical medicine compared to, 68–69
attitudinal healing methodologies, 110–111, 119, 126, 131
Auden, W. H., 63, 132
"autonomy," 164n60
awakenings, unorthodox health movements facilitating religious, 33–34
Ayanian, John, 179n75
Ayurvedic medicine, 5, 34, 108, 110
azidothymidine (AZT; Retrovir) (zidovudine; ZDV), 97, 134; Callen on, 104–107,

194n109, 194n111, 194n113, 194n116; controversy over, 103–107; critiques of, 193–194n107, 194n109, 194n111, 194n113, 194n116, 195n126–127; failure to adhere to treatment regimes, 148; FDA acknowledging therapeutic dose too high, 129; HEAL's outreach activities and, 138; holistic health activism and, 122; Navarre on, 193n106; rejection of, 2–3; toxicity of, 104–106

bacteriology, imperialist ideology and, 170n56
Bactrim, 105, 112, 129
Baltimore, David, 177n49
Barber, Charles, 41
barbiturates, 64
Barkins, Evelyn, 179n77
Barnes, Patricia, 19, 143
Barton, Clara, 31
Bayer, Ronald, 40
Ben Casey (television program), 65
benzodiazepines, 63
Berkowitz, Richard, 103, 185n18, 191n88, 192n97
Berliner, Howard S., 203n74
Berman, Edgar, 66, 69–70, 178n67, 178n68
Bernard, Claude, 172n70
Berndt, John, 185n24
Berwick, Donald, 179n75
Beshada v. Johns-Manville Products Corp., 176n44
Beveridge Plan, 171n61
Beyond the Germ Theory (Galdston), 45
bias towards action model, 67, 179–180n85, 179n74, 179n75
Bible, AIDS imagery and rhetoric and, 38–39
biblical scourge, AIDS portrayed as, 38
bioethicists: Illich and, 77; Rothman on, 173n4, 174n14
bioethics, 174n13; accused of ignoring structural abuses in system, 55–56; development of, 53–65, 164n58; feminist, 174n11; feminist critique of, 174n15; Illich and, 78–79; patients and, 53; power and, 54–56; professionalization of, 28, 29; Rosenberg on, 173n2; scope of, 54; view of patients, 28, 29
biological homeostasis, holistic movement and, 172n70
biomedical authority, COVID-19 response and, 151
biomedical model: AIDS activism challenging, 2; definition, function, and influence of, 7; hegemony of, 16; PWAs exploring treatment options outside of, 2
biomedical orthodoxy, PWAs self-organizing to challenge, 110
biomedicine: AIDS dissidence and, 136–137; alternative health systems views as reductionist and dogmatic, 108–109; dehumanization of patients and, 52; distrust of, 53, 57, 138–139; embrace of complementary medicine, 146; fear of overmedicated society in United States and, 57–65; funding for war on cancer and, 45–46; HEAL's criticism of, 123; health holism as remedy for broken, 109–110, 125; heroic medicine and response to AIDS, 162–163n34; HIV as cause of AIDS and, 99–103; lessons for, 145–149; power of science in, 170n53; as purveyor of fatality narratives regarding AIDS, 94–95; PWAC's critical view of, 92–93; Sonnabend on, 188n59; structural racism and, 181n105. *See also* AIDS research; medicine
biopsychosocial model, 45, 132–134, 171n64
Birth of Bioethics, The (Jonsen), 56
Bivins, Roberta, 25, 163n41, 209n3
Black, David, 38
Black Liberation Army, 140
body: health holism and gaining control over, 126; medicine accused of policing, 72–73; metaphysical approach to re-mystify the, 48; PWA activism and, 184n3; resistance at level of the, 86–87
Bolton, Herbert Eugene, 18
borderland model: African American communities and, 210n9; People with AIDS Coalition and, 88; social history and, 143, 145; understanding unorthodox health activism and, 17–20
borderlands of health paradigms, 51
Boston Women's Health Collective, 73, 82, 90
Bourdieu, Pierre, 133, 178n70, 206n103
Brandt, Allan, 15, 45; "AIDS in Historical Perspective," 39
Brave New World (Huxley), 64
bread, Graham and, 30–31
Brewin, Thurstan B., 161n15
Brier, Jennifer, 193n99
Brink, Anthony, 162–163n34

British Broadcasting Corporation (BBC), unorthodox views on climate change and, 8–9
British Medical Journal, 78
Brother to Brother (Harris), 145
Brown, E. Richard, 181n107
Brown, Raymond K., 101, 202n57
Brown, Tony, 139
Broyard, Anatole, 76
Bryant, Anita, 39
bubonic plague, AIDS as plague and, 38
Buianouckas, Frank, 127, 128
Burke, Bill, 185n18
Burnham, John C., 178n64, 179n77
Burns, Alan, 110, 120
Burroughs, Carola, 195n138
Burroughs Wellcome, 105, 122, 200n30, 204n78
Butler, Kurt, 172n73
By Prescription Only . . . Use of Prescription Drugs that May Be Worthless, Injurious, or Even Lethal (Mintz), 59, 60

Caisse, Rene, 22
Callahan, Daniel, 54
Callen, Michael, 124, 163–164n52, 185n18; AIDS etiology and, 27, 99, 100–103, 190n78, 190n80, 191n84, 191n88, 192n90–91; on AIDS panic, 191n86; on alternative medicine and long-term AIDS survival, 166n81; on AZT, 104–107, 194n109, 194n111, 194n113, 194n116; call for PWA to actively engage with disease, 92, 93; challenging fatality narratives, 93–96, 188n53, 188n56; criticism of AIDS research, 97; criticism of drug trials, 98; critique of biomedicine, 193n101; defense of editorial diversity and, 107; on Denver Principles, 88–89; on dogmatism of biomedicine, 144; as editor of *Newsline,* 89–90, 92; embrace of alternative therapies, 111–112; on Gallo, 27, 190n80, 191n81; on "gay AIDies," 184n8; GMHC and, 194n119; on Hay, 111–112; HEAL and, 120; Illich and, 193n98; leadership of, 116; Marxist principles and, 91; medical history, 188–189n62, 192n90; on medication prophylaxis, 129; multifactorial theory of AIDS etiology and, 101–103; on naltrexone, 197n163; on owning one's body and surviving AIDS, 103; on politics of sex and intimacy, 103; on Popper, 191n83; on promiscuous sex, 192–193n97; on PWA activism, 92; PWAC board and, 185n11; on PWA Health Group, 198n165; refusing to print "AIDS virus" in *Newsline,* 189n75; relationship with media, 188n53, 188n54; on repeated STI infection and AIDS, 127; resignation from PWAC, 113–114; on responsibility for illness, 192n96; safer sex manual and, 191n88; on society's hatred of homosexuality, 192n93; Sonnanbend on, 187n44; teaching how to make egg lipid mixture, 198n167; on treatment trials, 189n72; women's health movement as influence on, 90–91; in *Zero Patience,* 189–190n76. See also *Surviving AIDS* (Callen)
calomel, 21–22, 162n21, 162n22
"calomel rebellion," 21
Cambre, Susan, 187n41
Cambridge Advanced Learner's Dictionary and Thesaurus, 5
Campbell, Bobbi, 91, 185n18
cancer: criticism of funds given to biomedicine for war on, 45–46; dominant medical response to, 162n33; focus of medical research on, 43; heroic medicine and, 22–23, 162n31; holistic health activism and, 202n48; lay framings of, 162n33; visualization as treatment for, 196–197n150
Caplan, Arthur, 54
Capra, Fritjof, 131, 205n88
Carson, Rachel, 44, 59–60
Carter, Richard, 72
Cartesian dualism, rejection of, 48, 132
cartoons, AIDS, 38–39
Carver, Bob, Jr., 148–149
Cayleff, Susan, 160n10
Cecchi, Bob, 185n18
Centers for Disease Control (CDC), 42–43
Chambré, Susan, 10, 88
Cheeks, Rainey, 210n9
Chicago Tribune (newspaper), 48–49, 50
childhood autism, unorthodox activism about, 162n31
children, exposure to environmental hazards, 169–170n43
children with AIDS, 137, 167n15, 208n125
chiropractic medicine, 119, 126, 143
chiropractors, 172n73

chloramphenicol, 59
chlordiazepoxide (Librium), 63
cholera, 39, 167n13
Christian fundamentalists, on origins of AIDS, 34
Christian Science, 32
Christopher Street (publication), 139
chronic disease: defining, 126; health holism and, 125; individual interactions with environment and, 46–47; multifactorial models for, 102; PWAs viewing AIDS as, 102; supplanting contagious diseases in twentieth-century United States, 42–43, 45–47
chronicity, alternative and holistic approaches to AIDS and, 202n55
Church of Christ, Scientist, 32
Church of Religious Science, 111
civil rights advocates, bioethicists compared to, 54
Clark, Mary Marshall, 199n4
climate change: BBC policy on airtime for unorthodox views on, 8–9; individual responses to, 152–153
clinical care, public fear of overmedication, 57–65
clinical gaze, 45
clinical iatrogenesis, 75
clinical interventions, proper aims of, 146–147
clinical medicine, compared to assembly line, 68–69
Cohen, Michael H., 130
Cold War: biomedicine and, 47; holistic etiological models and, 172n71; science and, 170n57
Coley, Christiopher M., 62
Colter, Marc, 195n127
Community Constituency Consortium, 198n168
community physicians, AIDS and experience of, 95
Community Research Initiative (CRI), 113, 198n168
complementary medicine: health holism: HEAL and, 119–120; mainstream medicine's embrace of, 146. *See also* alternative therapies
Compound Q, 157n8
"Condomania" (HEAL), 203n63
conspiracy theories, about AIDS, 140
consumer rights movement: influence on Illich, 76; risks of useless medications and, 61–63
Consumers Union, The, 58
contagious diseases, supplanted by chronic diseases in twentieth-century U.S., 42–43, 45–47
Continuum Magazine, 136
contrarian health movements, ethical considerations in study of, 8–9
Cooke, John Esten, 162n21
Cordtz, Dan, 181n105
Cort, Andrew, 126, 135, 202n56, 207n114
COVID-19 etiology, 149–151
COVID-19 pandemic, 149–152; Trump and, 150, 151, 211n22; unorthodox health activism and, 10, 12, 212n25–27
Cox, Harvey, 74, 78
Crawford, Robert, 48, 173n78, 193n100
Crosby, Alfred, 169n30
cultural iatrogenesis, 75, 182n118
culture, as empowering and constraining force, 160n2
Cumming, William Fullerton, 21
Cunningham, Tom, 120, 197n155, 199n18
cure, objection to using for AIDS treatment, 105–106
current, historical, 20
cyclosporine, 164n59

Daily Mirror (newspaper), 39
Davidovitch, Nadav, 28
Davis, Joseph E., 125, 126
Defoe, Daniel, 38
denialist etiological debate over AIDS, 99–103
Dennett, Mary Ware, 28
Denver Principles, 88–89, 186n34; elided versions of, 89, 116; nursing practice philosophies and, 91
Descartes, René, 33
deviant sick role, 47
DeVoto, Bernard, 71–72, 180n93
dextran sulfate (Gentran; LMD), 113, 198n167
dextropropoxyphene (Darvon), 63, 177n53
diazepam (Valium), 63, 177n54
didanosine (ddI; Videx), 109, 122, 134
die-ins, 1, 85, 93, 184n2
diethylstilbestrol (Apstil), 61

DiFerdinando, Tom, 130, 204n84, 208n129
dimethyl sulfoxide, 59
Dirkson, Everett, 180n99
Discipline and Punish (Foucault), 206n103
Discover (magazine), 190n78
disease: AIDS and change in way to think about and respond to, 37; Dubos on modern life and, 44–45; Graham on, 31; history as guide to responding to, 15–16; how societies conceive of, 166n1; Mather on explanations for, 33; personal responsibility for, 103, 144, 202–203n57; seed *vs.* soil argument and, 165n67; transformations in constructions of, 42–51. *See also* illness
disease causality, 171n64
disease etiology, 11–12, 42; environmental stress-based model, 45, 172n70; multiple-cause model, 171–172n65; specific, 171–172n65. *See also* AIDS etiology
disease narratives, patient behavior and, 146
disease paradigm, changes in, 42–44
disestablishment philosophy of Illich, 74–75
dissident activism, Ellner and, 136–137
dissident etiological debate over AIDS, 99–103
Distinction, La (Bourdieu), 206n103
divine retribution, AIDS depicted as expression of, 39
Doctor Business, The (Carter), 72
Doctor's Case Against the Pill, The (Seaman), 60
Doctor's Dilemma, The (Shaw), 70
dogma, Callen's HIV denialism and, 100–101
dogmatism of physicians, popular perception of, 23–27
Donahue, Phil, 62
Dopacz, David, 78
Douglass, Frederick, 31
Dowling, Harry F., 67
Dr. Kildare (television program), 65
drugs: fear of overmedicated society, 57–65; HEAL attacks on, 128; history of regulation of, 59–61; ineffective, 61–63; psychotropic, 60, 63–65; self-help manual directing what to avoid, 62; that do not work, 176n47
"drugs into bodies," 1, 2, 85, 106, 157n8, 201n34
drug trials: Community Research Initiative and, 113; PWAC criticism of, 98–99
drug use, gay men and recreational, 106, 127, 128, 195n126, 206n104
Duberman, Martin, 10, 105, 193n101
Dubos, René, 44–45, 46, 48, 169–170n43, 170n55
Duesberg, Peter: Callen on, 193n101; HEAL and, 117, 141; HIV/AIDS denialism and, 100, 124, 136, 148, 159n22, 190n77, 190n78, 208n120, 211n14
Dulbecco, Renato, 177n49
Dunne, Richard, 122
Dunton, Lese, 129
Dvarackas, Peter, 110

Eaklor, Vicki Lynn, 184n7
echo chamber effects of social media, 151–152, 153
Eclectic medicine, 28, 163n43
Eddy, Mary Baker, 32
egg lecithin extract, 198n165
egg lipids, 105, 112, 113
Ehrenreich, Barbara, 81, 181n107
Ehrenreich, John, 45–46, 48, 81, 170n55, 171–172n65, 179n76, 181n107
Ehrlich, Paul, 22, 32, 65, 105
Eichelberger, Ethyl, 200n34
Eigo, Jim, 184n3
Eisenberg, David, 19, 143
Ellner, Michael, 166n82, 195n137, 199n4, 204n81; on AIDS as genocide, 208n130; on AIDS hysteria, 206n106; AIDS Zone and, 134; anti-HIV presentations, 138, 140; on biomedical response to AIDS, 135; condemnation of HIV/AIDS model and antiretrovirals, 134; on cultural hypnosis, 207n110; dissident activism and, 136–137; on HEAL's later work, 207n116; holistic interdependency and, 131–132; on medication prophylaxis, 129–130, 204n78; mind and AIDS, 131; mind's role in AIDS and, 132–134; multifactoriality and, 127–128; oral interviews with, 117; Schmidt and, 133–134
Emmanuel Movement, 32, 165n72
emotional habitus of a group, 199n11
empirical *vs.* rational medicine, 23–27
empiricism, physicians and, 163n38
empowerment: dissent and, 153–154; free availability of ideas and, 152; infectious disease and limits of individual, 149–152; metric of, 148, 153; morality of, 154;

multifactorial theory of AIDS etiology and, 102–103
energy healing, 161n16
Engel, George, 45, 46, 171n64, 195n136
environment: chronic disease and, 46–47; health and, 44
environmental hazards, exposure of children to, 169–170n43
environmental stress-based model of disease, 45, 172n70
"epidemic," 167n6
epidemics: communities resisting state efforts for protection during, 147–148; public response to, 3; study of past, 40–41, 168n23, 168n36, 168n37
Epstein, Steven, 3, 29, 98, 100, 184n3, 187n48, 190n79, 209n5
Epstein, Susan Fuchs, 158n19
Erickson, Daniel W., 212n25
Essex, Max, 148, 211n14
ethynerone (MK-665), 59
everyday forms of resistance, 2, 4, 6; African American communities and, 145; feminist scholarship on, 184n5
evolution, public acceptance/rejection of theory of, 153

falsification principle, Popper's, 191n83
Falwell, Jerry, 39, 167n13
family: Graham and changes in structure and function of, 30–31, 34–35; unorthodox AIDS activists and, 34–35
Farber, Leslie, 64
fatality narratives, 144, 199n9; AIDS Zone and, 134–135; Callen on, 93–96, 188n53, 188n56; Martin on, 188n61; PWAC and challenge to universal, 93–96
Fauci, Anthony, 150, 188n58
FDA (Food and Drug Administration): acknowledging therapeutic dose of AZT too high, 129; AIDS activism and changes in drug review at, 1; criticism for allowing useless medication, 61–62; failure to comply with Kefauver-Harris Amendment, 178n66; protests at, 1, 85; PWA distrust of, 93
Federal Trade Commission (FTC), AMA ban on advertising and, 70–71
Fedorko, Eugene: AZT and, 122, 200n30; on HEAL members, 122–123; on homocracy, 201n37; resignation from HEAL, 130, 204n83
Fee, Elizabeth, 39, 102, 167–168n18
Feldman, Mark, 185n18
Felson, Artie, 185n18
feminist activists: influence on Illich, 76; on marketing of psychotropic drugs to women, 64; support for PWAC by, 186n36
feminist bioethics, 174n11
feminist critique of bioethics, 174n15
feminist movement: criticism of mainstream medicine and physicians, 72–73; criticism of systems around women's health, 43–44; discourse on safety of pharmaceuticals, 60–61; politics of sex and intimacy and, 103
feminist scholarship: on activism, 5; on bioethics, 55; everyday forms of resistance and, 184n5; heroic medicine and cancer treatment and, 23
fermented foods, PWAs pursuing curative potential of, 158n10
Fifth National Lesbian/Gay Health Conference, 185n17
financial gain, charge physicians sacrificed patient care for, 68, 69–70
Firestone, John M., 58
Fisher, Sally, 197n151
Flannery, Michael, 27
Fogel, Robert, 39, 167n12
folk remedies, 24, 161n16
forgiveness, visualization practices and, 111
Fortune Magazine, 73
Foucault, Michel, 206n103; on clinical gaze, 45; Illich and, 77; on knowledge linked to power and truth, 168n19; microphysics of power and, 6, 133, 143, 159n21, 209n5; on power, 30, 55, 133; self-empowerment and, 209n6; on somatocracy, 47; on state's involvement in health, 171n61; on truth's links with power, 30
Fouratt, Jim: on ACT UP and new drugs, 200–201n34; on AIDS fatalism, 119; on debates between accomodationist and radical AIDS activists, 91; fatality narrative and, 199n9; on gay liberation, 186–187n37; resistance from ACT UP, 122
four horsemen of the apocalypse, AIDS personified as, 38
Fourth Great Awakening, 39, 167n12

Fox, Daniel, 39, 102, 167–168n18
Fox, Renee, 174n14
France, David, 138
Frank, Arthur W., 55
Freidson, Eliot, 67, 179n74, 179n75, 179n76
Friedan, Betty, 64–65
Friedman, Milton, 77
fringe medicine, defined, 161n15
fringe metaphor, study of alternative health movements and, 19
Fuller, Robert, 33, 166n78
Funkhouser, G. Ray, 43

Galdston, Iago, 45, 172n70
Galen, 24, 163n39
Gallo, Robert, 189n69; HTLV-III (HIV)/AIDS etiology and, 23, 27, 127, 163n50, 190–191n81, 190n80, 191n82, 202n48; rejection of multifactorial models, 203n58; theory that AIDS caused by cancer-causing virus and, 102
Gamson, William A., 181n106
Gannett, Lynn, 138
Gardner, Martha, 45
garlic pills, 105
Gay Activists Alliance (GAA), 91, 186–187n37, 201n37
Gay and Lesbian Community Center, 107
Gay and Lesbian Health Conference (1983), 88
gay liberation, 186–187n37; multifactorial theory and, 103
Gay Liberation Front (GLF), 91, 119, 186n37, 201n37
gay media, collaboration with African American media, 138–140
Gay Men's Health Crisis (GMHC), 116, 118, 187n41, 192n88, 194n119; accused of promoting fatality narrative, 95; as AIDS service organization, 87; criticism of, 88, 108; HEAL and, 120, 122–123; study of, 82; view of PWAC activism as radical, 92
Gay Men with AIDS (New York), 185n14
"gay plague," 38
gay recreational drug use, multifactorial model and, 128
gay sex: as agent of communion, 184n6; AIDS etiology and, 127–128; Callen on, 192–193n97
Geiger, H. Jack, 77, 175n20, 182n129
germanium, 105
germ theory: denigration of, 108–109; disillusion with, 46; focus on individual in disease and, 45; heroic medicine and, 22; physicians and, 26
Gerson, Michael, 150
Getting Well Again, 110
Gevitz, Norman, 17
Gilbert, David, 140
Giordano, Tony J., 87, 184n9
Giraldo, Roberto, 208n129
globalization, 130, 205n87
Gold, Griffin, 186n27
Goldsmith, Jeff, 42, 43, 169n37
Good Housekeeping (magazine), 64
Good Intentions (Nussbaum), 90
Goodman, Cliff, 138, 208n129
Google searches for disease etiologies, 11
Gordon, Arthur, 64
Gordon, James S., 49, 172n77, 202n56
Gould, Deborah, 93, 187–188n50, 199n11
Graham, Sylvester, 30–31, 34–35, 165n64
Graham bread, 31
Graham cracker, 165n65
gramicidin, 44
Gramsci, Antonio, 8
Greenberg, Jon, 196n139
"Group-Fantasy Origins of AIDS, The" (Schmidt), 132–133
group hysteria AIDS paradigm, 132–134, 206n102
Guccione, Bob, 23
Guinness Book of World Records, 64
Gurin, Joel, 50

habitus, 178n70
Hahnemann, Samuel, 166n77; coining term allopath, 25; on patient describing symptoms, 163n41; on vital spirit, 33
Hammond, William A., 21
Hannan, Tom, 198n165
Hannaway, Caroline, 168n23
Haring, Keith, 200n34
harm, Illich's iatrogenesis counts and medical, 75
HarperCollins, 105
Harrington, Michael, 44, 92
Harris, Craig G., 145
Harris, Richard, 72

Hartch, Todd, 182n112
Hastings Center, 174n16
Hastings Center Report, 55, 56
Hay, Louise, 108, 110–111, 131, 144, 197n155, 200n19, 205n90–91
HEAL Info Page, 128
healing, personal power and, 197n152
HEAL Los Angeles, 136
health: ethical obligation to maintain one's, 49–50; patient empowerment and, 147; personal responsibility for, 47–48, 103, 144, 171n59, 172–173n77, 173n78, 202–203n57; power and, 147; state involvement in, 171n61; transformations in construction of, 42–51
health activist movements: AIDS epidemic and, 85; rise in in postwar years, 82. *See also* unorthodox health activism
"health as praxis," 203n74
Health Care in America (Rosner & Reverby), 142
health care model, bioethics' effect on, 56
health care systems: doubts about American, 81–82; physicians blamed for broken, 69–70
Health Education AIDS Liaison (HEAL), 9, 10, 82–83, 116–141; advertisement for, 199n13; AIDS activists' view of early, 119–120; AIDS dissidence movement, 136–137; AIDS etiology and, 127, 131–137; alienation from larger PWA community, 135; alternative health methods and, 116–117; anti-AZT position, 122; archives, 159n28; collaboration and, 137–140; complicated history of, 140–141; contesting HIV as cause of AIDS, 99; criticism of pharmaceutical solutions, 128, 129–130; early years, 118–137; embrace of complementary medicine, 119–120; embrace of holistic interdependency, 131–132; health holism, multifactoriality, and, 125–130; health holism and, 118–119, 122, 125–130, 172–173n77, 173n78, 199n17; Kalichman on, 190n77; lack of scholarship on, 117–118, 123–124; lifestyle modification campaigns and, 129; macrobiotics and, 30; membership, 122–123; mission of, 119; moralistic tone of PWA empowerment, 128–129; multifactorial model and, 126–128; outreach events in Harlem, 137–138; outreach to prisoners, 138; public support for from other AIDS organizations, 120–121, 122; PWAC and, 120, 129; radicalization of health holism and, 123–124, 130–137; relationship with AIDS service organizations, 118; resignation of members, 130; rift with GMHC, 122–123; urging PWAs to take charge of their health, 202–203n57
health holism, 48–51; ACT UP and, 195–196n139; broken biomedical system and, 109–110; defining, 125, 201n46; HEAL and, 118–119, 122, 125–130, 172–173n77, 173n78, 199n17; interdependency and, 124; nature and, 49; PWAC and, 114–115, 196n146; social development theories and, 130–131. *See also* Health Education AIDS Liaison (HEAL)
"HEAL this Week" (television program), 130, 208n119
health legislation, AMA and universal health care debate, 71–72
Health Policy Advisory Center, 61, 67, 81
Health Research Group, 62
health services, concern AIDS patients victimized by, 88–89
Healthy People (U.S. Surgeon General), 47, 49
Heckler, Margaret, 40, 121
hegemony, 160n3
Helquist, Michael, 184n6, 185n18
herbalism, 49, 107, 110, 118, 119, 126, 161n16
herd immunity, 150
Herman, Bob, 92–93, 187n49
Herman, Tom, 108
heroic medicine, 20–23; effect of homeopathy on, 18; history of term, 161n19; response to AIDS and, 162–163n34
Hershey, Paul Turner, 159n26
Hess, David J., 22
Heywood, Mark, 183n3
Hippocratic Oath, 57
Hirsch, Michael, 105, 110, 111, 196n46, 197n154
historians, on AIDS and origins of public health measures, 39–40
historical currents, 20
historical memory: AIDS and, 37–38; existential threats and appeal to, 36–37
historiography, social history and, 142–145
history: meanings of, 41–42; as toolkit for aiding and informing actions, 15–16

HIV (human immunodeficiency virus): discovery of as HTLV-III/LAV, 40, 121; efforts to create vaccine for, 40; progress narrative for, 40; rejection of role for in AIDS, 3; SARS-CoV-2, 212n27; as target of pharmaceutical research, 103
HIV denialism, 23, 99–103, 124, 159n22
HIV vaccines, 168n21
Hobbes, Thomas, 33, 44, 49
Hoffman-La Roche, 63
Hofstadter, Richard, 153, 158–159n20
holistic health models, Hirsch on, 197n154
holistic health movement, 125; Illich and, 78–79
holistic interdependency, HEAL and, 131–132
Holistic Medical Association, 110
holistic medicine, 110. *See also* health holism
"Holistics 101" (Idavoy), 109
Hollinger, David A., 171n57
Holmes, Oliver Wendell, 165n75
home health kits, homeopathy and, 25
Homeopathic Envoy (journal), 28
homeopaths: approach to patients, 25; emphasizing flexibility of their system, 24–26
homeopathy, 119, 143, 161n16, 201–202n46, 201n38; anti-authoritarianism and, 28; bridging physical and spiritual worlds, 33; effect on heroic medicine, 18; extolled for AIDS, 108; institutionalization of, 29; regular medicine and, 160n10; Transcendentalists and, 166n77; vital force and, 32; women clinicians and, 25
homocracy, 201n37
homophobia, AIDS etiology and, 132–134
hope, 120; empowerment predicted on, 93–94; Fouratt and need for, 119
hopelessness, AIDS and, 94, 108, 120, 134, 199n18
How to Have Sex in an Epidemic (Callen, Sonnabend & Berkowitz), 103
"How to Talk to Your Doctor" (Herman), 92–93
Hoxsey, Harry, 22
Hoxsey health tonic, 202n48
HPA-23, 187n49
HTLV-III, 27, 191n82
HTLV-III/LAV, 40, 121
hucksters, health and disease and, 151–152
Humphrey, Hubert, 66, 178n66
hundred LEGENDS, a (Northern Lights Alternatives/Design Industries Foundation for AIDS), 211n16
Huxley, Aldous, 64
hydrogen peroxide, 105
hydropathy, 143, 162n25; anti-authoritarianism and, 28; religion and, 31–32; Twain on spirituality and, 32; women clinicians and, 18, 160n10
hypnoimmunotherapy, 131
hypnotherapy, 126, 131, 206–207n108
hysterectomies, overuse of, 72–73

iatrogenesis: clinical, 75; cultural, 75, 182n118; social, 75, 182n118
Idavoy, Alex, 109, 110
identity, subselves and, 158n19
Illich, Ivan, 55–57, 135, 181–182n111, 181n108, 182n11, 182n112, 182n119, 182n125, 204n84; Callen and, 103, 107, 193n98; clinical iatrogenesis, 75; cultural iatrogenesis, 75, 182n118; decline in popularity of arguments, 76–78; dissident philosophy of, 74–79; historical influence, 78; on medicine as social control, 73; on Mintz, 59; self-care society and, 76; social iatrogenesis, 75, 182n118; technology and, 75–76; work branded as polemical, 175n20
illness: biopsychosocial model of, 45; emotional and psychological sources of, 109; public health model of, 45; vital force and, 32. *See also* disease
Impure Science (Epstein), 3, 98, 100
individual: AIDS activism and individual acts of protest, 86; Illich on suppression of, 75–76; syncretizing health practices, 143–144
individual autonomy, bioethics and empowerment of, 55–56
individual interaction with environment, chronic disease and, 46–47
individual responses to climate change, 152–153
individual responsibility: for one's own health, 47–48, 172–173n77, 173n78; structural inequities and, 171n58

individual rights, public response to AIDS and, 41–42
individual right to challenge experts, arguing is obligation, 92–93
individual risk behaviors, focus on, 136
individual treatment decisions, lack of scholarly analysis of unorthodox AIDS activism and, 4–5
infectious disease: AIDS and infectious disease narratives, 167–168n18; individual empowerment and, 149–152; supplanted by chronic disease in twentieth-century United States, 42–43, 45–47
influenza pandemic of 1918–1920, 169n30
information, empower and free availability of, 152
informed consent, 28, 29, 55
Ingelfinger, Franz J., 71, 164n59, 180n89
"Ingelfinger rule," 164n59
inoculation debates, 165n75
Institute of Medicine, 143
Institute of Medicine Report, 19, 63
interdependency, AIDS etiology and, 124, 130–137
International Committee on the Taxonomy of Viruses, 163n50
International Journal of Feminist Approaches to Bioethics, 174n11
International Monetary Fund, 205n87
interventions, physician preference of aggressive, 67–68
intimacy, multifactorial model and, 103
itraconazole, 112

Jackson, Charles O., 62
Jackson, James Caleb, 31
Jackson, Mark, 172n71
Jacksonian era, anti-intellectualism during, 27
James, John S., 97, 189n68
James, Steven, 110, 112, 197n152
Jennings, Bruce, 55
Joint United Nations Programme on HIV/AIDS (UNAIDS), 89
Jones, Michael J., 91
Jones, Therese, 55
Jonsen, Albert, 56
Joseph, Stephen, 94
Journal of New Drugs, 176n35
Journal of Psychohistory, 132
Journal of the American Bar Association, 69
Journal of the American Medical Association, 160n8
Journal of Zoophily, 28

Kahn, Otto H., 57
Kalichman, Seth C., 190n77, 205n96
Kallaugher, Kevin, 167n7
Kaposi's sarcoma, 37, 188n54
Kaufman, Martin, 160n10
Kefauver, Estee, 59
Kefauver-Harris Amendment of 1962, 61, 178n66
Kellogg, C. W., 22
Kellogg, James Harvey, 165n69
Kelsey, Frances Oldham, 60
Kennedy, Edward M. "Ted," 177n54
Kenneth, Irving, 183n136
killer virus etiological model, 99, 108
Kirschmann, Anne Taylor, 32
Kline, Wendy, 18
knowledge: health professionals and borders of, 145–146; linked to power and truth, 168n19; power and rejection of codified systems of, 153; unorthodox health activism and methods of, 144
Knowles, John H., 47, 48, 49–50, 52–53, 171n57, 171n59, 180–181n99
Koch, Edward I., 139
Koch, Robert, 22, 32, 46
Koch's postulates, 208n120
Koop, C. Everett, 39, 167n15
Kramer, Larry, 118–119, 121, 167n15, 194n124, 201n34
Krebiozen, 202n48
Kruger, Steven F., 38
Kushi, Michio, 119

laetrile, 202n48
Laing, R. D., 72
Lalonde Report, 47, 49
Lancet (journal), 64
Lande, Paul, 104, 197n155
Lanzaratta, Phil, 185n18
Lasagna, Louis, 57–58
Latinx communities, AIDS cases in, 137
Lauritsen, John, 106, 109, 128, 133, 195n126–127, 204n81, 206n104

LAV (lymphadenopathy-associated virus), 40, 101, 121, 163n50, 190n78, 190n81, 191n82, 191n85
Lawrence, Sean, 139
Lears, Jackson, 30, 31, 33
Lederer, Bob, 110, 122, 130
Lee, Philip R., 58, 66
Leonard, Ralph B., 21
Lerner, Barron H., 29, 164n59
Lerner, Louise, 67
Lesbian and Gay Community Center, HEAL and, 118
LeVay, Simon, 184n7
Levin, Lowell S., 78
Librium, 63
Life Magazine, 191n86
lifestyle modification campaigns, HEAL and, 129
Linds, Justin Abraham, 158n10
lobelia, 162n25
Lorenzini, John, 104
Los Angeles Sentinel (newspaper), 139
Los Angeles Times (newspaper), 43, 64, 167n7
Love, Medicine and Miracles (Siegel), 110
Love Canal Tragedy, 44
Luther, Martin, 24
lymphadenopathy associated virus (LAV), 163n50

macrobiotics, 5, 6, 106, 110, 112, 118, 122, 126, 199n13
Madar, Chase, 74–75
Maggiore, Christine, 136, 138, 140, 208n131
"magical thinking," 50
magic bullets, 22, 65, 104, 125, 135, 194n124, 196n145
"Magna Mortalitas," 166n3
Mahapatra, Jayanta, 16
Malinowski, Bronislaw, 206n101
malpractice cases, rise in number of, 176n44, 179n79
Marcellus, Jane, 172n68
marginalized health movements, study of, 143
marginalized people, medicine accused of policing bodies of, 72–73
Markoff Asistent, Niro, 202n55
Martin, Cass, 188n61
Marx, Karl, 135
Marxism, influence on PWA movement, 91
Maryland Medical Journal, 25
massage, 161n16, 199n19
Massih, Artin, 212n25
Mather, Cotton, 33, 165n74
Mbeki, Thabo, 136, 211n14
McKeown, Thomas, 46, 170n55
McKinnie, Michael, 174n13
Meade, Margaret, 132
media: collaboration between gay and African American, 138–140; coverage of chronic diseases, 43; on dangers of psychotropic drugs, 63–64; on dangers of Valium use, 65–66; on fear of overmedication, 58; highlighting public protests, 184n4; portrayal of physicians in, 65; as purveyor of fatality narratives regarding AIDS, 94; use of "plague" to described AIDS, 38; whitewashing AIDS in, 188n53
Medic (television program), 65
medical history, bias for sectarianation in, 5–6
"Medical Industrial Complex," 81
medicalization: ethical status of, 55; of life and death, 182n118; of women's lives and bodies, 72
Medical Liberty News (journal), 28
Medical Matters section of *Newsline,* 92, 187n46
Medical Nemesis (Illich), 75, 78–79, 204n84
medical sectarianism, 160n8
Medical Talk for the Home (journal), 28
Medicare, AMA and, 72
medicine: boundary between public health and, 45; heroic, 18, 20–23, 161n19, 162–163n34; Illich on deprofessionalization of, 182n125; resistance to in U.S. history, 18–20; as social control, 73–79; specific disease etiology and, 171n65; study of alternative health movements and modernization of, 17–18. *See also* biomedicine
medicine, history of in United States: AIDS and, 37–38; anti-authoritarian sentiment and, 27–30; antimodern sentiment and, 30–35; heroic medicine, 20–23; rational *vs.* empirical medicine, 23–27
Medicines for Man (Dowling), 67
megavitamins, 161n16
Mesmer, Franz, 207n108
Mesmerism, 206–207n108
methodological considerations, 7

Michaelson, Michael G., 67, 72, 180n88, 180n98, 181n105
microphysics of power, 133, 143, 159n21, 209n5
Mikulski, Barbara, 64
Miles, Michael Wayne, 203n57
Mill, John Stuart, 159n26, 171n64
Millennium Approaches (Kushner), 200n31
Mills, Sara, 160n3
mind: AIDS etiology and, 131–134; role in AIDS treatment, 131
mind-body dualism, health holism *vs.*, 48
"Mind-Body Link and 'Heal Thyself' are New Medicine 'Miracle Drugs,'" 50
Mintz, Morton, 59–60, 61
Montagnier, Luc, 163n50, 191n82
moralistic tone, HEAL and, 128–129, 135
morality: alternative healing and, 110; of empowerment, 154
Moral Majority, war waged against gay men by, 133
moral obligation, for one's own health, 171n59
moral responsibility narratives, health officials and, 146, 147
Morbidity and Mortality Report (CDC), 43
Morgan, John P., 58
"Mother's Little Helper" (Rolling Stones), 65, 177n62
Muller, Charlotte, 66
multi-causal etiology of disease, 183n136
multifactoriality of health and disease, 124, 125–130
multifactorial model of AIDS etiology, 101–103, 109, 126–128, 192n90, 192n91; health holism and, 125–130; Sonnabend and, 101–103, 109, 124, 191n87, 193n102
Mycobacterium tuberculosis, 11, 32
"My Doctor and My Chiropractor" (Peck), 112

Nader, Ralph, 60, 62, 76
Nalbandian, Peter, 185n24
naltrexone, 112, 197n163
Naraindas, Harish, 7
Nasrallah, Tom, 185n18
Nassaney, Louis, 111
National Action Network, 138
National Cancer Act, 43
National Cancer Institute (NCI), 23
National Institutes of Health (NIH): AIDS drugs and, 194n124; AZT and, 104; Office of Alternative Medicine, 210n11; PWA distrust of, 93
National Women's Health Network, 61
nature, health holism and, 49
Navarre, Max, 197n155; on AL721, 196n148; on AZT, 104, 193n106; challenging fatality narratives, 93–96; criticism of drug trials, 98; on HIV and AIDS, 164n52
Needleman, Jacob, 67–68, 182–183n130
New England Journal of Medicine, 71
"New Perspective on the Health of Canadians, A" (Lalonde Report), 47
Newsweek, 64
New York City Department of Health, 121
New Yorker (magazine), 72
New York Gay and Lesbian Experimental Film Festival, 117
New York Magazine, 192n93
New York Native (newspaper), 6, 119, 121, 138–139, 191n86, 200n27, 209n138
New York Review of Books, 75
New York Times (newspaper), 38, 43, 64, 77, 132, 138, 188n53
New York Times Magazine, 64
Nichols, John Benjamin, 160n8
"nishmath-chajim," 33, 165n75
Nissenbaum, Stephen, 31
Nixon, Richard, 43, 180n99
Noble Sage, 182n129
"noble savage" imagery, 49, 172n68
Nonas, Elisabeth, 184n7
"noncompliance," 29, 146, 164n60
Northern Lights Alternatives, 113, 148; AIDS Mastery workshop, 110–111, 131, 144, 148, 200n19
Null, Gary, 23
nursing philosophies, Denver Principles and progressive, 91
Nussbaum, Bruce, 90

obesity, public health campaigns on, 147, 210n12
oral history interviews, with Ellner, 117
orthodox *vs.* unorthodox, 178n70
Osler, William, 12
osteopathy: institutionalization of, 29; Twain's defense of, 28

Other America, The (Harrington), 44
Otis, Laura, 170n56
Our Bodies, Ourselves, 44, 72–73, 90, 181n103
Out Magazine, 122
Overall, Christine, 55
overmedication: charge that physicians' guilty of, 66–67; discourse, 177n51; fear of, 57–65
Over the Counter Pills that Don't Work (Kaufman), 177n48, 177n50

Pain Medicine (journal), 201n38
pandemic science, 150–151, 211n22
Parachini, Allan, 183n136
Parsons, Talcott, 47, 181n107
Pasteur, Louis, 22, 46
paternalism, 159n26
patient autonomy, 28, 29
patient behavior, disease narratives and, 146
patient empowerment: health and, 147; holistic medicine and, 196n146; limits to, 145; reconceptualizing with borderland concept, 143; Thomsonian medicine and, 27
patient engagement model, HEAL and, 118
patient rights movement, 54, 92
patients: biomedical ethics and, 28, 29, 53, 54; biomedical system and dehumanization of, 52; history of unorthodox health activism and focus on, 16, 18–20; homeopaths approach to, 25; Illich's charge that medical system disempowered, 73, 76; noncompliant, 29, 146, 164n60; physician relationship with, 25; physicians' financial gain at expense of, 68, 69–70; as subject of historical analysis, 142; use of alternative therapies, 19
Patton, Cindy, 103, 193n99
Peck, Larry, 112, 197–198n164
pediatric AIDS cases, 137, 167n15, 208n125
Pellegrino, Edmund, 66, 178n71
pentamidine, 194n124
Penthouse Magazine, 23
people with AIDS (PWAs): alternative healing approaches used by long-term, 199–200n19; concern victimized by health service community, 88–89; desire to reframe AIDS as chronic condition, 126; focusing on lives and perspectives of, 6; furious living and, 148–149; health holism and, 114–115; HEAL urging them to take charge of their health, 202–203n57; infectious disease narratives, AIDS, and, 167–168n18; treatment options outside dominant biomedical model and, 2; women's health movement and, 90–91
People with AIDS (San Francisco), 185n14
People with AIDS Coalition (PWAC), 10, 82–83, 85–115, 185–186n26; acceptance of wide range of opinion, 107; AIDS etiology and, 99–103; birth of, 88–107; as borderline model in action, 88; Callen resignation from, 113–114; challenges to universal fatality narratives and, 93–96; compared to ACT UP, 89; conclusions about, 114–115; contributors' embrace of alternative health systems, 107–114; core mission, 87; cures and criticism of AZT use, 103–107; defined by gay white men, 87; end of, 115; focus on empowerment of PWAs, 91–93; formation of, 89; HEAL and, 120, 129; health holism and, 114–115; HIV, AIDS, and the "unholy holy war," 99–103; leadership turnover at, 185n11; operating within borderlands of unorthodoxy, 113; print publications, 89–90; PWAC activism and allegations of "fourth or fifth rate" science, 96–99; PWA empowerment and, 114; PWA Health Group, 113, 198n165–166
People with AIDS Coalition Newsline (PWAC Newsline), 6, 87–88, 89–90, 121; Callen as editor, 92, 195n137; challenging fatality narratives, 96; on complementary medicine, 120; debate over AZT in, 96–99, 104, 106–107; featuring alternative health systems, 107–114; as lifeline, 91; unorthodox AIDS healing systems and, 103
People with AIDS Coalition of New York (PWAC/NY), 186n26
personal responsibility for health and disease, 47–48, 103, 144, 171n59, 172–173n77, 173n78, 202–203n57
Pertschuk, Michael B., 71
Pew Research Poll, 153
pharmaceutical corporations: AZT toxicity and concern of motives and methods of, 105; charge concerned with profit over patients, 97; physicians' ties to, 67

pharmacological solutions: fear of overmedicated society, 57–65; HEAL's criticism of, 129–130; magic bullets, 22, 65, 104, 125, 135, 194n124, 196n145. *See also* antiretrovirals
physicians: ban on advertising lifted, 70–71, 180n89; bias towards action model, 67, 179–180n85, 179n74, 179n75; blamed for broken healthcare system, 69–70; character of, 68; charged with selective provisioning of care, 72; charge overprescribing drugs, 66–67; charge prioritized profits over patients, 68, 69–70; distrust of, 53; feminist framing of, 72–73; germ theory and, 26; national health care legislation and, 71–72; perception of dogmatism associated with, 23–27; post-war critiques of, 65–74; public attitudes toward, 178n64, 181n106; questioning motives and competence of, 66; relationship with patient, 25, 70–72; secularization of medicine and decline in trust in, 34; specialization and, 69; as victim, 68, 69; victimization narratives and, 73
Pier, Nathaniel, 189n63
Pieters, Stephen, 95
pill, birth control, 60, 176n36, 176n37
Pills That Don't Work (Health Research Group), 62
plague, AIDS described as, 38, 40, 119
"plague," 167n6
"Plague Years, The" (Black), 38
Planned Parenthood, 60, 176n37
Pneumocystis carinii, 37, 166n2
Pneumocystis jirovecii, 166n2
pneumocystis pneumonia (PCP), 16
"Politics of Medication, The" (Morgan), 58
Popper, Karl, 191n83
Porter, Roy, 6, 18, 32, 142
poverty, disease and, 44
power: bioethics and, 54–55; biomedicine and accumulation of, 54; Foucault and, 30, 133, 143; health and, 147; knowledge linked to truth and, 168n19; microphysics of, 133, 143, 159n21, 209n5; rejection of codified systems of knowledge and, 153; unorthodox AIDS activism and Foucault' micro-physics of, 6
Powles, John, 170n43
Praxis Pharmaceuticals, 198n165
prayer, to treat disease, 161n17
prestige surveys, physicians and, 181n106
principles, unorthodox AIDS activism's failure to mobilize around core set of, 5. *See also* Denver Principles
prisoners, HEAL's outreach to, 138
Profession of Medicine (Freidson), 67
progress, AIDS tragedy as cost of, 41
Project Inform, 193n107
prophylaxis to prevent AIDS, 129–130
protease inhibitors, 115
"Psychological Genocide: The Push for AIDS Testing," 134
psychophysical energy, curing illness and, 182–183n130
psychotherapy, Emmanuel Movement and, 165n72
psychotropic medications, 60, 63–65
public health: boundary between medicine and, 45; lessons for, 145–149
public health campaigns, 210n12; moral responsibility narratives and, 47, 146, 147
public health emergencies, unorthodox COVID-19 activism and, 151
public health interventions/measures: history of those recommended early in AIDS pandemic, 39–40; proper aims of, 146–147
public health model of illness, 45
Public Opinion Quarterly, 43
public protests by AIDS activists, 85–86, 93. *See also* die-ins
Purdy, Laura M., 174n11
PWA-New York, 185n26
PWA organizations, formation of PWA-New York, 89. *See also* AIDS service organizations
PWArcs (people with AIDS-related complex), 185n15

Quack, Johannes, 7
"quackery," 83, 114, 120, 131, 163n38, 196n145, 201n38, 209n3
Quarterly Bulletin (HEAL), 120
queer rights movement in New York City, 86
Quimby, Phineas, 196–197n150

racism, orthodox medicine and structural, 181n105
R.A.C. pills, 21, 162n21
radical monopolies, Illich's, 74–75
radical ontology, 48
Rasmussen, Nicolas, 63
rational *vs.* empirical medicine, 23–27
Rawlinson, Mary C., 174n11
Reagan, Ronald, 40, 151
recreational drugs, gay men's use of, 206n104
Reiki, 110, 119, 126, 131
Relationship (Mahapatra), 16
religion: AIDS etiology and, 34; alternative health movements and, 31–35; Callen and HIV etiological theory and, 100–101
religious imagery, AIDS and, 38–39
research scientists, biomedical ethics and abuse by, 53–54
resistance: emotions catalyzing, 93–94; everyday forms of, 2, 4, 6, 145, 184n5
resistance movements, radicalization of, 6–7
"Responsibility of the Individual, The" (Knowles), 52–53
Reverby, Susan M., 6, 18, 47, 142
reverse transcriptase, 177n49
Reynolds, Bobby, 185n18
rhubarb, in R.A.C. pills, 162n21
ribavirin, 164n59
ribavirin drug trial, 98–99
Robinson, Marty, 97
Rockefeller Foundation, 47, 50
Rolling Stone (periodical), 38
Rolling Stones, 65, 177n62
Room of One's Own, A (Woolf), 17
Rosenberg, Charles, 45, 167n6, 170–171n57, 173n2
Rosett, Jane, 94, 107, 113
Rosner, David, 6, 18, 47, 142
Ross, Loretta, 61
Rothman, David, 54, 73, 173n4, 174n14
Rothstein, William, 22
Rousseau, Jean-Jacques, 182n129
Rowe, Ed, 39
Rubin, Gayle, 91
Rush, Benjamin, 21, 24

safer sex manual, Callen, Berkowitz, and Sonnabend and, 191–192n88
Salk, Jonas, 40, 168n21
Salmon, J. Warren, 203n74
Salvarsan, 32
Sarason, Seymour, 70, 180n87
Sarner, Matthew, 185n18
SARS-CoV-2. *See* COVID-19
Saturday Review (magazine), 75
Schick, Rob, 102, 163–164n52, 195n127
Schmidt, Casper G., 132–134, 204n81, 206n97, 206n101–102, 206n104
Schuman, Howard, 181n106
science: opposition to Cold War and, 170n57; power in medicine, 170n53; PWAC activism and allegations of poor, 96–99
Science (journal), 149
science deniers, 153
Science Newsletter, 66
scientific empiricism, 24, 26–27
scientific expertise, COVID-19 and attacks on, 150
scientific findings, AIDS activists access to, 164n59
Scott, James C., 2, 4, 86
Scott-Hartland, Bree, 105
Scutero, James, 201n41
Seaman, Barbara, 60, 176n36
secularization, antimodernism in the late nineteenth-century and, 31–32
seed and soil metaphor, unorthodox AIDS activism and, 9–10, 159n3
seed *vs.* soil argument, disease and, 165n67
self-care for AIDS, 105
self-care society, Illich and, 76, 79
self-empowerment: Foucault and, 209n6; as HEAL's mission, 119, 120, 203n57; PWAC goal of, 91–93
self-help groups, 161n16
self-help movement, Illich and, 78
self-hypnosis, for AIDS, 108
self-interest, physicians and, 69–70
Seventh Day Adventists, 31
sexism of medical practice, 72–73
sexually transmitted diseases, multifactorial theory of AIDS etiology and repeated infection with, 101–103, 127, 191n87
sexual practices of gay men, multifactorial theory of AIDS etiology and, 101–103
sexual revolution, AIDS depicted as punishment for, 39
Sharpton, Al, 138

Shaw, George Bernard, 70
Sheff, Timothy J., 179n74
Shryock, Richard, 23–24, 163n39
Sikov, Ed, 184n4
Silent Spring (Carson), 44, 60
Siplon, Patricia, 186n34
Sirois, Francois, 206n101
skeleton harassing sick image, AIDS and, 39
smallpox, 33, 165n75
Smith, Meredith, 148
Smith, Richard, 182n118
social and political dimensions of individual treatment decisions, 4–5
social change, antimodernism and, 30–31
social control, 72; medicine as, 73–79
social development theories, health holism and, 130–131
social epidemiology, 131–132, 135–136
social history, study of health movements and, 142–145
social iatrogenesis, 75, 182n118
social issues, health and disease and, 44
social media, echo chamber effect of, 151–152, 153
social medicine, 131–132, 135–136, 180n99
social norms, unorthodox health activism and, 148–149
socioeconomic differences, between HEAL and GMHC, 122–123
socioeconomic status, unorthodox healing systems and, 145, 209–210n8
So Human an Animal (Dubos), 44
soil and seed metaphor, unorthodox AIDS activism and, 9–10, 159n3
Solid Gold Stethoscope, The (Berman), 69–70
somatocracy, 47
Sonnabend, Joseph, 206n97; accusing mainstream physicians of dogmatic thinking, 27; on AZT, 104; Callen and, 129, 187n44; challenging fatality narratives regarding AIDS, 95; criticism of AIDS research, 96–97; critique of biomedicine, 188n59; on Fauci, 188n58; multifactorial model and, 101–103, 109, 124, 191n87, 193n102; on repeated infections and AIDS, 191n87; on safer sex manual, 191–192n88; structural dimension so illness and, 192n93
Sontag, Susan, 162n33
soul sickness, 31, 33
Speaker, Susan Lynn, 65–66, 72, 178n64, 179–180n85
specialization, of physicians, 69
specificity, biomedicine and popularization of, 45
Spindell, Gail, 108
SPIN Magazine, 23, 203n58
spiritualism, alternative health movements and, 32
spiritual meaning, efforts to find in everyday life, 31–32
Staley, Peter, 183–184n1
state: involvement in individual health, 171n61; role as scientific entrepreneur, 81
Stevens, M. L. Tina, 56, 170n53, 174–175n16, 174n13
Stevens, Rosemary, 69
Stonewall Riots, 86, 119
Strangers at the Bedside (Rothman), 54
stress, AIDS and stress experienced by gay men, 133
Stress, Immunity and Aging (Cooper), 172n70
Strub, Sean, 185n21
structural abuses in clinical system, bioethics and, 55–56
structural factors in etiology of disease, 12
Sturken, Marita, 189–190n76
sulfamethoxazole/trimethoprim (Bactrim), 105, 112, 129
Summers, David, 108
Sunday Telegram (newspaper), 167n7
Surviving AIDS (Callen), 87, 184n10, 187n45, 195n136; Callen on multifactorial theory and empowerment, 102–103; challenging fatality narratives for AIDS and, 94–96, 188n53; critique of AZT in, 105
Surviving and Thriving with AIDS, 87, 89–90, 194n119; controversy over AZT and, 104, 122; criticism of AIDS research in, 98; featuring alternative health systems, 107–114; as safe space for debate, 93, 107
syphilis, 11, 32
Szasz, Thomas, 72, 181n107

Taylor, J. M., 26, 27, 163n48
Temin, Howard, 177n49
Temin, Peter, 62, 177n49
Tesh, Sylvia Noble, 168n27, 171n58, 171n64
thalidomide (Thalomid), 59, 60, 65, 176n35

Therapeutic Touch, 202n48
Thomas, Lewis, 50
Thompson, Dick, 194n124
Thomson, Samuel, 21
Thomsonian medicine, 21; anti-authoritarianism and, 27; institutionalization of, 29; study of, 5, 143; treatments, 162n25
Time Magazine, 43, 65, 194n124
tobacco use, public health campaigns on, 147, 210n12
To Fix or to Heal (Davis), 125
Tomes, Nancy, 18, 169n30
Tomycz, Nestor D., 71
tonsillectomies, overuse of, 67, 179n75
Tony Brown's Journal (television program), 128, 129
toxicity of AZT, 104–106
traditional Chinese medicine, 110
"Traffic in Women, The" (Rubin), 91
Transcendentalists, homeopathy and, 166n77
Traynor, Gar, 185n18
treatment activism, AIDS and twentieth-century, 3
treatments: individual decisions about, 2, 4–5; physicians and unnecessary, 67. *See also* alternative therapies
Treichler, Paula, 190n79
Treponema pallidum, 11
Trump, Donald, 150, 151, 211n22
truth, links with power, 30, 168n19
Tuana, Nancy, 186n30
tuberculosis, etiology of, 11, 12
Turner, Dan, 88, 185n18
Turning Point, The (Capra), 131
Tuskegee syphilis experiment, AIDS epidemic and, 139
Twain, Mark, 22, 28, 32, 165n71, 180n93

underrepresented voices, including in historical narrative, 8
Union of Concerned Scientists, 150
U.S. Civil War, heroic medicine and, 21
U.S. Department of Health and Human Services, 137–138
U.S. Department of Justice, 176n44
U.S. National Center for Health Statistics, 126
universal health care, AMA opposition to, 71–72
University of California, San Francisco magazine, 50
"unorthodox": choice of term, 157n7; "orthodox" vs, 178n70
unorthodox AIDS activism: acceptance of multiple perspectives and opinions within, 112; accusations of dogmatic thinking by physicians and, 27; anti-authoritarianism and, 28–30; antimodern sentiment and, 34–35; echoes of historical arguments between regular and irregular medical leaders, 26–27; emergence of, 81–83; ethical considerations in studying, 8–9; everyday forms of resistance and, 2, 4, 6; factors contributing to elision from scholarly analysis, 4–7; heterogeneity of, 5; historical examination of, 2–4; Illich and, 78, 79; methodological considerations in studying, 7; networks of support and, 4–5; preventable deaths and, 148; redefining and recreating the family and, 34–35; societal benefits of studying, 8; soil and seed metaphor in studying, 9–10, 159n3; transformation of activists into lay experts, 29–30; utilitarian considerations in studying, 8
unorthodox COVID-19 activism, 149–152, 212n25–27
unorthodox health activism, 3; borderland model, 17–20; focus on patient in study of, 16, 18–20; study of, 142–145
unorthodox health interventions: as complementary to mainstream medicine, 120–121; PWAC and, 103
unorthodox medicine, characterizing physicians as dogmatic, 24–25
Us Helping Us, 210n9

vaccines, efforts to create HIV, 40
Valium, 64, 65
Valley of the Dollas (Suzanne), 63–64
venereal disease campaigns, 39
victim, PWA as, 199n18
violence, 135; mind, disease, and structural, 131–132, 133
visualization, as AIDS therapy, 105, 108, 110–111, 196–197n150, 205n90

Visualization Workshop, 198n169
vital force/vital spirit, healthcare movements and, 32–33
vitamin therapy, 50, 110, 112, 113, 161n16

Waitzkin, Howard, 181n107
Wall Street Journal (newspaper), 188n53
Walters, Ray, 62
Warner, Margaret Humphreys, 33
Washington Post (newspaper), 150, 153
Waterman, Barbara, 181n107
Way of the Physician, The (Needleman), 67–68
Weber, Max, 165n66
Weiss, Barnett, 208n125, 208n129
Weston, Anthony, 54
White, Ellen, 31, 165n69
white bread, Graham and, 30–31
White House, AIDS protests at, 1
Whooley, Owen, 24–25
Whorton, James C., 78
Wiegmann, Wendy, 178n70
Williams, A. J. Roosevelt, 104–105
Williams, Rhys, 5
Willner, Robert E., 128, 203n69
Wipe Out AIDS (WOA), 119, 185n14, 187n37. *See also* Health Education AIDS Liaison (HEAL)
Wolfe, Sidney M., 62, 176n47
women: hydropathy and female clinicians, 18, 160n10; marketing of psychotropic drugs to, 64–65
women's health, feminist critiques of systems around, 43–44
women's health movement, 186n30; anti-authoritarianism, alternative medicine, and, 28; PWA movement and, 90–91; on safety of pharmaceuticals, 60–61
Woolf, Virginia, 17
Wordsworth, William, 41
World Review (magazine), 165n71
Wright, Joe, 91

yoga, 50, 108, 110, 161n17
You Can Heal Yourself (Hay), 205n91
Young, Ian, 206n102

zalcitabine (ddC; Hivid), 109
Zappa, Frank, 130, 205n86
"zaps," 122
Zero Patience (film), 189–190n76
zidovudine (ZDV). *See* azidothymidine (AZT; Retrovir) (zidovudine; ZDV)
Zola, Irving Kenneth, 181n107
zoxazolamine (Flexin), 59

ABOUT THE AUTHOR

MATTHEW KELLY earned his PhD in sociomedical sciences and his MPH from Columbia University, where he was honored with the Marisa de Castro Benton Award. Prior to that, he graduated from Brown University. Currently, he is pursuing a medical degree at the Johns Hopkins University School of Medicine.

Available titles in the Critical Issues in Health and Medicine series:

Emily K. Abel, *Prelude to Hospice: Florence Wald, Dying People, and Their Families*
Emily K. Abel, *Suffering in the Land of Sunshine: A Los Angeles Illness Narrative*
Emily K. Abel, *Tuberculosis and the Politics of Exclusion: A History of Public Health and Migration to Los Angeles*
Marilyn Aguirre-Molina, Luisa N. Borrell, and William Vega, eds. *Health Issues in Latino Males: A Social and Structural Approach*
Anne-Emanuelle Birn and Theodore M. Brown, eds., *Comrades in Health: U.S. Health Internationalists, Abroad and at Home*
Karen Buhler-Wilkerson, *False Dawn: The Rise and Decline of Public Health Nursing*
Susan M. Chambré, *Fighting for Our Lives: New York's AIDS Community and the Politics of Disease*
Stephen M. Cherry, *Importing Care, Faithful Service: Filipino and Indian American Nurses at a Veterans Hospital*
James Colgrove, Gerald E. Markowitz, and David Rosner, eds., *The Contested Boundaries of American Public Health*
Elena Conis, Sandra Eder, and Aimee Medeiros, eds., *Pink and Blue: Gender, Culture, and the Health of Children*
Cynthia A. Connolly, *Children and Drug Safety: Balancing Risk and Protection in Twentieth-Century America*
Cynthia A. Connolly, *Saving Sickly Children: The Tuberculosis Preventorium in American Life, 1909–1970*
Brittany Clair, *Carrying On: Another School of Thought on Pregnancy and Health*
Brittany Cowgill, *Rest Uneasy: Sudden Infant Death Syndrome in Twentieth-Century America*
Patricia D'Antonio, *Nursing with a Message: Public Health Demonstration Projects in New York City*
Kerry Michael Dobransky, *Managing Madness in the Community: The Challenge of Contemporary Mental Health Care*
Tasha N. Dubriwny, *The Vulnerable Empowered Woman: Feminism, Postfeminism, and Women's Health*
Edward J. Eckenfels, *Doctors Serving People: Restoring Humanism to Medicine through Student Community Service*
Julie Fairman, *Making Room in the Clinic: Nurse Practitioners and the Evolution of Modern Health Care*
Jill A. Fisher, *Medical Research for Hire: The Political Economy of Pharmaceutical Clinical Trials*
Lori Freedman, *Bishops and Bodies: Reproductive Care in American Catholic Hospitals*
Asia Friedman, *Mammography Wars: Analyzing Attention in Cultural and Medical Disputes*
Charlene Galarneau, *Communities of Health Care Justice*
Alyshia Gálvez, *Patient Citizens, Immigrant Mothers: Mexican Women, Public Prenatal Care and the Birth Weight Paradox*

Laura E. Gómez and Nancy López, eds., *Mapping "Race": Critical Approaches to Health Disparities Research*
Janet Greenlees, *When the Air Became Important: A Social History of the New England and Lancashire Textile Industries*
Gerald N. Grob and Howard H. Goldman, *The Dilemma of Federal Mental Health Policy: Radical Reform or Incremental Change?*
Gerald N. Grob and Allan V. Horwitz, *Diagnosis, Therapy, and Evidence: Conundrums in Modern American Medicine*
Rachel Grob, *Testing Baby: The Transformation of Newborn Screening, Parenting, and Policymaking*
Mark A. Hall and Sara Rosenbaum, eds., *The Health Care "Safety Net" in a Post-Reform World*
Laura L. Heinemann, *Transplanting Care: Shifting Commitments in Health and Care in the United States*
Rebecca J. Hester, *Embodied Politics: Indigenous Migrant Activism, Cultural Competency, and Health Promotion in California*
Laura D. Hirshbein, *American Melancholy: Constructions of Depression in the Twentieth Century*
Laura D. Hirshbein, *Smoking Privileges: Psychiatry, the Mentally Ill, and the Tobacco Industry in America*
Timothy Hoff, *Practice under Pressure: Primary Care Physicians and Their Medicine in the Twenty-first Century*
Beatrix Hoffman et al., eds., *Patients as Policy Actors*
Ruth Horowitz, *Deciding the Public Interest: Medical Licensing and Discipline*
Powel Kazanjian, *Frederick Novy and the Development of Bacteriology in American Medicine*
Matthew Kelly, *The Sounds of Furious Living: Everyday Unorthodoxies in an Era of AIDS*
Claas Kirchhelle, *Pyrrhic Progress: The History of Antibiotics in Anglo-American Food Production*
Rebecca M. Kluchin, *Fit to Be Tied: Sterilization and Reproductive Rights in America, 1950–1980*
Jennifer Lisa Koslow, *Cultivating Health: Los Angeles Women and Public Health Reform*
Jennifer Lisa Koslow, *Exhibiting Health: Public Health Displays in the Progressive Era*
Susan C. Lawrence, *Privacy and the Past: Research, Law, Archives, Ethics*
Bonnie Lefkowitz, *Community Health Centers: A Movement and the People Who Made It Happen*
Ellen Leopold, *Under the Radar: Cancer and the Cold War*
Barbara L. Ley, *From Pink to Green: Disease Prevention and the Environmental Breast Cancer Movement*
Sonja Mackenzie, *Structural Intimacies: Sexual Stories in the Black AIDS Epidemic*
Stephen E. Mawdsley, *Selling Science: Polio and the Promise of Gamma Globulin*
Frank M. McClellan, *Healthcare and Human Dignity: Law Matters*
Michelle McClellan, *Lady Lushes: Gender, Alcohol, and Medicine in Modern America*
David Mechanic, *The Truth about Health Care: Why Reform Is Not Working in America*

Richard A. Meckel, *Classrooms and Clinics: Urban Schools and the Protection and Promotion of Child Health, 1870–1930*

Terry Mizrahi, *From Residency to Retirement: Physicians' Careers over a Professional Lifetime*

Manon Parry, *Broadcasting Birth Control: Mass Media and Family Planning*

Alyssa Picard, *Making the American Mouth: Dentists and Public Health in the Twentieth Century*

Heather Munro Prescott, *The Morning After: A History of Emergency Contraception in the United States*

Sarah B. Rodriguez, *The Love Surgeon: A Story of Trust, Harm, and the Limits of Medical Regulation*

David J. Rothman and David Blumenthal, eds., *Medical Professionalism in the New Information Age*

Andrew R. Ruis, *Eating to Learn, Learning to Eat: School Lunches and Nutrition Policy in the United States*

James A. Schafer Jr., *The Business of Private Medical Practice: Doctors, Specialization, and Urban Change in Philadelphia, 1900–1940*

Johanna Schoen, ed., *Abortion Care as Moral Work: Ethical Considerations of Maternal and Fetal Bodies*

David G. Schuster, *Neurasthenic Nation: America's Search for Health, Happiness, and Comfort, 1869–1920*

Karen Seccombe and Kim A. Hoffman, *Just Don't Get Sick: Access to Health Care in the Aftermath of Welfare Reform*

Leo B. Slater, *War and Disease: Biomedical Research on Malaria in the Twentieth Century*

Piper Sledge, *Bodies Unbound: Gender-Specific Cancer and Biolegitimacy*

Dena T. Smith, *Medicine over Mind: Mental Health Practice in the Biomedical Era*

Kylie M. Smith, *Talking Therapy: Knowledge and Power in American Psychiatric Nursing*

Matthew Smith, *An Alternative History of Hyperactivity: Food Additives and the Feingold Diet*

Paige Hall Smith, Bernice L. Hausman, and Miriam Labbok, *Beyond Health, Beyond Choice: Breastfeeding Constraints and Realities*

Susan L. Smith, *Toxic Exposures: Mustard Gas and the Health Consequences of World War II in the United States*

Rosemary A. Stevens, Charles E. Rosenberg, and Lawton R. Burns, eds., *History and Health Policy in the United States: Putting the Past Back In*

Marianne Sullivan, *Tainted Earth: Smelters, Public Health, and the Environment*

Courtney E. Thompson, *An Organ of Murder: Crime, Violence, and Phrenology in Nineteenth-Century America*

Barbra Mann Wall, *American Catholic Hospitals: A Century of Changing Markets and Missions*

Frances Ward, *The Door of Last Resort: Memoirs of a Nurse Practitioner*

Jean C. Whelan, *Nursing the Nation: Building the Nurse Labor Force*

Shannon Withycombe, *Lost: Miscarriage in Nineteenth-Century America*